RENAL FAILURE

DEVELOPMENTS IN NEPHROLOGY

Volume 37

The titles published in this series are listed at the end of this volume.

Renal Failure

Diagnosis & Treatment

Edited by

J. GARY ABUELO, M.D.
Associate Professor of Medicine
Brown University School of Medicine
Associate Physician
Division of Renal Diseases, Department of Medicine
Rhode Island Hospital Providence, Rhode Island, U.S.A.

Springer Science+Business Media, B.V.

Library of Congress Cataloging-in-Publication Data

```
Renal failure : diagnosis & treatment / edited by J. Gary Abuelo.
      p.   cm. -- (Developments in nephrology ; v. 37)
   Includes index.
   ISBN 978-94-010-4026-6     ISBN 978-94-011-0047-2 (eBook)
   DOI 10.1007/978-94-011-0047-2
   1. Chronic renal failure.  2. Acute renal failure.  I. Abuelo, J.
Gary.  II. Series.  III. Series: Developments in nephrology ; 37.
   [DNLM: 1. Kidney Failure, Acute--diagnosis.  2. Kidney Failure,
Acute--etiology.  3. Kidney Failure, Acute--therapy.   W1 DE998EB
v.37 1995 / WJ 342 R3925 1995]
RC918.R4R452  1995
616.6'14--dc20
DNLM/DLC
for Library of Congress                                   95-7920
```

ISBN 978-94-010-4026-6

Table of contents

Contributors vii

Preface ix

Acknowledgements xi

PART I   Introduction and causes
Chapter 1. Introduction 3
Chapter 2. Causes of Renal Failure 7

PART II   The evaluation
Chapter 3 History 11
Chapter 4 Physical Examination 21
Chapter 5 Initial Laboratory Studies 25
Chapter 6 Additional Laboratory Tests 35

PART III   The various causes of renal failure and their diagnosis
Chapter 7 False Renal Failure and Chronic Renal Failure 49
Chapter 8 Prerenal Renal Failure 55
Chapter 9 Postrenal Renal Failure 59
Chapter 10 Vascular Causes of Renal Failure 65
Chapter 11 Glomerular Causes of Renal Failure 93
Chapter 12 Tubular Causes of Renal Failure 117
Chapter 13 Interstitial Causes of Renal Failure 131

PART IV   The differential diagnosis
Chapter 14 Review of Diagnostic Practices 145
Chapter 15 The Undiagnosed Patient 149

PART V   Management of renal failure
Chapter 16 General Management of the Patient with Acute Renal Failure 153
Chapter 17 General Management of the Patient with Chronic Renal Failure 169
Chapter 18 Treatment of Specific Causes of Renal Failure 187

PART VI   Problem cases 233

APPENDIX – LIST OF NEPHROTOXINS 255
    A. Medications that may cause renal failure with proper use 255
    B. Nephrotoxins other than properly used ligitimate drugs 260

Index 269

Contributors

J. Gary Abuelo, M.D.,   Associate Professor of Medicine, Brown University School of Medicine, Associate Physician, Division of Renal Diseases, Department of Medicine, Rhode Island Hospital, Providence, Rhode Island, USA.

Rex L. Mahnensmith, M.D.,   Associate Professor of Medicine and Clinical Director of Nephrology, Yale University School of Medicine, Medical Director of Dialysis, Yale New Haven Hospital, New Haven, Connecticut, USA.

Douglas Shemin, M.D.,   Clinical Assistant Professor of Medicine, Brown University School of Medicine, Associate Physician, Division of Renal Diseases, Department of Medicine, Rhode Island Hospital, Providence, Rhode Island, USA.

Aaron Spital M.D.,   Associate Professor of Medicine, University of Rochester School of Medicine, Division of Nephrology, Genesee Hospital, Rochester, New York, USA.

August Zabbo, M.D.,   Assistant Professor of Surgery, Brown University School of Medicine, Staff Urologist, Department of Urology, Rhode Island Hospital, Providence, Rhode Island, USA.

Preface

The most common and most important clinical problem in the field of nephrology is the diagnosis and treatment of renal failure. In many cases, the cause of the patient's illness is obvious and its management is straightforward. However, sometimes either the diagnosis or the treatment is difficult, and demands all the physician's knowledge and judgment. *Renal Failure, Diagnosis and Treatment* is a guide to the care of such challenging patients.

The intended readers are clinicians who wish to improve their competence in this area. They might include medical house officers, internists, renal fellows and nephrologists. Although *Renal Failure, Diagnosis and Treatment* contains much practical information about the various diseases that impair renal function, and can serve as a reference source, it is not intended to be used in that way. The first section on the diagnostic process (Parts I–IV) should ideally be read from beginning to end, while the second section on treatment can be consulted when necessary for the problem at hand.

This book focuses on potentially reversible causes of acute and subacute renal failure in which serum creatinine concentration rises over days to weeks, but more chronic diseases will be mentioned when appropriate.

The first step in the diagnostic process is addressed in Part II of the book, The Evaluation. It involves *gathering basic information* about the case through a history, physical examination, and initial laboratory studies (Chapters 3–6). The second diagnostic step is *syndrome recognition*. Here the physician looks at the clinical picture and attempts to recognize the patient's disease. This calls for a substantial fund of knowledge about the clinical manifestations of the disorders that cause renal failure. The signs and symptoms of these disorders are described in Part III, The Various Causes of Renal Failure and Their Diagnosis (Chapters 7–13). The third diagnostic step, also covered in Part III, is the *confirmation of the diagnosis* through specific testing or through a period of judicious observation.

While these three steps usually are successful, a rare patient may still be undiagnosed at this point and additional investigation is necessary. This fourth step of *broad scale but selective testing* for difficult cases is discussed in Part IV of the book (Chapter 15, The Undiagnosed Patient).

Since the reader is encouraged to read the diagnostic section of the book completely, detailed information that is not absolutely necessary for the understanding of the subject has been set in small print. It is available for interested individuals, but need not be read by everyone.

Part V describes the general management of patients with renal failure (Chapters 16 and 17), and the specific treatment of the individual diseases (Chapter 18).

Finally, to illustrate the application of the diagnostic principles described, in Part VI twenty cases are presented for analysis by the reader. They are followed by the diagnoses and discussions of the cases.

Acknowledgements

I am grateful to my wife, Dianne N. Abuelo, M.D. and to the following colleagues for reviewing and commenting on various sections of the book: Darrell Abernethy, M.D., Jaime S. Carvalho, M.D., Richard A. Cottiero, M.D., James P. Crowley, M.D., Lance D. Dworkin, M.D., Reginald Y. Gohh, M.D., Edward Lally, M.D., Michael J. Maher, M.D., John Maynard, M.D., Charles E. McCoy, M.D., Michael D. Plager, M.D., Jack Schwartzwald, M.D., Francis H. Scola, M.D., Douglas Shemin, M.D., Mark S. Siskind, M.D., Adam Ming Sun, M.D., August Zabbo, M.D., and Stephen B. Zipin, M.D.

I thank Mrs. Charlene McGloin for her patience and the countless hours spent preparing this manuscript. Dr. Alfredo Esparza graciously provided photomicrographs of various renal diseases, and Milton H. Lipsky, the medical illustrator at the Rhode Island Hospital, advised me during preparation of the diagrams. The photographs of the urine sediment were a gift of Frances Andrus, Registered Laboratory Technologist, Division of Nephrology, Department of Medicine, Victoria Hospital, London, Ontario, Canada.

PART ONE

Introduction and causes

1. Introduction

INCIDENCE OF RENAL FAILURE

Renal failure is a familiar diagnostic problem to practicing physicians. Acute renal failure has an incidence in the general population of 5 to 14 cases per 100,000 per year [1–3], and in general hospitals occurs in about one of 20 patients [4]. In certain situations almost one of four individuals may be affected. This includes patients in intensive care units [5, 6], those with community-acquired bacteremia [7] and individuals after elective surgery [8]. In severe burn cases three out of four patients develop azotemia [5]. In addition, 17 new cases of chronic renal failure per 100,000 general population reach end stage each year [9], and often need to be distinguished from cases of acute renal failure.

IMPORTANCE OF MAKING A DIAGNOSIS

Renal failure is usually discovered fortuitously in an asymptomatic phase. Consequently, there may be a tendency to put off investigations into its cause, especially if a patient has other serious problems that require attention. However, even slight degrees of azotemia are worthy of evaluation. First, only small changes in serum creatinine concentration (Scr) may result from significant falls in glomerular filtration rate (GFR) due to the mathematical relationship: GFR is proportional to 1/Scr (Figure 1.1). For example, a rise in Scr from 0.8 to only 1.6 mg/dl (71 to 141 μmol/L) reflects the loss of *half* of total renal function, which is equivalent to that of one entire kidney! Second, if a treatable cause is identified, appropriate therapy may prevent further damage or even reverse renal impairment. Finally, the search for an etiology of the renal disease may uncover an unsuspected con-

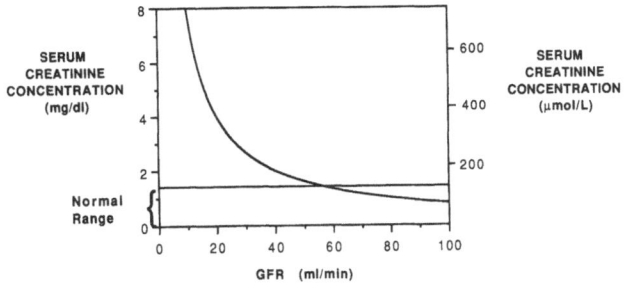

Fig. 1.1. Relation between GFR and steady state Scr in a hypothetical individual during gradual loss of renal function.

dition, such as multiple myeloma, vasculitis or other multisystem disease, whose extrarenal manifestations had been eluding diagnosis.

OBVIOUS VERSUS OBSCURE DIAGNOSES

Fortunately in most cases of renal failure, diagnosis is not difficult. Patients usually either have evidence of a chronic irreversible process or have acute renal failure with an obvious cause. In one study, almost 80% of hospital acquired renal failure could be attributed to four easily recognized conditions: reduced renal perfusion, postoperative renal insufficiency, contrast medium-induced renal failure, and aminoglycoside nephrotoxicity [4]. In some cases there were multiple causes [4]. However, in other situations the diagnosis is not so apparent. Primary renal diseases such as idiopathic crescentic glomerulonephritis often present with azotemia, an abnormal urinalysis, and no clues to a specific etiology. Even with renal dysfunction secondary to urinary obstruction or poor renal perfusion the patient may have few or none of the usual clinical manifestations. Finally, the physi-

3

J.G. Abuelo (ed.), Renal Failure, 3–5.
© 1995 *Kluwer Academic Publishers.*

cian may be unfamiliar with the responsible condition, if it is a rare disease such as essential mixed cryoglobulinemia or is a common disease with renal failure as a rare complication such as infectious mononucleosis with interstitial nephritis [10, 11].

DEFINITIONS

It is worthwhile at the outset to define renal failure and some common qualifying terms like *severe, chronic or oliguric.*

Renal Failure. This is a loss of renal function leading to a fall of GFR to below 80 ml/min[1] and to an accumulation of creatinine, urea and other nitrogenous wastes.

> *Severity.* The degree of renal failure may be roughly divided into mild, moderate and severe. In *mild* renal failure, the GFR is 50 to 79 ml/min. Enough renal function remains to minimize the accumulation of waste products so that the patient has no symptoms and Scr levels off at 2.5 mg/dl or less (<221 μmol/L). In *moderate* renal failure, the GFR is 20 to 49 ml/min and Scr between 2.6 and 6 mg/dl (230 and 530 μmol/L). Loss of concentrating ability may produce nocturia, and with time reduced erythropoietin production and red cell survival may cause anemia. In *severe* renal failure, the GFR is less than 20 ml/min and Scr more than 6.0 mg/dl (530 μmol/L). The high levels of nitrogenous wastes usually produce uremic symptoms and the low GFR may lead to retention of salt and water as manifested by hypertension, pulmonary congestion and peripheral edema. Hyperkalemia, hyponatremia and metabolic acidosis may occur. With time anemia worsens and renal bone disease, amenorrhea and other endocrine abnormalities can develop.

Terms like acute, chronic or rapidly progressive are used to describe the tempo of the disease process:

Acute Renal Failure. Here a *rapid* loss of renal function reduces waste excretion rate well below production rate so that a daily rise in Scr and blood urea nitrogen level (BUN) results. The process may be relatively benign and cause only a transient and asymptomatic fall in GFR. In other cases complete loss of renal function leads to life threatening uremia in less than a week. Of the many possible causes, reduced renal perfusion and nephrotoxic agents are the most common. In most cases of acute renal failure, the damage is *reversible* if the underlying cause resolves.

Chronic Renal Failure. The loss of renal function is *slow and progressive* in chronic renal failure. The rise in Scr is not apparent from one week to the next, but becomes evident over months to years. Indeed, patients with very slow progression may appear to have stable renal impairment for a year or more. The disease process is insidious and usually continues unnoticed for months or years. Ultimately, most patients develop uremic symptoms unless they die of another cause. In most cases of chronic renal failure, the damage is *irreversible.*

Subacute or Rapidly Progressive Renal Failure. These terms indicate renal failure with a loss of renal function that is occurring at a tempo intermediate between that of acute and chronic renal failure. The rise in Scr is apparent from one week to another.

Acute-on-Chronic Renal Failure. An intercurrent process such as volume depletion may produce a rapid worsening of renal failure with a daily rise in BUN and Scr in individuals with chronic renal failure. This acute deterioration is often reversible if the underlying cause resolves.

The following definitions may also be helpful:

Oliguric Renal Failure. This is renal failure accompanied by a fall in urine output to less than 500 ml/day.

> Adults usually have urine outputs of 1 to 2 liters/day, but, if water is scarce, normal individuals concentrate their urine and reduce urine output to as low as 500 ml/day. Since the kidneys need 500 ml/day to excrete the daily load of salts and metabolic wastes, a urine volume less than this indicates renal failure.

Anuric Renal Failure. This is renal failure accompanied by a fall in urine output to less than 50 ml/day.

Nonoliguric Renal Failure. This is renal failure with a urine output greater than 500 ml/day. Most patients with renal failure maintain a urine volume in the *nonoliguric* range (one half to two liters/day) [12].

Azotemia ("nitrogen in the blood"). This is the accumulation of nitrogenous wastes in the blood, when the renal excretion of these products of protein and nucleic acid metabolism is impaired. It is reflected by an increase in BUN and Scr.

Uremia ("urine in the blood"). This is the complex of symptoms produced by severe renal failure.

> The GFR is usually less than 20% of normal when uremic manifestations start, but the onset of symptoms does not correlate well with level of GFR, Scr or BUN. Uremia is a result of the excretory, regulatory and hormonal failure of the kidney. *Excretory failure* leads to the buildup of organic degradation products, enzymes, hormones and peptides in the body. Although urea and creatinine are measured as an index of this waste accumulation, these substances are not toxic at the levels they attain. The identity of the uremic toxins is still under investigation. *Regulatory failure* is the inability of the kidney to maintain the pH, ion concentrations and fluid volume of the body due to retention of water, sodium, hydrogen, potassium, phosphate and other electrolytes. *Hormonal failure* includes the inadequate renal production of erythropoietin and activated vitamin D which, along with other factors, lead to anemia and renal osteodystrophy.

Renal Insufficiency. Some authorities use *renal insufficiency* to describe any reduction in GFR and reserve the term *renal failure* for severe azotemia. In this book these terms are used interchangeably and refer to a fall in GFR below 80 ml/min/1.73m^2 and accumulation of nitrogenous wastes.

NOTES

1. The lower limit of normal GFR is more properly given corrected for standard adult body surface area: 80 ml/min/1.73m^3. While clinicians should consider the patient's size in looking at GFR, a formal correction for body surface area is rarely necessary.

REFERENCES

1. Eliahou HE, Modan B, Leslau V, Bar-Noach N, Tchiya P and Modan M. Acute renal failure in the community: an epidemiological study. In: Friedman EA and Eliahou HE, editors. Proceedings Acute Renal Failure Conference DHEW Publication No.(NIH) 74–608 1974:143–63.
2. Feest TG, Round A and Hamad S. Incidence of severe acute renal failure in adults: results of a community based study. BMJ 1993; 306:481–3.
3. Abbas EET, Mohammed AO, Abdelgadir EI and Wafa AM. Pattern of acute renal failure in a general hospital in Saudi Arabia. Saudi Kid Dis Transplant 1990; 1:89–93.
4. Hou SH, Bushinsky DA, Wish JB, Cohen JJ and Harrington JT. Hospital-acquired renal insufficiency: a prospective study. Am J Med 1983; 74:243–8.
5. Wilkins RG and Faragher EB. Acute renal failure in an intensive care unit: incidence, prediction and outcome. Anaesthesia 1983; 38:628–34.
6. Groeneveld ABJ, Tran DD, van der Meulen J, Nauta JJP and Thijs LG. Acute renal failure in the medical intensive care unit: predisposing, complicating factors and outcome. Nephron 1991; 59:602–10.
7. Rayner BL, Willcox PA and Pascoe MD. Acute renal failure in community-acquired bacteraemia. Nephron 1990; 54:32–5.
8. Charlson ME, MacKenzie CR, Gold JP and Shires T. Postoperative changes in serum creatinine. Ann Surg 1989; 209:328–33.
9. U.S. Renal Data System, USRDS 1993 Annual Data Report, The National Institutes of Health, National Institute of Diabetes and Digestive and Kidney Diseases, Bethesda, MD, March 1993, page xvi.
10. Kopolovic J, Pinkus G and Rosen S. Interstitial nephritis in infectious mononucleosis. Am J Kidney Dis 1988; 12:76–7.
11. Lee S and Kjellstrand CM. Renal disease in infectious mononucleosis. Clin Nephrol 1978; 9:236–40.
12. Dixon BS and Anderson RJ. Nonoliguric acute renal failure. Am J Kidney Dis 1985; 6:71–80.

2. Causes of renal failure

J. GARY ABUELO

This chapter outlines the traditional etiologic categories of renal failure and their prevalence in azotemic patients.

MAIN CATEGORIES

Renal failure may be caused by: (1) any general circulatory disturbance that reduces renal perfusion, such as volume depletion, or cardiogenic shock, (2) any impediment to the excretion of urine formed by the kidney, such as urinary tract obstruction, or neurogenic or ruptured bladder and (3) any disease of the renal blood vessels or parenchyma. Traditionally these pathophysiologic categories come under the rubrics of *prerenal, postrenal* and *intrinsic or parenchymal* renal failure. The intrinsic renal diseases may be further classified anatomically as primarily *vascular, glomerular, tubular or interstitial* in nature. In addition, a category of *false* renal failure should be added to this overall schema to cover patients with falsely elevated Scr.

FACTORS AFFECTING THE OCCURRENCE OF DIFFERENT CAUSES

The incidence of the different causes of renal failure varies with geographic, ethnic and socio-economic factors [1].

In certain countries, a disease that is uncommon elsewhere may be responsible for many cases of renal failure. Such is true of septic abortion in Ghana [2], Southeast Asia [3], India [1] and South Africa [4], intravascular hemolysis in India and Ghana [1, 2], leptospirosis in Singapore, Thailand and the Philippines [5–7], nephrotoxic herbal remedies in South Africa [4, 8], snake bites and malaria in Thailand [5], and severe gastroenteritis in India [1, 9], Indonesia [10], and South Africa [4].

Patient age is also a factor. Myeloma kidney, renal artery stenosis and atheromatous renal emboli are causes of renal failure limited to older adults. Also, acute tubular necrosis is far less common in children after infancy than in adults [11–16].

INCIDENCE OF DIFFERENT CAUSES IN DEVELOPED NATIONS

Adults. In the United States and other industrialized countries prerenal conditions account for about 15% of cases of acute renal failure, postrenal conditions account for about 5% of cases, and intrinsic renal disease for the rest (Table 2.1). There are no data on false renal failure, which is rare. Of the intrinsic renal diseases (Table 2.2), acute tubular necrosis (ATN) is the most common (about 75% of patients) with three cases of ATN due to ischemia for every case due to nephrotoxins [17, 22, 23]. Glomerulonephritis and vascular disorders each account for roughly 10% and interstitial nephritis for about 5% of cases of intrinsic forms of renal failure (Figure 2.1).

Table 2.1. Pathophysiologic categories of acute renal failure and prevalence in various studies (17–21)

Category	Approximate % of cases (range)
False renal failure	< 1 (?)
Prerenal renal failure	15 (4–32)
Postrenal renal failure	5 (4–11)
Intrinsic renal disease	80 (59–87)

J.G. Abuelo (ed.), Renal Failure, 7–9.
© 1995 *Kluwer Academic Publishers.*

Table 2.2. Intrinsic renal causes of acute renal failure and prevalence in various studies (17–18, 22–24)

Category	Example	Approximate % of cases (range)
Vascular	ACE inhibitors	10 (3–19)
Glomerular	Glomerulonephritis	10 (0–22)
Tubular	Acute tubular necrosis	75 (61–82)
Interstitial	Allergic interstitial nephritis	5 (0–8)

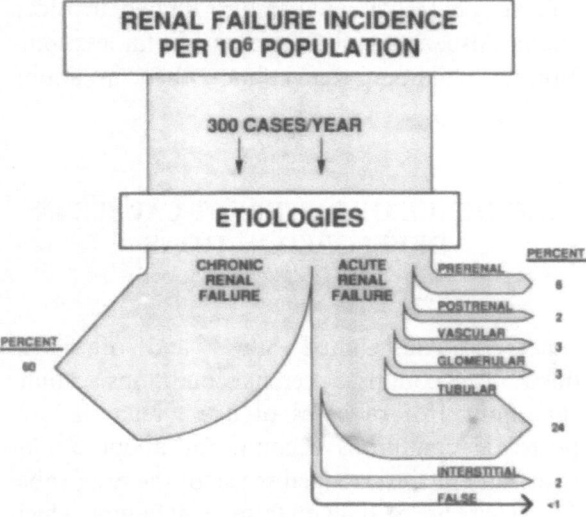

Fig. 2.1. The incidence and causes of renal failure.

Infants and Children. ATN comprises only 50% of cases of intrinsic renal disease, while hemolytic uremic syndrome, a thrombotic condition of the renal arteries and arterioles that is rare in adults, accounts for about 25% of cases [11–16, 25].

REFERENCES

1. Chugh KS, Singhai PC, Nath IVS, Tewari SC, Muthesethupathy MA, Yiswanathan S et al. Spectrum of acute renal failure in north India. J Ass Phys Ind 1978; 26:147–54.
2. Adu D, Anim-Addoy, Foli AK, Yeboah ED, Quartey JKM and Riberio BF. Acute renal failure in tropical Africa. Brit Med J 1976; 1:890–2.
3. Chugh KS and Singhal PC. Acute renal failure in the tropics. In: Takeuchi T, Sugino N and Ota K, editors. Asian manual of nephrology. Tokyo: Southeast Asian Medical Information Center, 1981;181–94.
4. Seedat YK and Nathoo BC. Acute renal failure in blacks and Indians in South Africa – Comparison after 10 years. Nephron 1993; 64:198–201.
5. Sitprija V. The kidney in acute tropical disease. Abstracts of the Int Congr Nephrol 1981:273.
6. Ku G, Lim CH, Pwee HS and Khoo OT. Review of acute renal failure in Singapore. Ann Acad Med (Singapore) Suppl 1975; 4:115–20.
7. Dela Cruz CM, Pineda L, Rogelio G and Alano F. Clinical profile and factors affecting mortality in acute renal failure. Renal Failure 1992; 14:161–8.
8. Seedat YK. Acute renal failure among Blacks and Indians in South Africa. S Afr Med J 1978; 54:427–31.
9. Chugh KS, Narang A, Kumar L, Sakhuja V, Unni VN, Pirzada R et al. Acute renal failure amongst children in a tropical environment. Int J Artif Org 1987; 10:97–101.
10. Oesman R, Markum MS, Rahardjo J and Sidabutar RP. Acute renal failure in General Hospital, Jakarta. Ann Acad Med (Singapore) Suppl. 1975; 4:121–3.
11. Niaudet P, Haj-Ibrahim, Gagnadoux M-F and Broyer M. Outcome of children with acute renal failure. Kidney Int 1985; 28:S148–51.
12. Offner G, Brodehl J, Galaske R and Rutt T. Acute renal failure in children: prognostic features after treatment with acute dialysis. Eur J Pediatr 1986; 144:482–6.
13. Hodson EM, Kjellstrand CM and Mauer SM. Acute renal failure in infants and children: outcome of 53 patients requiring hemodialysis. J Pediatr 1976; 93:756–61.
14. Shapiro SR, Stratton ML and Adelman RD. Anuria in infants and children. J Urol 1978; 120:227–8.
15. Counahan R, Cameron JS, Ogg CS, Spurgeon P, Williams DG, Winder E et al. Presentation, management, complications and outcome of acute renal failure in childhood: Five years' experience. Br Med J 1977; 1:599–602.
16. Rengel M, Caro P, Fdez-Llebrez J, Vargas-Z F, Gomes F and Garcia L. Acute renal failure in children. Kidney Int 1985; 28:299.
17. Manis T, Heneghan W, Charles G and Friedman EA. Acute renal failure in a municipal hospital. In: Eliahou HE, editor. Acute renal failure. London: John Libbey, 1982;129–32.
18. Miller TR, Anderson RJ, Linas SL, Henrich WL, Berns AS, Gabow PA et al. Urinary diagnostic indices in acute renal failure. Ann Intern Med 1978; 89:47–50.
19. Kleinknecht D and Ganeval D. Preventive hemodialysis in acute renal failure. Its effect on mortality and morbidity. In: Friedman EA and Eliahou HE, Proceedings Acute Renal Failure Conference. DHEW Publication No. (NIH) 74–608 1973:165–86.
20. Eliahou HE, Modan B, Leslau V, Bar-Noach N, Tchiya P and Modan M. Acute renal failure in the community: an epidemiological study. In: Friedman EA and Eliahou HE, editors. Proceedings Acute Renal Failure Conference. DHEW Publication No. (NIH) 74–608, 1974;146–64.
21. Thomas MAB, Ibels LS. Rhabdomyolysis and acute renal failure. Aust NZ J Med 1985; 15:623–8.
22. Hou SH, Bushinsky DA, Wish JB, Cohen JJ and Harrington JT. Hospital-acquired renal insufficiency: a prospective study. Am J Med 1983; 74:243–8.

23. Bonomi V, Baldrati L, Scolari MP, Stefoni S and Vangelista A. Acute renal failure: ten years' experience. In: Eliahou HE, editor. Acute renal failure. London: John Libbey & Company Limited, 1982;129–32.

24. Biesenbach G, Zazgornik J, Kaiser W, Grafinger P, Stuby U and Necek S. Improvement in prognosis of patients with acute renal failure over a period of 15 years: An analysis of 710 cases in a dialysis center. Am J Nephrol 1992; 12:319–25.

25. Gallego N, Gallego A, Pascual J, Liano F, Estepa R and Ortuno J. Prognosis of children with acute renal failure: a study of 138 cases. Nephron 1993; 64:399–404.

PART TWO

The evaluation

The first step in the diagnosis of renal failure is the gathering of basic information about the case. The physician must take a medical history, perform a physical examination and obtain laboratory studies with a view to understand the cause of renal failure. The special concerns to be addressed in evaluating the azotemic patient are covered in this part of the book.

3. History

J. GARY ABUELO

In most cases of renal failure the diagnosis will be made or at least suspected from the patient's history and his medical record. Certain information is particularly important.

CHIEF COMPLAINT

The presenting symptoms of individuals with renal failure vary greatly.

No Symptoms. In early or mild renal disease the patient often feels well and the renal failure is accidentally discovered during a routine medical check-up or evaluation of an unrelated illness.

Symptoms of a Primary Illness. Non-renal conditions, such as sepsis or systemic lupus erythematosis, commonly cause renal failure, and symptoms of these diseases bring patients to medical attention. Scr may be elevated initially or may rise later in the illness.

Uremic Symptoms. Many patients with renal failure first feel sick when advanced renal failure produces frank uremia (see next section, History of Present Illness).

Other Renal or Urological Symptoms. Edema, gross hematuria, or another complaint originating in the urinary tract may be the heralding symptom in patients with renal failure (see next section).

HISTORY OF PRESENT ILLNESS

Onset and Duration of Illness

First, it is paramount to date the beginning of the renal disease. If the renal failure is new, this allows the physician to focus on the onset of the patient's illness and to identify potential renal insults. If the renal failure is longstanding, a different diagnostic approach is indicated as discussed in Chapter 7, Chronic Renal Failure.

Uremic Symptoms. In patients with chronic renal failure, the long duration of azotemia may be suggested by a protracted history of *uremic manifestations.* In contrast, uremia of recent onset does not help establish the duration of disease, since it comes after an asymptomatic stage that can vary from days to years.

Uremic patients may have one or many of the following complaints: easy fatigability, anorexia, nausea, sporadic vomiting, weight loss, insomnia, hiccoughs, impotence, amenorrhea, loss of libido, muscle cramps, bad breath, dysgeusia,[1] pruritus, anemia, neuropathy, somnolence, decreased attention span, irritability and symptoms of volume overload, including hypertension, pulmonary or peripheral edema. Such hypervolemia can manifest as congestive heart failure, but is usually caused by renal fluid retention rather than by primary heart disease. Defects in urinary concentration may produce nocturia or rarely polyuria and polydipsia, especially if chronic renal disease is due to partial urinary obstruction or interstitial renal diseases.

Uremic patients often minimize or do not admit to symptoms because of denial or uremic encephalopathy. Corroboration of the history by a close relative or friend can be helpful.

13

J.G. Abuelo (ed.), Renal Failure, 13–19.
© 1995 *Kluwer Academic Publishers.*

Other Renal or Urologic Symptoms. These complaints may also indicate the onset of the illness as well as suggest the diagnosis. The nephrotic syndrome may produce *edema* or occasionally a *fall in urine output.* The patient may note *gross hematuria,* which can accompany an acute (glomerulo-) nephritic process, obstructive uropathy, or less often atheroembolic renal disease, acute interstitial nephritis, malignant hypertension, thrombotic thrombocytopenic purpura, or renal infarction. The sudden onset of *pain* over the back, flank, abdomen or even the chest can be seen with renal failure caused by acute pyelonephritis, renal embolism, renal vein thrombosis, or acute ureteral obstruction by a stone or sloughed papilla. The pain of ureteral obstruction may also be felt in the inguinal or genital region.

> Various glomerulonephritides [1–6], atheroembolic renal disease [7] malacoplakia,[2] xanthogranulomatous pyelonephritis,[2] and acute interstitial nephritis [8], especially following rifampin [9], can produce lumbar pain. Gradual ureteral obstruction by retroperitoneal fibrosis or tumor and replacement of a single kidney by a tumor can give rise to an ill-defined chronic aching pain of the flank or back.

Failure to empty the bladder completely either due to neurogenic impairment or bladder outlet obstruction can produce a weak or intermittent urinary stream, hesitancy in starting urination, straining, frequent voiding, nocturia, terminal dribbling, urgency, incontinence, the sensation of incomplete emptying or even acute urinary retention.

Azotemia or fall in urine output

The physician may not always be sure of the temporal relation between the uremic and other symptoms just discussed and the loss of renal function. Therefore, to identify the onset of renal failure accurately one must search the medical record for the first rise in Scr or fall in urine output. In chronic renal failure, the gradual progression of the renal disease will be appreciated from the steadily rising BUN or Scr over time.

Clinical Example. *A 59-year-old woman is admitted to the hospital with congestive heart failure, new atrial fibrillation and a Scr of 5.0 mg/dl (442 μmol/L). The patient had been healthy except for occasional palpitations and for a left nephrectomy for* renal cell carcinoma ten years ago. One week ago she went to an emergency room for epigastric pain and nausea. Vital signs, abdominal examination, electrocardiogram, complete blood count, serum bilirubin, amylase and aminotransferase levels, and right upper quadrant and right renal sonogram were normal. The patient vomited once, reported relief of the pain and was sent home with a diagnosis of gastroenteritis.*

The physician should be suspicious that this episode of abdominal pain is related to the renal failure. An examination of the emergency room record shows a normal Scr, indicating that the azotemia developed over the past week. It also shows an unexplained elevation in lactic dehydrogenase level (602 U/L) and low grade hematuria (8 to 12 red blood cells per high power field). With this added information, the clinical picture suggests that the patient has intermittent atrial fibrillation and one week ago had a right renal artery embolism and infarction of a solitary kidney. This produced abdominal pain, nausea, hematuria, high lactic dehydrogenase concentration and renal failure. A computed tomography of the abdomen with contrast media will confirm this diagnosis.

Causes of Renal Failure

Poor renal perfusion

Fall in Blood Pressure. Cardiac disease, volume depletion and vasodilation[3] all may reduce arterial pressure and, as a result, renal perfusion. Since, about half of cases of renal failure are caused by prerenal azotemia or acute tubular necrosis due to decreased renal perfusion, one should note any conditions that may reduce blood pressure and examine the records of patients' blood pressures for hypotension of even brief duration.

Occasionally a fall in pressure within the normal range (or from above into the normal range) will be sufficient to produce renal ischemia and a fall in GFR. This occurs most commonly in the elderly or in patients with chronic renal insufficiency [10–13] or severe hypertension [14–16], especially renovascular hypertension [17].

Fluid Losses. Volume depletion is the leading cause of poor renal perfusion and, when due to hemorrhage or gastrointestinal fluid losses, is usually easily recognized. However, when volume depletion is due to urinary salt loss as seen with diuretics, Addison's disease, or "salt-losing nephropathy" [12, 18, 19], the renal losses may go unnoticed. Also, the physician may not appreciate fluid losses in patients with weight-losing behavior who hide self-induced vomiting, and abuse of diuretics and laxatives [20].

Evidence of such occult salt and water losses can appear as negative daily fluid balances on the intake and output sheets or an unexplained weight loss recorded in the hospital or detected by the difference between the weight at home and the weight in the hospital.

Finally, the patient may report symptoms of salt depletion, including weakness or lightheadedness on standing, constant thirst, muscle cramps, muscle weakness, apathy, fatigue, salt craving, anorexia, and nausea [21].

Nephrotoxins

Drugs Used Therapeutically. Twenty to 30% of acute renal failure due to intrinsic renal disease is caused by radiographic contrast media, aminoglycosides or other drugs [22–25]. Medications may also lead to chronic renal failure. Drug-induced renal damage comes about through a variety of mechanisms (Table 3.1). The appendix lists the nephrotoxic drugs by their pathogenic action.

Unfortunately, the causal role of drugs in renal failure may be overlooked. For example, commonly used medications, such as cimetidine [26, 27] or cephalosporins [28, 29] may be nephrotoxic only in rare cases. Furthermore, drugs taken for long periods of time may be erroneously assumed not to cause renal failure. In fact, while renal function may fall almost immediately following agents like rifampin [30, 31] or contrast media [32], with other drugs nephrotoxicity may only be noted weeks (aminoglycosides [33, 34], β-lactams [29]), months (diuretics [35–37], cisplatin [38], mitomycin [39]), years (nitrosoureas [40–43]) or decades (analgesics [44, 44a, 44b, 44c]) after starting therapy. Moreover, renal insufficiency may even begin *after* the causative agent has been stopped (nitrosourea, mitomycin). Still another way nephrotoxic drugs can be missed is that the physician may not be aware that a patient has received the causative agent. This can happen with contrast media given during computerized tomography [32, 45] or with

Table 3.1. Nephrotoxic mechanisms of drugs

Mechanism	Illustrative drug
Acute tubule necrosis	
Nephrotoxic	Aminoglycoside
Hemoglobinuric	Chloroquine
Myoglobinuric	Lovastatin
Allergic interstitial nephritis	β-lactams
Chronic interstitial nephritis	Nitrosoureas
Renal vasomotor reaction	NSAIDS
Glomerulonephritis	Penicillamine
Tubular obstruction	Sulfonamides
Retroperitoneal fibrosis	Methysergide
Hemolytic uremic syndrome	Mitomycin C
Vasculitis	Sulfonamides

medications recorded not on the medication record, but on the intake and output sheet or on special forms used in the operating suite, emergency room or intensive care unit. Also, patients may not reveal their longstanding excessive use of medications, such as diuretics or laxatives taken for weight loss, and analgesics. Patients may obtain excess diuretics by seeing multiple physicians or by pilfering from their workplace in a pharmacy or hospital. Chronic headaches, backache or arthralgias can be a clue to analgesic abuse.

Thus, a complete listing of the patient's past and present medications must be assembled and the nephrotoxic potential of each agent must be considered. For newer drugs, this may require consulting with a nephrologist, searching the literature, or contacting the drug company.

One must never assume that a medication is not nephrotoxic without looking it up. An extensive list of nephrotoxic drugs is provided in Table A in the Appendix.

Drugs Used Improperly and Other Toxins. Nephrotoxic renal damage may sometimes occur by means other than the therapeutic use of drugs.

These other nephrotoxins may be divided into four general categories:

(1) Overdose of legitimate drugs or abuse of illicit drugs. These cases usually involve patients who attempt suicide with an overdose of medication or take mood altering "street" drugs.
(2) Ingestion of nephrotoxic chemicals, foods or plants. Renal failure from the ingestion of chemicals is usually

observed after suicide attempts. The substances involved are mainly agricultural and industrial chemicals. Nephrotoxic chemicals such as rat poison can also be found around the house.

Renal failure from foods is rare and usually is seen in mentally ill patients who ingest such extraordinary amounts of a food, e.g. rhubarb, or drink that one component reaches nephrotoxic levels.

Poisonous plants, like toxic mushrooms, are usually ingested because they are mistaken for edible plants.

(3) Inhalation or cutaneous absorption of toxic chemicals. Nephrotoxicity usually occurs after excessive exposure at work due to carelessness, accident or ignorance of the toxicity of the substance.

(4) Envenomization by poisonous stings or bites. Renal failure following snakebites is not unusual in rural areas of tropical countries. Nephrotoxicity is a rare complication of spider bites or bee and wasp stings.

The physician, therefore, should query the patient about the illicit use of drugs, exposure to dust, fumes or chemicals at work or elsewhere, and in appropriate circumstances about suicide attempts by ingestion of drugs or chemicals. Table B in the Appendix is an extensive list of nephrotoxins other than properly used drugs.

Extrarenal or systemic diseases

Acute renal failure usually is a sequela of some other illness, and rarely occurs "out of the blue" in an otherwise healthy individual. It is a common postoperative complication; it may be associated with cardiovascular (renal emboli), pulmonary (Goodpasture's syndrome), hepatic (hepato-renal syndrome), rheumatologic (lupus nephritis), oncologic (ureteral obstruction), hematologic (thrombotic thrombocytopenic purpura), endocrine (Addison's disease), or infectious disease (post-infectious glomerulonephritis). Therefore, the diagnosis of the renal insufficiency will often depend on eliciting a history of predisposing disorders. In particular, one should ask about fever, rash, arthralgias, sinusitis and other manifestations of systemic diseases that can affect the kidneys.

On rare occasion the precipitating illness or condition will have resolved before the onset of renal insufficiency. Some examples of this are postpartum renal failure weeks or months after delivery [46], embolization of mural thrombi one to several weeks after myocardial infarction, hemolytic uremic syndrome one to ten days after a bout of vomiting or diarrhea [47], and various forms of glomerulonephritides days or weeks after an upper respiratory infection [48–50].

SOCIAL HISTORY

Abuse of Drugs. As noted above, many illegal drugs can produce acute or chronic renal failure. Also, parenteral drug abuse with shared needles transmits human immunodeficiency virus (HIV) infection, which can cause or even present with renal disease [51]. As drug use occurs in every socioeconomic group, virtually all patients should be asked about drug use.

Occupational Exposure. A rare cause of acute or chronic renal failure is occupational exposure to hydrocarbons, heavy metals or other substances. Such exposure usually involves inadvertent ingestion or absorption through the skin or lungs, and occurs due to carelessness, accident or ignorance of the danger of the chemical involved [52]. Similar exposures may rarely occur during pursuit of a hobby or in tasks like cleaning or painting at home. The history should include questions about exposure to dust, fumes or chemicals at work and elsewhere.

Sexual Lifestyle. Sexual contact with many partners or with someone who has had many partners is a risk factor for HIV infection. Prostitutes and promiscuous homosexual men appear most vulnerable to become infected in this way, but heterosexual spread is becoming more important.

FAMILY HISTORY

Two hereditary diseases, adult polycystic kidney disease and hereditary nephritis (Alport's syndrome), are common causes of chronic renal failure. Chronic renal failure can also be the principal manifestation or a component of several rare familial disorders. Therefore, one needs to ask if any relatives have kidney disease. The medical records of the affected relatives should be obtained, and any renal biopsy or autopsy material reviewed.

One should also ask about other illnesses that run in the family. This may reveal a hereditary disease like tuberous sclerosis that presents with renal failure in the patient being evaluated, even though other affected family members may not have renal involvement [53, 54].

Table 3.2. Examples of hereditary disorders that can cause chronic renal failure

Cystic diseases
Autosomal dominant polycystic kidney disease (mainly adults)*
Autosomal recessive polycystic kidney disease (pediatric age group)
Juvenile nephronophthisis
Medullary cystic disease
Tuberous sclerosis

Metabolic diseases
Type II diabetes mellitus*
Hereditary hyperoxaluria
Angiokeratoma corporis diffusum universale (Fabry's disease)
Cystinosis

Glomerular diseases
Hereditary nephritis (Alport's syndrome)*
Hereditary osteo-onychodysplasia (Nail-Patella syndrome)
Laurence-Moon-Biedl syndrome
Congenital nephrotic syndrome
Familial Mediterranean fever (Causes amyloidosis)
Familial form of IgA nephropathy
Sickle cell disease

Vascular diseases
Familial hemolytic-uremic syndrome
Fibromuscular dysplasia

* Common cause of chronic renal failure.

Table 3.2 lists some more common hereditary disorders that may affect the kidney. Other less common conditions may be found in published lists [55–57] and texts [58].

NOTES

1. Dysgeusia – perversion of the sense of taste, bitter, metallic or disagreeable taste in the mouth, abnormal or reduced taste of food.
2. These chronic infectious processes are discussed in Chapter 13, Interstitial Causes of Renal Failure.
3. Sepsis is the most common cause of hypotension due to vasodilation.

REFERENCES

1. Kincaid-Smith P and Nicholls K. Severe flank pain as the predominant symptom of IgA nephropathy. Am J Kid Dis 1989; 14:532.
2. Paller MS, Daniels BS and Hostetter TH. Severe flank pain as the predominant symptom of IgA nephropathy. Am J Kid Dis 1989; 13:494–6.
3. Nortman DF, Rever BL, Stanley TM and Kurokawa K. The loin pain-hematuria syndrome in two cases of IgA and IgM nephropathy. Arch Intern Med 1981; 141:1782–4.
4. Rodrigues-Iturbe B. Epidemic poststreptococcal glomerulonephritis. Kidney Int 1984; 25:129–36.
5. Sibley RK and Kim Y. Dense intramembranous deposit disease: New pathologic features. Kidney Int 1984; 25:660–70.
6. Galle P and Mahieu P. Electron dense alteration of kidney basement membranes. Am J Med 1975; 58:749–64.
7. Dahlberg PJ, Frecentese DF and Cogbill TH. Cholesterol embolism: experience with 22 histologically proven cases. Surgery 1989; 105:737–46.
8. Simenhoff ML, Guild WR and Dammin GJ. Acute diffuse interstitial nephritis. Review of literature and case report. Am J Med 1968; 44:618–25.
9. Pereira A, Sanz C, Cervantes F and Castillo R. Immune hemolytic anemia and renal failure associated with rifampicin-dependent antibodies with anti-I specificity. Ann Hematol 1991; 63:56–8.
10. Wilkinson R, Luetscher JA, Dowdy AJ, Gonzales C and Nokes GW. Studies in the mechanism of sodium excretion in uremia. Clin Sci 1972; 42:711–23.
11. Schrier RW and Regal EM. Influence of aldosterone on sodium, water and potassium metabolism in chronic renal failure. Kidney Int 1972; 1:156–68.
12. Peer G, Wigler I and Aviram A. Prolonged volume depletion imitating end-stage renal failure. Am J Med Sci 1987; 30:214–7.
13. Nickel JF, Lowrance PB, Leifer E and Bradey SE. Renal function, electrolyte excretion and body fluids in patients with chronic renal insufficiency before and after sodium deprivation. J Clin Invest 1953; 32:68–79.
14. Pohl JEF, Thurston H and Swales JD. Hypertension with renal impairment: Influence of intensive therapy. Quart J Med 1974; 43:569–81.
15. Mroczek WJ, Davidov M, Gavrilovich L and Finnerty FA. The value of aggressive therapy in the hypertensive patient with azotemia. Circulation 1969; 15:893–904.
16. Green TP, Nevins TE, Houser MT, Sibley R, Fish AJ and Sinaiko AR. Renal failure as a complication of acute antihypertensive therapy. Pediatrics 1981; 67:850–4.
17. Ying CY, Tifft CP, Gavras H and Chobanian AV. Renal revascularization in the azotemic hypertensive patient resistant to therapy. N Engl J Med 1984; 311:1070–5.
18. Polak A. Sodium depletion in chronic renal failure. J Roy Coll Phycns Lond. 1971; 5:333–43.
19. Uribarri J, Oh MS and Carroll HJ. Salt-losing nephropathy. Am J Nephrol 1983; 3:193–8.
20. Mira M, Stewart PM and Abraham SF. Hypokalaemia and renal impairment in patients with eating disorders. Med J Aust 1984 140:290–2.
21. McCance RA. Experimental sodium chloride deficiency in man. Proc Roy Soc (London) 1936; 119:245–268.
22. Jacobs D, Vonlanthen M, Agrafoitis A, Degaichia A and Rottembourg J. Acute renal failure of medical origin:

clinical and therapeutic aspects in 126 cases. In: Eliahou HE, editor. Acute renal failure. John Libbey, London, 1982;299.

23. Manis T, Heneghan W, Charles G and Friedman EA. Acute renal failure in a municipal hospital. In: Eliahou HE, editor. Acute renal failure. John Libbey, London, 1982; 129–32.

24. Bonomi V, Baldrati L, Scolari MP, Stefoni S and Vangelista A. Acute renal failure: ten years' experience. In: Eliahou EH, editor. Acute renal failure. John Libbey & Company Limited, London, 1982;129–32.

25. Hou SH, Bushinsky DA, Wish JB, Cohen JJ and Harrington JT. Hospital-acquired renal insufficiency: a prospective study. Am J Med 1983; 74:243–8.

26. Kaye WA, Passero MA, Solomon RJ and Johnson LA. Cimetidine-induced interstitial nephritis with response to prednisone therapy. Arch Intern Med 1983; 143:811–1.

27. Watson AJS, Dalbow MH, Stachura I, Fragola JA, Rubin MF, Watsons RM et al. Immunologic studies in cimetidine-induced nephropathy and polymyositis. N Engl J Med 1983; 308:142–5.

28. Nemati C and Abuelo JG. Cephalosporin induced hypersensitivity nephritis: report of a case caused by cefazolin. RI Med J 1981; 64:91–4.

29. Appel GB and Neu HC. Acute interstitial nephritis induced by beta-lactam antibiotics, In: Fillastre J-P, editor. Nephrotoxicity. INSERM, France, 1981;195–212.

30. Mauri JM, Fort J, Bartolome J, Camps J, Capdevila L, Morlans M et al. Antirifampicin antibodies in acute rifampicin-associated renal failure. Nephron 1982; 31:177–9.

31. Minetti L, Barbiano di Belgioioso G and Busnach G. Immunohistologic diagnosis of drug induced hypersensitivity nephritis. Contr Nephrol 1978; 10:15–29.

32. Byrd L and Sherman RL. Radiocontrast-induced acute renal failure: a clinical and pathophysiological review. Medicine 1979; 58:270–9.

33. Gary NE, Buzzeo L, Salaki J and Eisinger RP. Gentamicin-associated acute renal failure. Arch Intern Med 1976; 136:1101–4.

34. Schentag JJ, Plaut ME and Cerra FB. Comparative nephrotoxicity of gentamicin and tobramycin: pharmacokinetic and clinical studies of 201 patients. Antimicrob Agents Chemother 1979; 16:468–74.

35. Lyons H, Pinn VW, Cortell S, Cohen JJ and Harrington JT. Allergic interstitial nephritis causing reversible renal failure in four patients with idiopathic nephrotic syndrome. N Engl J Med 1973; 288:124–8.

36. Fuller TJ, Barcenas CG and White MG. Diuretic-induced interstitial nephritis. Occurrence in a patient with membranous glomerulonephritis. JAMA 1976; 235:1998–9.

37. Magil AG. Drug-induced acute interstitial nephritis with granulomas. Human Pathol 1983; 13:36–41.

38. Womer RB, Pritchard J and Barratt TM. Renal toxicity of cisplatin in children. J Pediatr 1985; 106:659–63.

39. Hamner RW, Verani R and Weinman EJ. Mitomycin-associated renal failure. Case report and review. Arch Intern Med 1983; 143:803–7.

40. Harmon WE, Cohen HJ, Schneeberger EE and Grupe WE. Chronic renal failure in children treated with methyl CCNU. N Engl J Med 1979; 300:1200–3.

41. Schacht RG, Feiner HD, Gallo GR, Lieberman A and Baldwin DS. Nephrotoxicity of nitrosoureas. Cancer 1981; 48:1328–34.

42. Micetich KC, Jensen-Akula M, Mandard JC and Fisher RI. Nephrotoxicity of semustine (methyl-CCNU) in patients with malignant melanoma receiving adjuvant chemotherapy. Am J Med 1981; 71:967–72.

43. Perry DJ and Weiss RB. Nephrotoxicity of streptozocin. Ann Intern Med 1982; 96:122.

44. Schwarz A, Keller F, Kunzendorf U, Kuhn-Freitag G, Heinemeyer G, Pommer W and Offermann G. Characteristics and clinical course of hemodialysis patients with analgesic-associated nephropathy. Clin Nephrol 1988; 29:299–306.

44a.Burry A. The evolution of analgesic nephropathy. Nephron 1968; 5:185–201.

44b.Dawborn JK, Fairley KF, Kincaid-Smith P and King WE. The association of peptic ulceration, chronic renal disease and analgesic abuse. Quart J Med 1966; 35:69–83.

44c.Murray RM. Genesis of analgesic nephropathy in the United Kingdom. Kidney Int 1978; 13:50–7.

45. Meeker TC, Ludwig S and Glimp R. Computerized axial tomography and acute renal failure. JAMA 1978; 240:2247–8.

46. Segonds A, Louradour N, Suc JM and Orfila C. Postpartum hemolytic uremic syndrome: a study of three cases with a review of the literature. Clin Nephrol 1979; 12:229–42.

47. Kaplan BS, Thompson PD and de Chadarevian J-P. The hemolytic uremic syndrome. Pediat Clin NA 1976; 23:761–77.

48. Lewis EJ and Schwartz MM. Idiopathic crescentic glomerulonephritis. Sem in Nephrol 1982; 2:193–213.

49. Habib R, Loirat C, Gulbler MC and Levy M. Morphology and serum complement levels in membranoproliferative glomerulonephritis. Adv Nephrol 1974; 4:109–136.

50. Levy M, Broyer M, Arsan A, Levy-Bentolila D and Habib R. Anaphylactoid purpura nephritis in childhood: natural history and immunopathology. Adv Nephrol 1976; 6:183–228.

51. Carbone L, D'Agati V, Cheng J-T and Appel GB. Course and prognosis of human immunodeficiency virus-associated nephropathy. Am J Med 1989; 87:389–95.

52. Abuelo JG. Renal failure caused by chemicals, foods, plants, animal venoms, and misuse of drugs. Arch Intern Med 1990; 150:505–10.

53. O'Callaghan TJ, Edwards JA, Tobin M and Mookerjee BK. Tuberous sclerosis with striking renal involvement in a family. Arch Intern Med 1975; 135:1082–7.

54. Stillwell TJ, Gomez MR and Kelalis PP. Renal lesions in tuberous sclerosis. J Urol 1987; 138:477–81.

55. Chantler C. Syndromes with a renal component. In: Rubin MI and Barratt TM, editors. Pediatric nephrology. The Williams & Wilkins Company, Baltimore, 1975;891–902.

56. Bernstein J. Hereditary renal disease. In: Churg J, Spargo BH, Mostoti FK and Abell MR, editors. Kidney disease: present status. The Williams and Wilkins Company, Baltimore, 1979;218–38.

57. Waldherr W. Familial glomerular disease. Contr Nephrol 1982; 33:104–21.

58. Crawfurd MD'A. The genetics of renal tract disorders. Oxford: Oxford University Press, 1988.

4. Physical examination

J. GARY ABUELO

A careful examination should include particular attention to certain physical findings.

VOLUME STATUS

Of foremost importance in both diagnosis and treatment is the clinical determination of volume status, since volume regulation is often disturbed in renal insufficiency.

Hypervolemia

Intravascular volume overload is usually caused by inadequate excretion of salt and water by kidneys with severely reduced GFR or, in some patients with acute glomerulonephritis, by kidneys with only mildly reduced GFR [1, 2]. In either situation, one finds some or all of the typical signs of congestive heart failure: tachycardia, inability to lie flat, neck vein distention, rales, laterally displaced cardiac apical impulse, a third heart sound, hepatomegaly and edema. Blood pressure is higher than normal for the patient or is clearly hypertensive.

Intravascular volume overload may also be present in patients with primary heart failure and secondary prerenal azotemia; blood pressure may be low due to low cardiac output, high due to adrenergic vasoconstriction or normal.

Hypovolemia

Volume depletion due to either renal or extrarenal fluid losses is a common cause of renal ischemia. The physical findings may include tachycardia, failure of neck veins to distend on lying flat, tenting of the skin, and dry mucous membranes and axillae. The extremities may be cool and pale or even cyanotic due to vasoconstriction. The blood pressure will be lower than its usual level or clearly hypotensive. If possible, euvolemic or questionably hypovolemic patients should be placed in the sitting position with their lower extremities dangling over the side of the bed or, even better, in the standing position to look for orthostatic changes in pulse and blood pressure. An increase in pulse by more than 15 beats per minute or a fall in systolic blood pressure by more than 15 mmHg is suggestive of volume depletion. However, orthostatic falls in blood pressure are seen in up to 24% of euvolemic elderly individuals. Risk factors include medical problems, medications and an elevated supine systolic blood pressure [3–9].

In euvolemic patients with serum albumin concentration less than 2.5 to 3.0 G/dl, edema will usually be present. Absence of edema in such a patient is suggestive of volume depletion, i.e. there is probably a sufficient degree of volume depletion present to counteract the edema producing effect of low intracapillary oncotic pressure.

Importance of Weight. A valuable physical finding often overlooked in the estimation of volume is the patient's weight. A weight gain or loss may confirm subtle physical signs of volume overload or depletion, or may even be the only evidence of a change in volume status. The patient's current weight should be compared with previous weights in the hospital or at home. Abrupt weight loss over a few days usually reflects fluid depletion, and is unlikely to be caused by malnutrition alone if the loss exceeds 0.5 to 1.0 kg per day. Chronic weight loss may be due to a wasting illness or uremia itself.

Clinical Example. A 71-year-old woman is admitted to the hospital because of nausea, anorexia, and fatigue for the past three days. She has had hypertension for thirty years controlled with hydrochloro-

21

J.G. Abuelo (ed.), Renal Failure, 21–24.
© 1995 *Kluwer Academic Publishers.*

thiazide. Scr was 1.4 mg/dl (124 μmol/L) one month ago. Physical examination is unremarkable; the blood pressure is 120/60 mmHg and the pulse 82 per minute. BUN is 73 mg/dl (26 mmol/L), Scr 3.8 mg/dl (336 μmol/L) and urinalysis: specific gravity 1.012, protein and sediment negative.

The blood pressure is somewhat low for a patient with hypertension and suggests the possibility of volume depletion. Further history reveals that the patient weighs herself frequently. The weight has been stable at 110 lb (50 kg), but three days ago she weighed 107 lb (48.6 kg). A weight is checked and is 97 lb (44 kg). The more than 1 kg weight loss per day over three days is evidence of fluid loss. The blood pressure and pulse are measured in the standing position and orthostatic changes are noted. Further history is then taken and reveals that after reading a public health pamphlet the patient started a low salt diet ten days ago while continuing the diuretic. This produced volume depletion as evidenced by resolution of the patient's azotemia with intravenous volume repletion over three days.

SPECIFIC FINDINGS

General appearance

The overall appearance and behavior of the patient do not usually point to a diagnosis, but can indicate the toll of disease on his or her health. With mild and moderate renal failure, patients usually look and act well. With advanced renal failure, the patient may show uremic manifestations like fatigue after little effort, continual scratching, hiccoughs, wandering attention, drowsiness, tremulousness or uremic breath. Puffiness of the face, extremities and torso due to anasarca or wasting due to chronic uremia or other illness may be noted at first glance. Discomfort from pain or dyspnea will also be apparent. Inappropriate behavior or affect might raise suspicion of nephrotoxicity from illegal drugs or from drugs ingested in a suicide attempt.

Vital signs

Pulse. As noted above, both hyper- and hypovolemia may produce tachycardia. An irregular pulse suggests atrial fibrillation and the possibility of renal emboli from left atrial thrombi.

Blood Pressure. Low blood pressure suggests that poor renal perfusion, producing either prerenal azotemia or acute tubular necrosis (ATN), is responsible for the renal failure. Volume depletion, cardiogenic shock and low peripheral resistance states like sepsis all will have to be considered in the diagnosis of the hypotension. In advanced renal failure, pericardial tamponade can lower blood pressure, so the physician must look for a paradoxical pulse, Kussmaul's sign and pericardial rub.

Normal blood pressure is not helpful in making a diagnosis; however, the blood pressure should be checked with the patient in the upright position to look for orthostatic changes. The blood pressures should also be compared to previous blood pressures to exclude a significant fall within the normal range.

High blood pressure is common in patients with renal failure. When it rises gradually and is mild to moderate, it usually reflects hypervolemia. Sudden rise in blood pressure may be seen with atrial thrombi or cholesterol crystals embolizing to the kidneys. Severe hypertension with diastolic BP of 140 mmHg or more raises the question of renal failure due to malignant hypertension. Isolated systolic hypertension is a sign of loss of arterial distensibility due to atherosclerosis. It raises the possibility of renal failure from cholesterol emboli or bilateral renovascular disease.

Temperature. Fever is usually due to infection which commonly produces renal failure due to ischemic ATN. Less often, infection produces renal failure through an immune complex type of glomerulonephritis, as in bacterial endocarditis, or through an interstitial nephritis as in leptospirosis. Rhabdomyolysis and myoglobinuric ATN may occur with extreme hyperpyrexia or with the viral myositis of influenza. Several non-infectious illnesses produce fever and renal failure including thrombotic thrombocytopenic purpura, collagen vascular diseases or drug-induced allergic interstitial nephritis.

Low body temperature is an early sign of sepsis, although fever is usually present by the time ATN appears. Extreme hypothermia due to exposure to the cold often in association with acute alcoholism may damage skeletal muscle and precipitate myoglobinuric ATN.

Skin

The combination of pallor from anemia and yellow discoloration from deposition of urochromes gives uremic patients a characteristic sallow appearance suggestive of chronic renal failure. Excoriations from pruritus and petechiae from platelet dysfunction can also be seen at this stage.

Other skin changes have diagnostic significance. I have mentioned the tenting, and dry axillae of volume depletion and the cool, cyanotic vasoconstricted extremities in individuals in shock. Ecchymoses or petechiae may reflect low platelet counts seen in hemolytic uremic syndrome or thrombotic thrombocytopenic purpura. Signs of liver failure such as jaundice, spider angiomata, palmar erythema suggest hepatorenal syndrome. The presence of ischemic changes of the feet and toes such as livedo reticularis or even frank areas of gangrene is suggestive of cholesterol emboli to the kidney. A dermatologist may be helpful in diagnosing cutaneous vasculitis and other skin findings, such as impetigo, scleroderma, and the drug rashes seen with allergic interstitial nephritis.

Eye findings

On funduscopic examination severe hypertensive changes such as flame-shaped hemorrhages, exudates, papilledema, retinal edema or localized serous detachments usually indicate malignant nephrosclerosis [10], while even mild diabetic changes suggest diabetic glomerulosclerosis.

Retinal vasculitis and a variety of other inflammatory changes in ocular tissues can be seen in connective tissue diseases [11–13]. Scleritis and anterior uveitis can be found in patients with glomerulonephritis [14] and idiopathic interstitial nephritis [15], respectively. Hollenhorst plaques (atheromatous emboli) in the retina should raise the question of cholesterol emboli to the kidney and Roth's spots in the retina may be found in bacterial endocarditis. Yellow retinal nodules are a specific finding in membranoproliferative glomerulonephritis [16–18]. An ophthalmologist can be of assistance in confirming these findings or in performing fluorescein retinography to find early diabetic changes. He or she may also help identify eye abnormalities found in hereditary diseases such as whorl-like corneal deposits in Fabry's disease, and the retinal white dots and lens malformations in Alport's syndrome [19–21].

Heart and lungs

The typical findings of volume overload will be noted. A pericardial rub can be heard in some uremic patients. New heart murmurs in a febrile patient raise the question of bacterial endocarditis.

Abdomen

On abdominal examination, enlarged kidneys may be found in patients with hydronephrosis or polycystic kidneys. Hepatomegaly, ascites and a *caput medusae* or collateral venous pattern suggest hepatorenal syndrome. Abdominal bruits might lead to a consideration of renal ischemia due to renal artery stenosis. Bladder outlet obstruction often will be associated with a palpable tender bladder.

Rectovaginal examination

A rectal examination in men and pelvic examination in women can detect prostatic enlargement or pelvic masses.

Peripheral pulses

Bruits or the absence of pulses in the lower extremities usually indicate advanced atherosclerosis which may also involve the renal arteries.

Joints

Acute arthritis is uncommon but, when present, suggests renal failure associated with bacterial endocarditis, collagen vascular disease, drug hypersensitivity or septic arthritis.

Neurological examination

Altered mental status is seen in advanced uremia, but alternatively can be a clue to the etiology of the renal failure, as changes in sensorium may occur in shock, hypercalcemia, thrombotic thrombocytopenic purpura, malignant hypertension, hepatorenal syndrome, vasculitis and certain nephrotoxins. Asterixis is usually due to hepatic or renal failure.

REFERENCES

1. Glassock RJ. Clinical aspects of glomerular diseases. Am J Kidney Dis 1987; 10:181–5.
2. Chita G and Milne FJ. Acute post-streptococcal glomerulonephritis (APSGN) with disproportionate circulatory volume overload. Kidney Int 1989; 35:915.
3. MacLennan WJ, Hall MRP and Timothy JI. Postural hypotension in old age: is it a disorder of the nervous system or of blood vessels? Age and Aging 1980; 9:25–32.

4. Editorial: postural hypotension in the elderly. Brit Med J 1973; 4:246–7.

5. Mader SL, Josephson KR and Rubenstein LZ. Low prevalence of postural hypotension among community-dwelling elderly. JAMA 1987; 258:1511–4.

6. Lipsitz LA, Storch HA, Minaker KL and Rowe JW. Intra-individual variability in postural blood pressure in the elderly. Clin Sci 1985; 69:337–41.

7. Myers MG, Kearns PM, Kennedy DS and Fisher RH. Postural hypotension and diuretic therapy in the elderly. CMA J 1978; 119:581–5.

8. Atkins D, Hanusa B and Sefcik T. Syncope and orthostatic hypotension. Am J Med 1991; 91:179–85.

9. Rutan GH, Hermanson B, Bild DE, Kittner SJ. LaBaw F and Tell GS. Orthostatic hypotension in older adults. Hypertension 1992; 19:508–19.

10. deVenecia G and Jampol LM. The eye in accelerated hypertension. II. Localized serous detachments of the retina in patients. Arch Ophthal 1984; 102:68–73.

11. Kanski JJ. The eye in systemic disease. Butterworth & Co., Stoneham, 1986.

12. Ferry AP. Ocular manifestations of rheumatic diseases. In: Kelley WN, Harris ED, Ruddy S, Sledge CB, editors. Text-book of rheumatology. W.B. Saunders Co., Philadelphia, 1985:2nd ed., 511–32.

13. Kinyoun JL, Kalina RE and Klein ML. Choroidal involvement in systemic necrotizing vasculitis. Arch Ophth 1987; 105:939–42.

14. Hurault de Ligny B, Sirbat D, Bene MC, Faure G and Kessler M. Scleritis associated with glomerulonephritis. Nephron 1983; 35:207.

15. Ten RM, Torres VE, Milliner DS, Schwab TR, Holley KE and Gleich GJ. Acute interstitial nephritis: immunologic and clinical aspects. Mayo Clin Proc 1988; 63:921–30.

16. Elzinga LW, Weleber RG, Muller D, Houghton DC and Bennett WM. Ocular manifestations of mem-branoproliferative GN Type II (MPGN-II). J Am Soc Nephrol 1992; 3:310.

17. DiMaggio A, Loperfido A and Scatizzi A. Retinal lesions specific for membranoproliferative glomerulonephritis type II: description of 2 cases. Nephron 1993; 63:365–6.

18. Kim DD, Mieler WF and Wolf MD. Posterior segment changes in membranoproliferative glomerulonephritis. Am J Ophthalmol 1992; 114:593–9.

19. Chantler C. Syndromes with a renal component. In: Rubin MI and Barratt TM, editors. Pediatric nephrology. The Williams & Wilkins Company, Baltimore, 1975;891–902.

20. Severin M. The diagnosis contribution of the ophthalmologist in renal insufficiency in childhood. In: Bulla M, editor. Renal insufficiency in children. Springer-Verlag, Berlin, 1982;81–5.

21. Dufier J-L. Ophthalmologic involvement in inherited renal disease. Adv Nephrol 1992; 21: 143.

5. Initial laboratory studies

J. GARY ABUELO

In ordering preliminary tests, the physician should investigate any extrarenal findings that might reveal diseases also affecting the kidneys. For example, back pain may be due to multiple myeloma which is producing myeloma kidney. The basic renal studies, Scr, BUN, serum electrolyte concentrations, and urinalysis are usually available at the outset. If not, these tests should be performed first and repeated as appropriate during the course of the disease.

SERUM CREATININE CONCENTRATION (SCR)

Best test of renal failure

Sudden partial loss of renal function increases Scr from the normal level to a new steady state concentration in a few days. Such a day-to-day rise in Scr is the most reliable indicator of acute renal failure used in clinical medicine. GFR can be accurately determined by the clearance of an infused marker, such as inulin, but the test is too impractical for clinical use. Endogenous creatinine clearance, while a less cumbersome measure of GFR, is often inaccurate in the setting of renal failure, because of increased tubular secretion of creatinine [1], difficulties in obtaining complete urine collections, and varying Scr [2, 3]. Although the blood concentrations of other substances such as urea and phosphate also increase in acute renal failure, these concentrations are affected by diet, volume status, drugs and other extrarenal factors to a far greater degree than Scr.

Creatinine is produced and released by muscle at a rate that varies little (10–15% from the mean value) from day-to-day. It is eliminated from the body largely by glomerular filtration, except at higher Scr when excretion and metabolism by the gut [4] and secretion by the renal tubules [1, 5] become important. Consequently, with few exceptions rises and falls in Scr reflect deterioration and improvement in renal function. In severe acute renal failure, the Scr will rise an average of 1.7 mg/dl (150 μmol/L) per day [6], although with milder renal impairment increments less than 1 mg/dl (88 μmol/L) per day are seen. The highest rates of rise of Scr, sometimes exceeding 5 mg/dl (442 μmol/L) per day [7], occur with release of creatinine from damaged muscle in some patients with rhabdomyolysis [7, 8].

A measure of GFR

Normal Scr. Scr is also used to estimate the GFR in patients with stable renal function (stable Scr). Scr within the normal range usually indicates normal GFR. The exact upper limits of normal vary slightly from one laboratory to another depending on the method used for the determination. Because of increasing creatinine production, the normal range increases over the first two decades of life from 0.3 to 0.5 mg/dl (27 to 44 μmol/L) at age one year [9] to 0.6 to 1.0 mg/dl (53 to 88 μmol/L) in young adult females and 0.8 to 1.3 mg/dl (71 to 115 μmol/L) in adult males. The upper limit of normal range then increases very little throughout life [10–13]. Muscular men and women may have even higher normal values, reaching 1.5 mg/dl (133 μmol/L), due to higher rates of creatinine production.

Low Scr. An above normal GFR may lead to low Scr. Pregnancy increases GFR, and decreases Scr to 0.4 to 0.8 mg/dl (35 to 71 μmol/L) by the third trimester [14, 15]. A similar increase in GFR occurs

25

J.G. Abuelo (ed.), Renal Failure, 25–34.
© 1995 *Kluwer Academic Publishers.*

in newly diagnosed Type I (juvenile onset) diabetics and may lead to Scr as low as 0.2 to 0.6 mg/dl (18 to 53 μmol/L) [16]. Low Scr in this range may also be seen with low creatinine production in individuals with muscle wasting due to cachexia, myopathies or total immobilization [16].

High Scr. Scr above the normal range indicates a reduced GFR. In fact, since Scr is inversely proportional to GFR, one may calculate a creatinine clearance in adults from the Scr (without the need of collecting a timed urine sample) by using the patient's age, weight and sex to estimate creatinine production, which is roughly equal to renal excretion. There are several empirically derived formulae for this [17, 18]. The most commonly used one is that of Cockcroft and Gault [10]:

creatinine clearance (ml/min) =
$$\frac{[140\text{-age (yrs)}] \times \text{weight(kg)} \times 0.85^* \times 88.4^\dagger}{72 \times \text{Scr (mg/dl)}}$$
* multiply by factor of 0.85 if patient is female
† multiply by factor of 88.4 if Scr is in μmol/L.

This formula overestimates creatinine clearance in pregnant women [19], and patients with muscle wasting, ascites or severe obesity [10, 20–22].

A formula to estimate creatinine clearance from Scr and length has also been proposed for children, adolescents and full-term infants [23]:

creatinine clearance (ml/min/1.73M^2) =
$$\frac{k^* \times \text{length (cm)} \times 88.4^\dagger}{\text{Scr (mg/dl)}}$$
* = 0.45 in infants up to 1 year of age
   = 0.55 in children and adolescent girls
   = 0.7 in boys between 13 and 21 years of age
† = multiply by 88.4 if Scr is in μmol/L.

Low GFR's with Normal Scr's. Occasionally, patients have a low creatinine clearance, but due to decreased creatinine production have a normal Scr. A 10% incidence of such false negatives occurs when using Scr to judge normal GFR [4]. Loss of muscle mass from muscle wasting [22] or surgical amputation of limbs [24] may reduce creatinine production and Scr, so that decreases in GFR for whatever reason may not raise Scr above normal. The physician must be mindful that a change in Scr, say from 0.6 to 1.2 mg/dl (53 to 106 μmol/L), in such patients although seemingly small and within the

normal range, indicates loss of half the patient's renal function! Thus, a normal or high normal Scr should prompt a comparison to previous Scr's. The same concern holds in other individuals with low baseline Scr, like young children, pregnant women and juvenile onset diabetics. (In pregnancy and diabetes mellitus, low Scr is caused by high GFR rather than reduced creatinine production.)

Some patients with low GFR and normal Scr may not have renal disease. This is commonly seen in old age where a reduced creatinine clearance, presumably due to "normal" senescent changes in the kidneys [25, 26], is accompanied by a proportional reduction in creatinine production, due to reduced muscle mass. Consequently, the Scr remains in the normal range, despite the fact that half of the normal creatinine clearance is lost between the third and eight decades of life [10, 12, 26]. Therefore, in the elderly patient a normal Scr, especially one that has not risen over many years of observation, probably indicates normal aging kidneys.

In some situations low GFR's with a normal Scr may represent physiologic down-regulation of renal function in response to a reduced load of metabolic waste or animal protein in the diet [27]. This is seen in vegetarians [28] or malnourished individuals [29], where a low protein diet induces a functional reduction in creatinine clearance to levels well below normal. Since there is a proportional fall in creatinine production, Scr remains in the normal range. This phenomenon may also explain the reports of cirrhotic patients who exhibit severely reduced GFR, to less than 20 ml/min in some cases [30], creatinine production well below predicted amounts [17], and normal Scr. Much of this reduction in GFR may be due to low protein intakes, since so many alcoholic patients with cirrhosis have protein malnutrition [31]. Cirrhotics also may have an increased tubular secretion of creatinine. The resulting reduction in Scr further diminishes its usefulness in gauging GFR in this population [30].

Misleading Elevations in Scr. The physician will occasionally encounter *false renal failure*, which is a rise in Scr not caused by a fall in GFR. Most often such elevated Scr's are seen in normal but very muscular individuals due to high production of creatinine by muscle tissue. Transient elevations in

Scr reaching 2 mg/dl (177 μmol/L), may also occur for three to eight hours after a meal containing a large amount (200–300G) of well-cooked meat [32], due to ingestion of creatinine formed from creatine during cooking [33]. False renal failure also may come about through the impairment of tubular secretion of creatinine by *salicylate* [34], *cimetidine* [35–38] or *trimethoprim* [39–42]. The rise in Scr will usually be less than 0.5 mg/dl (22 μmol/L) in normals, but can be more than 2 mg/dl (177 μmol/L) in chronically azotemic individuals whose tubular secretion of creatinine may account for up to half of creatinine clearance [1, 5, 38, 42].

Certain drugs such as *acetohexamide* [43, 44], *cefoxitin* [45, 46] and *methyldopa* [47] give a false positive test for creatinine in the commonly used Jaffe method for measuring creatinine, and false elevations of 0.7 mg/dl (62 μmol/L) or more are possible. *5-Flucytosine* may cause a false elevation of up to 5 mg/dl (442 μmol/L) with the creatinine imidohydralase method (Ektachem, Eastman Kodak Company, Rochester, NY) [48, 49]. In some disease states, endogenous substances may appear in the serum that also interfere with the Jaffe reaction. Acetoacetate may produce a false rise in the Scr of about 0.7 mg/dl (62 μmol/L) during fasting and of 2 to 3 mg/dl (177 to 265 μmol/L) in severe alcoholic or diabetic ketoacidosis [50–55]. In contrast, in jaundiced patients negative interference by bilirubin and other substances may falsely lower Scr by as much as 1.8 mg/dl (159 μmol/L) when kinetic Jaffe creatinine methods are used [56].

UREA

In many laboratories the BUN is still used as a screening test for renal insufficiency despite the superiority of Scr. Although BUN is rarely affected by false elevations due to drugs [57], it is influenced by several factors other than GFR.

BUN to Creatinine Ratio. In renal failure the BUN (mg/dl) is generally between 10 and 20 times the Scr, when both are expressed in mg/dl (between 0.40 and 0.80 times the Scr, when BUN is in mmol/L and Scr in μmol/L) [58]. However, a BUN to creatinine ratio above this range may be seen in certain circumstances due to either a fall in urea clearance out of proportion to the fall in GFR or to

augmented urea production. Such excessive rises in BUN in relation to the fall in GFR have led to the abandonment of BUN as a single test to estimate renal function. However, when exaggerated rises in BUN are considered together with the clinical picture, they can suggest unsuspected conditions that merit investigation. Therefore, one should order a BUN along with the Scr and look at the BUN to Scr ratio.

High Ratios (BUN : Scr of 20 : 1 or Greater)[1]. These are most commonly seen in prerenal azotemia [58]. Here, the decreased renal perfusion and secondary renal hemodynamic changes, not only reduce GFR, but also disproportionately increase BUN due to *increased tubular reabsorption of urea* [59]. The excessive rise in BUN in prerenal azotemia due to diuretic-induced sodium depletion or to heart failure may be further exaggerated by an increased production of urea [60, 61].

> An increased BUN to Scr ratio may occur in patients with acute urinary tract obstruction because of high tubular urea reabsorption [62], or in patients with surgical diversion of the urine into the colon or a segment of the ileum because of intestinal reabsorption of urea [63, 64].

Increased urea production can induce an exaggerated rise in BUN in some patients with renal failure not caused by prerenal azotemia. This occurs with stimulation of protein catabolism by glucocorticoids, inhibition of protein synthesis by tetracyclines, and increased absorption of protein from the intestine due to a high protein diet or bleeding into the gut [65, 66]. Patients with acute myocardial infarctions may also have augmented urea production [67].

Finally, some individuals with acute tubular necrosis may have an increased BUN to creatinine ratio [58]. The mechanism for this has not been elucidated, but these patients have renal ischemia and may well have the same pathophysiologic changes that increase tubular reabsorption of urea in prerenal azotemia.

> *Low Ratios (BUN : Scr of 10 : 1 or Less).[2]* Renal insufficiency with a decreased BUN to Scr ratio may be due to reduced urea production in patients on a low protein diet [68], to increased elimination of urea in voluminous vomitus or diarrheal stools [63], to spurious elevations of Scr (see *Misleading Elevations in Scr* above), or to increased

creatinine production in patients with rhabdomyolysis [7]. This latter occurrence may be rare, since Gabow et al. failed to find low BUN:Scr ratios in patients with rhabdomyolysis [8]. The high urine flow rate in untreated central diabetes insipidus increases urea clearance and may cause dehydration [69]. Theoretically, this could also lead to prerenal azotemia with low BUN to Scr ratios.

URINALYSIS

The urinalysis is a combination of several urine tests and can provide a variety of diagnostic clues to the cause of renal failure.

Appearance

Bloody urine with a brown or reddish-brown color, resembling Coca-Cola or tea, is typical of an acute glomerulonephritis, while pink or bright red bloody urine is usually seen with post-glomerular processes such as polycystic kidneys, renal infarction and urinary tract obstruction. Gross hematuria may also occur in occasional patients with malignant hypertension, thrombotic thrombocytopenic purpura and allergic interstitial nephritis due to beta-lactam antibiotics [70, 71]. In hemoglobinuric and myoglobinuric acute tubular necrosis, hemoglobin or myoglobin may give a reddish-brown color to the urine [72].

Concentration

A urine specific gravity of 1.015–1.020 or above is suggestive of prerenal azotemia and hepato-renal syndrome, since reduced arterial blood pressure or flow stimulates vasopressin secretion and other mechanisms that increase urine concentration. Some elderly patients [73] or individuals with underlying chronic renal disease are unable to concentrate their urine and may develop prerenal azotemia without a high urine specific gravity. Poorly nourished subjects may have concentrated urine (high urine *osmolality*) without a high specific gravity due to reduced urea production and excretion in the urine [74].

Qualitative protein test

This is typically negative or trace in conditions with little or no glomerular or tubular damage such as prerenal azotemia, postrenal azotemia and renal failure caused by drugs that alter renal hemodynamics (angiotensin converting enzyme in-

hibitors [75] or non-steroidal anti-inflammatory drugs [76]). The qualitative protein test is negative to 2+ (100 mg/dl) in conditions with predominantly tubular or interstitial changes such as acute tubular necrosis [77–79] or acute interstitial nephritis [80, 81]. Presumably, this is tubular proteinuria, i.e. the poorly functioning tubules fail to reabsorb the low molecular weight proteins that are normally filtered by the glomeruli. Qualitative protein values of 3+ to 4+ (300 to 1000 mg/dl) are seen with primary or secondary glomerulopathies, and are almost always due to increased glomerular permeability to proteins. Small vessel diseases like malignant hypertension can also produce heavy proteinuria presumably through secondary glomerular involvement (see Chapter 10).

Application of these general rules can be helpful, but many exceptions must be kept in mind. Patients with volume depletion or dehydration often make small quantities of concentrated urine (S.G. ~ 1.030) in which normal amounts of protein may be concentrated enough to give a 1+ (30 mg/dl) qualitative test. Transient proteinuria may be seen with burns [82, 83], pancreatitis [84], fever, congestive heart failure, seizures and extreme physical exercise [85, 86]. This or proteinuria from underlying chronic renal disease may confuse the diagnosis in prerenal, postrenal or vasomotor types of renal failure. Also a false positive urine dipstick test for protein may be caused by phenazopyridine, urinary infection with urea splitting organisms, and contamination of the urine with antiseptic [85]. On the other hand, occasional patients with severe glomerulonephritis for unknown reasons have little (1+) or no proteinuria [87, 88]. Also falsely low or negative dipstick tests for protein may occur when high urine volumes (suggested by urine specific gravity below 1.010) dilute urine protein concentration.

Multiple myeloma causes renal failure in older subjects in whom the monoclonal immunoglobulin light chains (Bence-Jones proteins) in the urine seem to be "nephrotoxic" and lead to myeloma kidney (cast nephropathy) [89]. Since the dipstick protein method is insensitive to light chains [90], patients over 50 years of age with renal failure and no proteinuria detected by dipstick should have their urine retested for protein with an alternate method, such as the sulfosalicylic acid test or the urine protein to creatinine ratio.

Sediment

Red Blood Cells. The microscopic examination of the urine sediment may detect various degrees of hematuria which is *defined as 5 or more red cells per high power field.* The finding of more than 50 to 100 red cells per high power field suggests the presence of the same conditions as seen with gross hematuria, while the absence of hematuria (less than 5 red cells per hpf) excludes an acute glomerulonephritic process. An intermediate number of red cells may be seen with any intrinsic renal disease, but is evidence against functional disorders such as prerenal azotemia or vasomotor disturbances (e.g. due to NSAIDs – see Chapter 10). The absence of red cells in the presence of a positive dipstick for "blood" suggests hemoglobinuric or myoglobinuric tubular necrosis.

> In patients with microscopic hematuria due to glomerular disease, many red cells are *dysmorphic*, i.e. irregular in outline, collapsed or devoid of hemoglobin. These "glomerular" red cells may be appreciated on routine microscopy of the urine sediment, but are more easily seen on a Wright stain of the urinary sediment [91] or with phase contrast microscopy of a freshly spun urine [92, 93]. Dysmorphic red cells may also be detected by their smaller size in an electronic particle-size analyzer [94]. In contrast to the diagnostic usefulness of dysmorphic red cells claimed in early reports, recent studies found their presence or absence in the urine to be unreliable in determining the cause of hematuria [95–98]. Also for some reason when patients with glomerulonephritis have gross hematuria [91, 99] or diuresis due to furosemide or water [100], only a small percentage of the red cells have a "glomerular" appearance.

White Blood Cells. The presence of increased numbers of white cells in the spun urine *(more than 3 to 5 per high power field)* suggests an interstitial nephritis such as acute pyelonephritis. A Wright stain of the urine sediment showing that more than 33% of these white cells are eosinophils is evidence for an allergic interstitial nephritis, although eosinophils are not always seen in this condition [80, 101]. One report claims that Hansel's stain for eosinophils in the urine sediment is more sensitive than Wright's stain. This stain showed 5 to 50% eosinophils in four and 1 to 5% in six of eleven patients with allergic nephritis. However, the presence of eosinophiluria in cases with prostatitis or glomerulonephritis showed the lack of specificity of urinary eosinophils regardless of the

stain used [102].

Urinary white blood cells may also be somewhat increased in glomerulonephritis and acute tubular necrosis, where an interstitial infiltrate frequently accompanies the glomerular or tubular lesions, respectively [103].

Casts, Epithelial Cells and Crystals. The presence of *red cell casts* is time honored evidence that hematuria is due to glomerulonephritis (Figure 5.1A).

> Exceptions include the rare finding of red cell casts in conditions such as atheroembolic renal disease [104], renal thromboembolism, diabetes mellitus [105, 106], strenuous exercise [107], malignant hypertension [108], hemolytic uremic syndrome [109, 110], thrombotic thrombocytopenic purpura [111], allergic interstitial nephritis [112] or acute cortical necrosis [113].

Tubular epithelial cells and *muddy brown coarse granular casts* (Figure 5.1B) are characteristic of the sediment in acute tubular necrosis, but may not be present in almost a quarter of cases [79, 114, 115]. *Uric acid crystalluria* is common in tumor lysis syndrome (Figure 5.1C) [116], and massive *oxalate crystalluria* can be seen in ethylene glycol intoxication (Figure 5.1D) [117]. *Crystals within leukocytes* occur in acyclovir induced renal failure [118].

Bland Urinary Sediment [115]. A normal urine sediment without proteinuria is typical of prerenal and vasomotor types of renal failure in which there is no intrinsic renal disease. A normal urinalysis is also common in postrenal renal failure and ischemic renal disease caused by renal artery stenosis. Small vessel diseases (e.g. atheroembolic disease), tubular diseases (e.g. acute tubular necrosis) and interstitial nephritis may occasionally cause renal failure with a bland urinary sediment.

SERUM ELECTROLYTES

Hyperkalemia, hyponatremia and low serum bicarbonate concentration due to metabolic acidosis are non-specific manifestations of advanced renal failure. *Hyperkalemia with less severe renal failure* (Scr less than 6 mg/dl) is unusual, but can be seen in obstructive uropathy [119] and in several low

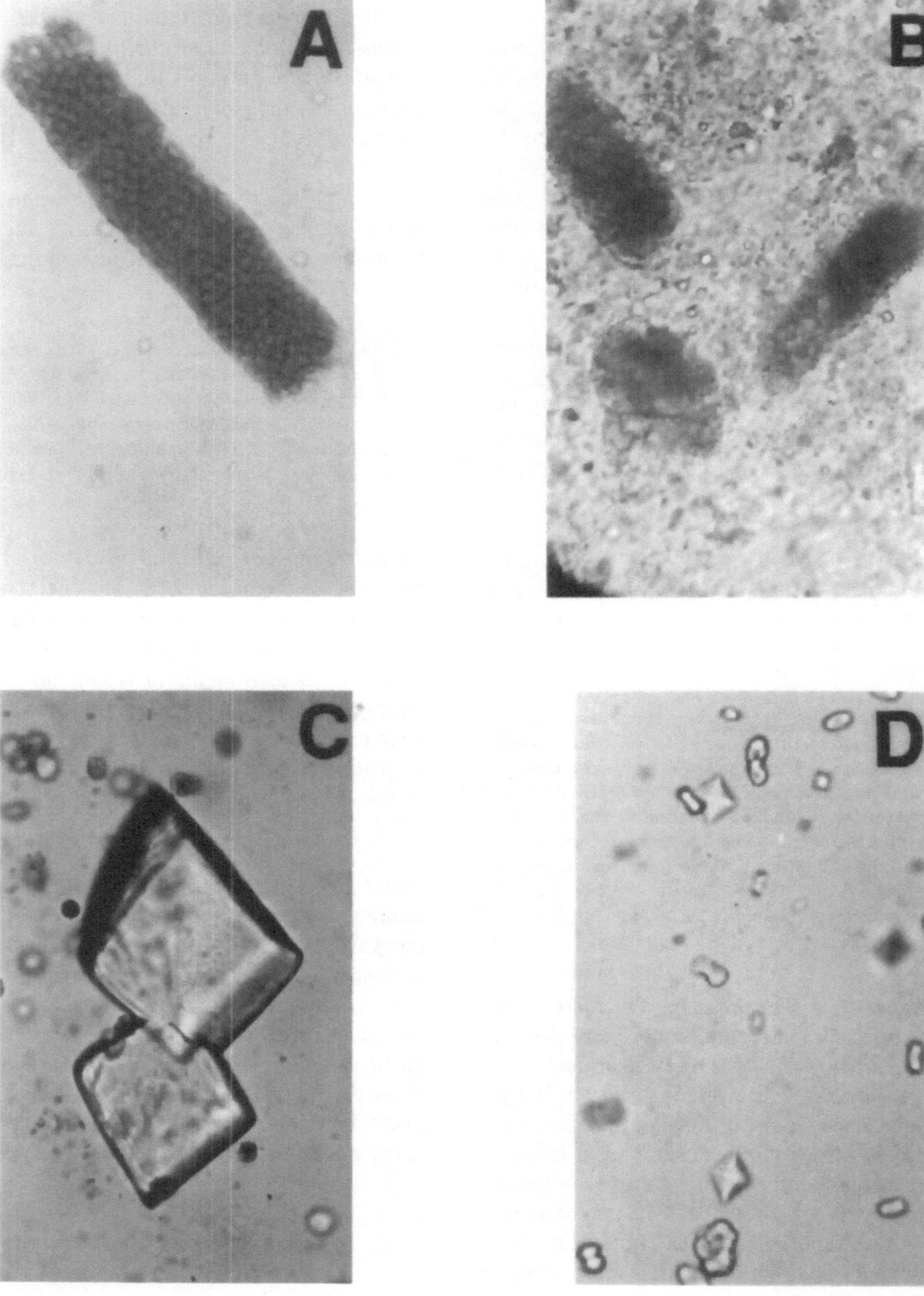

Fig. 5.1A-D. Certain findings in the urinary sediments have diagnostic importance. (A) red cell cast in GN; (B) muddy brown granular casts in acute tubular necrosis; (C) rhomboid shaped uric acid crystals in tumor lysis syndrome; and (D) calcium oxalate crystals in ethylene glycol toxicity. The envelope form is a calcium oxalate dihydrate crystal; the ovoid and dumbbell forms are calcium oxalate monohydrate crystals. (Courtesy of Frances Andrus, B.A.)

aldosterone states: prerenal azotemia due to adrenal insufficiency, vasomotor type renal failure due to angiotensin converting enzyme inhibitors [120] or nonsteroidal anti-inflammatory drugs [121], and hyporeninemic hypoaldosteronism due to diabetic nephropathy or interstitial nephritis [122]. Hyperkalemia can also be due to potassium supplements or potassium sparing diuretics. *Hypokalemia* is unusual in patients with azotemia and may be a clue to the cause of renal failure. Most common would be prerenal renal failure or ischemic acute tubular necrosis resulting from diarrhea, vomiting or excess diuretics. The less common causes of renal failure with hypokalemia are shown on Table 5.1. *Hypernatremia* reflects dehydration (water deficit) and suggests prerenal azotemia, since many dehydrated patients have hypovolemia as well. An *elevated serum bicarbonate concentration* often indicates metabolic alkalosis and raises the question of prerenal azotemia due to vomiting or diuretics, or possibly hypercalcemia due to milk-alkali syndrome (see Chapter 10) [123].

Table 5.1. Causes of renal failure with hypokalemia

Diarrhea
Vomiting
Diuretics
Nephrotoxins
    Aminoglycosides
    Amphotericin
    Cisplatin
    Ifosfamide
High renin state
    Malignant hypertension
    Renal artery stenosis
Cystinosis
Medullary and other cystic disease

NOTES

1. 0.80 or greater in SI units.
2. 0.40 or less in SI units.

REFERENCES

1. Bauer JH, Brooks CS and Burch RN. Clinical appraisal of creatinine clearance as a measure of glomerular filtration rate. Am J Kidney Dis 1982; 2:337–46.

2. Payne RB. Creatinine clearance: a redundant clinical investigation. Ann Clin Biochem 1986; 23:243–250.

3. Wharton WW III, Sondeen JL, McBiles M, Gradwohl SE, Wade CE, Ciceri DP et al. Measurement of glomerular filtration rate in ICU patients using ^{99m}Tc-DTPA and inulin. Kidney Int 1992; 42:174–8.

4. Duarte CG, Elveback LR and Liedtke RR. Creatinine in renal function tests. In: Duarte CG, editor. Clinical laboratory procedures and diagnosis. Little, Brown and Company, Boston, 1980;1–28.

5. Shemesh O, Golbetz H, Kriss JP and Myers BD. Limitations of creatinine as a filtration marker in glomerulopathic patients. Kidney Int 1985; 28:830–8.

6. Lordon RE and Burton JR. Post-traumatic renal failure in military personnel in Southeast Asia. Am J Med 1972; 53:137–47.

7. Grossman RA, Hamilton RW, Morse BM, Penn AS and Goldberg M. Nontraumatic rhabdomyolysis and acute renal failure. N Engl J Med 1974; 291:807–11.

8. Gabow PA, Kaehny WD and Kelleher SP. The spectrum of rhabdomyolysis. Medicine 1982; 61:141–52.

9. Schwartz GJ, Haycock GB, Edelman CM and Spitzer AA. A simple estimate of glomerular filtration rate in children derived from body length and plasma creatinine. Pediatrics 1976; 58:259–63.

10. Cockcroft DW and Gault MH. Prediction of creatinine clearance from serum creatinine. Nephron 1976; 16:31–41.

11. Rowe JW, Andres R, Tobin JD, Norris AH and Shock NW. The effect of age on creatinine clearance in men: A cross sectional and longitudinal study. J Gerontology 1976; 31:155–63.

12. Kampmann J, Siersback-Nielsen K, Kristensen M and Hansen JM. Rapid evaluation of creatinine clearance. Acta Med Scand 1974; 196:517–20.

13. Tietz NW, Shuey DF, Wekstein DR. Laboratory values in fit aging individuals – Sexagenarians through centenarians. Clin Chem 1992; 38:1167–85.

14. Moniz CF, Nicolaides KH, Bamforth FJ and Rodeck CH. Normal reference ranges for biochemical substances relating to renal, hepatic, and bone function in fetal and maternal plasma throughout pregnancy. J Clin Pathol 1985; 38:468–72.

15. Ezimokhai M, Davison JM, Philips PR and W Dunlop. Non-postural serial changes in renal function during the third trimester of normal human pregnancy. Br J Obstet Gynaecol 1981; 88:465–71.

16. Hagemann P and Kahn SN. Significance of low concentrations of creatinine in serum from hospital patients. Clin Chem 1988;34:2311–2.

17. Cocchetto DM, Tschanz C and Bjornsson TD. Decreased rate of creatinine production in patients with hepatic disease: Implications for estimation of creatinine clearance. Ther Drug Monit 1983; 5:161–8.

18. Gates GF. Creatinine clearance estimation from serum creatinine values: an analysis of three mathematical models of glomerular function. Am J Kidney Dis 1985; 5:199–205.

19. Parker RA, Bennett WM and Porter GA. Clinical estimate of creatinine clearance without urine collection. Dialysis and Transplantation 1980; 9:251–2.

20. Mohler JL, Barton SD, Blouin RA, Cowen DL and Flanigan RC. The evaluation of creatinine clearance in spinal cord injury patients. J Urol 1986; 136:366–9.

21. Salazar DE and Corcoran GB. Predicting creatinine clearance and renal drug clearance in obese patients from estimated fat-free body mass. Am J Med 1988; 84:1053–60.

22. Boers M, Dijkmans BAC, Breedveld FC and Mattie H. Errors in the prediction of creatinine clearance in patients with rheumatoid arthritis. Brit J Rheumatol. 1988; 27:233–5.

23. Schwartz GJ, Brion LP and Spitzer A. The use of plasma creatinine concentration for estimating glomerular filtration rate in infants, children, and adolescents. Pediat Clin N Amer. 1987; 34:571–90.89

24. Charlson ME, MacKenzie CR, Gold JP and Shires T. Postoperative changes in serum creatinine. Ann Surg 1989; 209:328–33.

25. McLachlan MSF. The aging kidney. Lancet 1978; 2:143–6.

26. Abrass CK. Glomerulonephritis in the elderly. Am J Nephrol 1985; 5:409–18.

27. Kontessis P, Jones S, Dodds R, Trevisan R, Nosadini R, Fioretto P et al. Renal, metabolic and hormonal responses to ingestion of animal and vegetable proteins. Kidney Int 1990; 38:136–44.

28. Bosch JP, Saccaggi A, Lauer A, Ronco C, Belledonne M and Glabman S. Renal functional reserve in humans. Effect of protein intake on glomerular filtration rate. Am J Med 1983; 75:943–50.

29. Klahr S and Alleyne GAO. Nutrition and the kidney. In: Suki WN and Eknoyan G, editors. The kidney in systemic disease. John Wiley Publishers, New York, 1981: 2nd ed, 307–46.

30. Caregaro L, Menon F, Angeli P, Amodio P, Merkel C, Bortoluzzi A et al. Limitations of serum creatinine level and creatinine clearance as filtration markers in cirrhosis. Arch Intern Med 1994; 154:201–5.

31. Mendenhall CL, Anderson S, Weesner RE, Goldberg SJ and Crolic KA. Protein-calorie malnutrition associated with alcoholic hepatitis. Veterans Administration Cooperative Study Group on Alcoholic Hepatitis. Am J Med 1984; 76:211–22.

32. Mayersohn M, Conrad KA and Achari R. The influence of a cooked meat meal on creatinine plasma concentration and creatinine clearance. B J Clin Pharmac 1983; 15:227–30.

33. Jacobsen FK, Christensen CK, Mogensen CE and Heilskov NSC. Evaluation of kidney function after meals. Lancet 1980; 1:319.

34. Burry HC and Dieppe PA. Apparent reduction of endogenous creatinine clearance by salicylate treatment. BMJ 1976; 2:16–17.

35. Larsson R, Bodemar G, Kagedal B and Walen A. The effects of cimetidine (Tagamet) on renal function in patients with renal failure. Acta Med Scand 1980; 208:27–31.

36. Burgess E, Blair A and Krichman. Inhibition of renal creatinine secretion by cimetidine in humans. Renal Physiol (Basel) 1982; 5:27–30.

37. Pachon J, Lorber MI and Bia MJ. Effects of H$_2$-receptor antagonists on renal function in cyclosporine-treated renal transplant patients. Transplantation 1989; 47:254–9.

38. Artz MA, Hilbrands LB, Wetzels JFM and Koene RAP. Reliability of creatinine as a marker of glomerular filtration after oral ingestion of cimetidine. Kidney Int 1991; 39:1051–6.

39. Shouval D, Ligumsky M and Ben-Ishay D. Effect of co-trimoxazole on normal creatinine clearance. Lancet 1978; 1:244–5.

40. Berglund F, Killander J and Pompeius R. Effect of trimethoprim-sulfamethoxazole on the renal excretion of creatinine in man. J Urol 1975; 114:802–8.

41. Brautigam M, Froese P, Baethke R and Kessel M. Zur Kreatininausscheidung beim Menschen nach Gabe von Co-Trimoxazol. Klin Wochenschrift 1979; 57:95–6.

42. Myre SA, McCann J, First MR and Cluxton RJ Jr. Effect of trimethoprim on serum creatinine in healthy and chronic renal failure volunteers. Ther Drug Monitor 1987; 9:161–5.

43. Roach NA, Kroll MH and Elin RJ. Interference by sulfonylurea drugs with the Jaffe method for creatinine. Clin Chem Acta 1985; 151:301–5.

44. Baba S, Baba T and Iwanaga T. Effect of acetohexamide (a sulfonylurea hypoglycemic agent) in blood plasma on creatinine assay in clinical laboratory tests. Chem Pharm Bull 1979; 27:139–43.

45. Saah AJ, Koch TR and Drusano GL. Cefoxitin falsely elevates creatinine levels. JAMA 1982; 247:205–6.

46. Durham SR, Bignell AHC and Wise R. Interference of cefoxitin in the creatinine estimation and its clinical relevance. J Clin Path 1979; 32:1148–51.

47. Maddocks J, Hann S, Hopkins M and Coles GA. Effect of methyldopa on creatinine estimation. Lancet 1973; 157:157.

48. Herrington D, Drusano GL, Smalls U and Standiford HC. False elevation in serum creatinine levels. JAMA 1984; 252:2962.

49. Mitchell RT, Marshall LH, Lefkowitz LB and Stratton CW. Falsely elevated serum creatinine levels secondary to the presence of 5-fluorocytosine. Am J Clin Pathol 1985; 84:251–3.

50. Gerard SK and Khayam-Bashi H. Characterization of creatinine error in ketotic patients. Amer J Clin Pathol 1985; 84:659–64.

51. Mascioli SR, Bantle JP, Freier EF and Hoogweaf BJ. Artifactual elevation of serum creatinine due to fasting. Arch Intern Med 1984; 144:1575–6.

52. Lebel RR, Gutmann FD, Mazumdar DC and Grzys M. Creatinine determination in ketosis. N Engl J Med 1974; 310:1671.

53. Molitch ME, Rodman E, Hirsch CA and Dubinsky E. Spurious serum creatinine elevations in ketoacidosis. Ann Intern Med 1980; 93:280–1.

54. Assadi FK, John EG, Fornell L and Rosenthal IM. Falsely elevated serum creatinine concentration in ketoacidosis. J Pediatr 1985; 107:562–4.

55. Glick MR, Moorehead WR, Oei TO and Moore GR. Acetoacetate and "ketone" interference in kinetic and continuous-flow methods for creatinine. Clin Chem 1980; 26:1626.

56. Bowers LD and Wong ET. Kinetic serum creatinine assays. II. A critical evaluation and review. Clin Chem 1980; 26:555–61.

57. Sher PP. Drug interferences with clinical laboratory tests. Drugs 1982; 24:24–63.

58. Morgan DB, Carver ME and Payne RB. Plasma creatinine and urea: creatinine ratio in patients with raised plasma urea. BMJ 1977; 2:929–32.

59. Baum N, Dichoso CC and Carlton CE. Blood urea nitrogen and serum creatinine. Physiology and interpretations. Urology 1975; 5:583–8.

60. Kamm DE, Wu L and Kuchmy BL. Contribution of the urea appearance rate to diuretic-induced azotemia in the rat. Kidney Int 1987; 32:47–56.

61. Thomas RD, Newill A and Morgan DB. The cause of the raised plasma urea of acute heart failure. Postgrad Med J 1975; 55:10–4.

62. Marshall S. Urea-creatinine ratio in obstructive uropathy and renal hypertension. JAMA 1964; 190:719–20.

63. Dosseter JB. Creatininemia versus uremia. The relative significance of blood urea nitrogen and serum creatinine concentrations in azotemia. Ann Intern Med 1966; 65:1287–99.

64. Gensten HG and Skjoldborg H. Changes in the composition of the urine after ileal loop urinary diversion. Scand J Urol Nephrol 1971; 5:37–40.

65. Cohn TD, Lane M, Zuckerman S, Messinger N and Griffith A. Induced azotemia in humans following massive protein and blood ingestion and the mechanism of azotemia in gastrointestinal hemorrhage. Am J Med Sci 1956; 231:394–401.

66. Shils ME. Renal disease and the metabolic effects of tetracycline. Ann Intern Med 1963; 58:389–408.

67. Moseley MJ, Sawminathan R and Morgan B. Raised plasma urea levels after myocardial infarction. Arch Intern Med 1981; 141:438–40.

68. Kopple JD and Coburn JW. Evaluation of chronic uremia. Importance of serum urea nitrogen, serum creatinine and their ratio. JAMA 1974; 227:41–4.

69. Comtois R, Bertrand S, Beauregard H and Vinay P. Low serum urea level in dehydrated patients with central diabetes insipidus. CMAJ 1988; 139:965–9.

70. Appel GB, Neu HC. Acute interstitial nephritis induced by beta-lactam antibiotics. In: Fillastre J-P, editor. Nephrotoxicity. INSERM, France, 1981;195–212.

71. Nemati C and Abuelo JG. Cephalosporin induced hypersensitivity nephritis: report of a case caused by cefazolin. RI Med J 1981; 64:91–4.

72. Grossman RA, Hamilton RW, Morse BM, Penn AS and Goldberg M. Nontraumatic rhabdomyolysis and acute renal failure. N Engl J Med 1974; 291:807–11.

73. Sporn N, Lancestremere RG and Papper S. Differential diagnosis of oliguria in aged patients. N Engl J Med 1962; 267:130–2.

74. Joekes S, Mowbray JF and Dormandy K. Oliguria with urine of "fixed" specific gravity. Lancet 1957; 2:864–7.

75. Dzau VJ, Hricik DE, Browning PJ, Kopelman RI, Goorno WE, and Madias NE. Captopril-induced functional renal insufficiency in patients with bilateral renal-artery stenoses or renal-artery stenosis in a "solitary" kidney. Amer Soc Nephrol 1982: abstract; 28A.

76. Blackshear JL, Davidman M and Stillman T. Identification of risk for renal insufficiency from nonsteroid anti-inflammatory drugs. Arch Intern Med 1983; 143:1130–4.

77. MacLean PR and Robson JS. Unselective proteinuria in acute ischaemic renal failure. Clin Sci 1966; 30:91–102.

78. Revillard JP, Manuel Y, Francois R and Traeger J. Renal diseases associated with tubular proteinuria. In: Manuel Y, Revillard JP and Betuel H, editors. Proteins in normal and pathological urine. Karger, Basel/New York, 1970;209–19.

79. Graber M, Lane B, Lamia R and Pastoriza-Munoz E. Bubble cells: renal tubular cells in the urinary sediment with characteristics of viability. J Am Soc Nephrol 1991; 1:999–1004.

80. Linton AL, Clark WF, Driedger AA, Turnbull I and Lindsay RM. Acute interstitial nephritis due to drugs. Review of the literature with a report of nine cases. Ann Intern Med 1980; 93:735–41.

81. Kida H, Abe T, Tomosugi N, Koshino Y, Yokoyama H and Hattori N. Prediction of the long-term outcome in acute interstitial nephritis. Clin Nephrol 1984; 22:55–60.

82. Yu H, Cooper EH, Settle JA and Meadows T. Urinary protein profiles after burn injury. Burns, Including Thermal Injury 1983; 9:339–49.

83. Lindquist J, Drueck C, Simon NM, Elson B, Hurwich D and Roxe D. Proximal renal tubular dysfunction in severe burns. Am J Kid Dis 1984; 4:44–7.

84. Meier PB and Levitt MD. Urine protein excretion in acute pancreatitis. J Lab Clin Med 1986; 108:628–34.

85. Abuelo JG. Proteinuria: diagnostic principles and procedures. Ann Intern Med 1983; 98:186–91.

86. Houser MT, Jahn MF, Kobayashi A and Walburn J. Assessment of urinary protein excretion in the adolescent: effect of body position and exercise. J Pediatr 1986; 109:556–61.

87. Beirne GJ, Wagnild JP, Zimmerman SW, Macken PD and Burkholder PM. Idiopathic crescentic glomerulonephritis. Medicine 1977; 56:349–81.

88. Neild GH, Cameron JS, Ogg CS, Turner DR, Williams DG, Brown CB et al. Rapidly progressive glomerulonephritis with extensive glomerular crescent formation. Quart J Med 1983; 52:395–416.

89. Hill GS, Morel-Maroger L, Mery J-P, Brouel JC and Mignon F. Renal lesions in multiple myeloma: their relationship to associated plasma associations. Am J Kidney Dis 1983; 2:423–38.

90. Clough G and Reah TG. A "protein error". Lancet 1964; 1:1248.

91. Chang BS. Red cell morphology as a diagnostic aid in hematuria. JAMA 1984; 252:1747–9.

92. Fairley KF and Birch DF. Hematuria: A simple method for identifying glomerular bleeding. Kidney Int 1982; 21:105–8.

93. DeSanto NG, Nuzzi F, Capodicasa G, Lama G, Caputo G, Rosati P et al. Phase contrast microscopy of the urine sediment for the diagnosis of glomerular and nonglomerular bleeding-data in children and adults with normal creatinine clearance. Nephron 1987; 45:3–9.

94. Pollock C, Pei-Ling L, Gyory AZ, Grigg R, Gallery EDM, Caterson R et al. Dysmorphism of urinary red blood cells-Value in diagnosis. Kidney Int 1989; 36:1045–9.

95. Piccoli G, Rotunno M, Quarello F and Piccoli GB. Urinary sediment analysis: A useful tool? Contrib Nephrol 1989; 70:157–62.

96. Raman GV, Pead L, Lee HA and Maskell R. A blind controlled trial of phase-contrast microscopy by two observers

for evaluating the source of hematuria. Nephron 1986; 44:304–8.

97. Kohler H, Wandel E and Brunck B. Acanthocyturia – a characteristic marker for glomerular bleeding. Kidney Int 1991; 40:115–20.

98. Gibbs DD and Lynn KL. Red cell volume distribution curves in the diagnosis of glomerular and non-glomerular hematuria. Clin Nephrol 1990; 33:143–7.

99. Van Iseghem P, Hauglustaine D, Bollens W and Michielsen P. Urinary erythrocyte morphology in acute glomerulonephritis. BMJ 1983; 287:1183.

100. Schuetz E, Schaefer RM, Heidbreder E and Heidland A. Effect of diuresis on urinary erythrocyte morphology in glomerulonephritis. Klin Wochenschr 1985; 63:575–577.

101. Galpin JE, Shinaberger JH and Stanley TM. Acute interstitial nephritis due to methicillin. Am J Med 1978; 65:756–65.

102. Nolan CR, Anger MS and Kelleher SP. Eosinophiluria – a new method of detection and definition of the clinical spectrum. N Engl J Med 1986; 315:1516–9.

103. Segasothy M, Fairley KF, Birch DF and Kincaid-Smith P. Sterile pyuria. Clin Nephrol 1991; 35: 87–8.

104. Ludmerer KM and Kissane JM. Progressive renal failure with hematuria in a 62 year old man. Am J Med 1981; 71:468–74.

105. O'Neill WM, Wallin JD and Walker PD. Hematuria and red cell casts in typical diabetic nephropathy. Am J Med 1983; 74:389–95.

106. Lopes De Faria JB, Moura LAR, Lopes De Faria SR, Ramos OL and Pereira AB. Glomerular hematuria in diabetics. Clin Nephrol 1988; 30:117–21.

107. Fassett RG, Owen JE, Fairley J, Birch DF and Fairley KF. Urinary red-cell morphology during exercise. BMJ 1982; 285:1455–7.

108. Mattern WD, Sommers SC and Kassirer JP. Oliguric acute renal failure in malignant hypertension. Am J Med 1972; 52:187–97.

109. Clarkson AR, Lawrence JR, Meadows R and Seymour AE. The haemolytic uraemic syndrome in adults. Quart J Med 1970; 39:227–44.

110. Dolislager D and Tune B. The hemolytic-uremic syndrome. Am J Dis Child 1978; 132:55–58.

111. Eknoyan G and Riggs SA. Renal involvement in patients with thrombotic thrombocytopenic purpura. Am J Nephrol 1986; 6:117–31.

112. Sigala JF, Biava CG and Hulter HN. Red blood cell casts in acute interstitial nephritis. Arch Intern Med 1978; 138:1419–21.

113. Goergen TG, Lindstrom RR, Tan H and Lilley JJ. CT appearance of acute renal cortical necrosis. AJR 1981; 137:167–7.

114. Gay C, Cochat P, Pellet H, Floret D and Buenerd A. Le sediment urinaire dans l'insuffisance renale aigue de l'enfant. Pediatrie 1987; 42:723–7.

115. Bouffet E, Laville M, Zanettini MC, Pellet H, Buenerd A and Traeger J. Le sediment urinaire dans l'insuffisance renale aigue. Valeur diagnostique et prognostique de l'examan en microscopie a contraste de phase. La Presse Medicale 1984; 13:2307–10.

116. List AF, Kummet TD, Adams JD and Chun HG. Tumor lysis syndrome complicating treatment of chronic lymphocytic leukemia with fludarabine phosphate. Am J Med 1990; 89:388–90.

117. Jacobsen D, Hewlett TP, Webb R, Brown ST, Ordinario AT and McMartin KE. Ethylene glycol intoxication: Evaluation of kinetics and crystalluria. Am J Med 1988; 84:145–52.

118. MH Sawyer, DE Webb, JE Balow and Straus SE. Acyclovir-induced renal failure. Am J Med 1988; 84:1067–71.

119. Battle DC, Arruda JAL and Kurtzman NA. Hyperkalemic distal renal tubular acidosis associated with obstructive uropathy. N Engl J Med 1981; 304:373–80.

120. Grossman A, Eckland D, Price P and Edwards CRW. Captopril: reversible renal failure with severe hyperkalemia. Lancet 1980; 1:712.

121. Clive DM and Stoff JS. Renal syndromes associated with non-steroidal anti-inflammatory drugs. N Engl J Med 1984; 310:563–72.

122. DeFronzo RA. Hyperkalemia and hyporeninemia hypoaldosteronism. Kidney Int 1980; 17:118–34.

123. Abreo K, Adlakha A, Kilpatrick S, Flanagan R, Webb R and Shakamuri S. The milk-alkali syndrome. Arch Intern Med 1993; 153:1005–10.

6. Additional laboratory investigation

J. GARY ABUELO

The initial laboratory evaluation that I have just outlined will suffice to diagnose individuals with an obvious etiology, who make up about half of cases with renal insufficiency. Many patients with prerenal azotemia, ischemic acute tubular necrosis, contrast media reactions or acute urinary retention have such easy diagnoses. Patients without a diagnosis after the initial laboratory tests require additional extrarenal and renal studies.

EXTRARENAL TESTS

General screening

Routine tests for systemic conditions with secondary renal involvement include a complete blood count, chest X-ray, stool guaiac, liver function tests, serum glucose, calcium, phosphorus and uric acid levels, and in patients over 50 years of age without proteinuria a non-dipstick urine test for protein to detect immunoglobulin light chains (see Qualitative Protein Test, Chapter 5).

Low platelets and red cell fragmentation on the peripheral smear suggest a small vessel disease like thrombotic thrombocytopenic purpura and should not be overlooked (see Chapter 10). Eosinophilia may be a clue to atheroembolic renal disease or allergic interstitial nephritis.

Indications for Specific Tests

Streptococcal Infections. Individuals with impetigo or a recent sore throat should have *serum complement levels (CH50, C3 and C4), skin or throat cultures*, and serum titers for *antibodies against several streptococcal enzymes* (e.g. antistreptolysin O titer).

Respiratory Symptoms. Cough, hemoptysis or lung infiltrates are indications for *antiglomerular basement membrane antibodies* to diagnose Goodpasture's syndrome, and *antineutrophil cytoplasmic antibodies (ANCA)* to look for Wegener's granulomatosis. Also, sinusitis, otitis media or other upper respiratory findings are compatible with the latter disease, and may be evaluated with *sinus X-rays* and *otolaryngological consultation.*

Vasculitis-Like Picture. Constitutional symptoms, multiorgan involvement, hematuria and proteinuria suggests a collagen vascular disease.

Systemic lupus erythematosus presents typically as fever, arthralgias and rash in a young woman, but in other patients it may have a highly varied onset and course, involving any of several organ systems and affecting any age and either sex. Thus, an *antinuclear antibody test* and *serum complement levels* must be done in patients with both classic and atypical presentations of systemic lupus erythematosus. In addition, patients with a picture suggesting collagen vascular disease should have *a sedimentation rate, ANCA, rheumatoid factor, cryoglobulins and complement studies* ordered, and may be candidates for *arteriography* [1] or for *biopsies of affected extra-renal tissues* (see Secondary Glomerulonephritis, Chapter 11). Because of the characteristic immunopathologic appearance of skin lesions in Henoch-Schonlein purpura [2], systemic lupus erythematosus, essential cryoglobulinemia [3], and hypocomplementemic vasculitis urticaria syndrome [4], any *skin biopsies* should be submitted for immunofluorescent studies as well as light microscopy [5, 6] and, if possible, should be examined by a dermatopathologist.

J.G. Abuelo (ed.), Renal Failure, 35–46.
© 1995 *Kluwer Academic Publishers.*

Note on Anti-Neutrophil Cytoplasmic Antibody (ANCA). ANCA is usually detected by indirect immunofluorescence on fixed neutrophils, and is present in most cases of active Wegener's granulomatosis, polyarteritis nodosa and idiopathic crescentic glomerulonephritis (7). ANCA also occurs in many other autoimmune diseases (Table 6.1). These antibodies are directed against neutrophil cytoplasmic enzymes such as proteinase 3 and myeloperoxidase. Immunoassays for antibodies specific for these major antigens have shown disease associations, such as that between antiproteinase 3 and Wegener's granulomatosis. However, these associations are not close enough for such assays to improve the disease sensitivity or specificity of ANCA testing to any practical extent (8-10).

Antiproteinase 3 antibodies produce a "cytoplasmic" pattern on immunofluorescence, which can be distinguished from the perinuclear pattern of antimyeloperoxidase antibodies. As with the immunoassays for specific antibodies, these patterns have not proved to be clinically useful.

Proteinuria. Older patients with proteinuria may have renal failure associated with multiple myeloma even in the absence of symptoms like bone pain. If proteinuria is found in a patient over 50 years of age, it is important to order serum and urine *protein and immuno-* (or even better) *immunofixation electrophoreses.* This will diagnose multiple myeloma, and will also detect most dysproteinemias that produce renal amyloidosis or light chain deposition disease [11]. These latter dysproteinemias may have serum and urine concentrations of monoclonal proteins below the level of detection of protein electrophoresis, so that immunoelectrophoresis or the more sensitive immunofixation electrophoresis should be done [12, 13]. The heat test for urinary Bence-Jones proteins is relatively insensitive and is not recommended [14].

Hematuria and Proteinuria. These urinary abnormalities suggest an acute (glomerulo-) nephritic process and are indications for an ANCA test and complement studies. A positive ANCA points towards idiopathic crescentic glomerulonephritis, or a systemic vasculitis. Depressed complement levels are commonly found in several glomerulonephritides and, on occasion, in other disorders (Table 6.2).

ADDITIONAL RENAL TESTS

In order to obtain further information about the nature of the renal lesion, the physician should quantitate protein losses in patients with proteinuria, assess renal salt avidity, order a renal ultrasound, and possibly other radiologic studies and, if indicated, obtain a renal biopsy.

Quantitation of Protein Excretion

Timed Urine Collection. A 24 hour urine sample for protein is performed to quantitate proteinuria. Timed collections over shorter periods may also be used.

In individuals with a stable Scr, the sample should also be tested for creatinine in order to assure the adequacy of the collection using the following rough guideline. In men a complete 24 hour urine contains 1.0 to 2.0 g (8.85 to 17.70 mmol) of creatinine depending on size and in women 0.7–1.4 g (6.20 to 12.40 mmol) of creatinine; however, between ages 45 and 80 years, creatinine excretion declines by about half in both men and women [16].

Table 6.1. Diseases associated with ANCA [7]

Pauciimmune crescentic GN common
    Wegener's granulomatosis
    Polyarteritis nodosa
    Idiopathic crescentic GN
Pauciimmune crescentic GN uncommon
    Systemic lupus erythematosus
    Rheumatoid and other arthritis
    Inflammatory bowel disease
    Autoimmune liver disease

Table 6.2. Causes of low serum complement levels [15]

Glomerulonephritis	Other conditions
Membranoproliferative GN	Atheroembolic renal disease
Post infectious GN	Severe sepsis
Lupus nephritis	Hemolytic uremic syndrome
Mixed essential cryoglobulinemia	Severe malnutrition
Hypocomplementemic vasculitis	Hepatic failure
Inherited C' deficiencies	Acute pancreatitis

A modification of the formula of Cockcroft and Gault [17] may also be used to calculate the amount of creatinine that one should have in an adequate 24 hour urine collection:

$$\text{creatinine excretion (mg/24 hours)} = \frac{[140-\text{age (years)}] \times \text{weight (kg)} \times 0.85^*}{5 \times 113 \,\dagger}$$

* multiply by factor of 0.85 if patient is female
† divide by factor of 113 if result desired in mmol creatinine/24 h.

Once the physician confirms that the urine sample has been properly collected, he may use the rate of protein excretion to draw conclusions about the nature of the renal disease. Normal urine protein excretion in adults is up to 150 mg per day [18]. Patients with less than 1 g protein per 24 hours usually have a non-glomerular disease, patients with greater than 2.5 g protein per 24 hours usually have a glomerular disease, and patients with intermediate values may have either. Several cases of non-glomerular disease with protein excretion greater than 2.5 g per day have been described, including malignant hypertension [19], thrombotic thrombocytopenic purpura [20], hemolytic uremic syndrome [21, 22], renovascular hypertension [23, 24], allergic interstitial nephritis due to methicillin [25], cholesterol emboli to the kidney [26, 27], and most importantly myeloma kidney with heavy excretion of Bence-Jones proteins. Patients with renal artery embolism may also have heavy proteinuria based on the 3 to 4+ qualitative proteinuria reported by Lessman et al. [28].

Protein to Creatinine Ratio. In some patients, it may be difficult to obtain an accurately collected 24 hour urine for quantitation of proteinuria because of incontinence, poor cooperation or logistical reasons. *An indwelling urethral catheter should never be placed just to collect such a specimen.* Instead, a random urine sample should be sent to the laboratory to determine the ratio of protein to creatinine concentrations. The value of this ratio expressed in mg protein/mg creatinine corresponds closely to the g protein excreted per 24 hours, particularly if the random sample is obtained after the first voided urine in the morning and before 6 PM. In fact, many feel that this ratio may replace the 24 hour urine for quantitation of protein [29–34]. A

ratio less than 0.2 mg/mg (0.023 g/mmol) is normal and greater than 3.0 mg/mg (0.34 g/mmol) corresponds to nephrotic range proteinuria [29].

Salt avidity
There has been interest in using urinary sodium and chloride content to assess renal salt avidity (tubular reabsorption of salt) in the evaluation of patients with renal failure. Sodium and chloride content is usually estimated by measuring sodium and chloride concentration or *fractional excretion of sodium or chloride* in a random ("spot") urine sample (see below). These tests should be ordered to diagnose hepatorenal syndrome, to help distinguish prerenal azotemia from ATN and to detect subclinical hypovolemia, especially in patients with acute-on-chronic renal failure.

Inappropriately Low Urinary Salt Content. A good example of the role of these tests is in *hepato-renal syndrome*, where increased tubular reabsorption of salt is an almost constant finding and leads to the production of urine poor in sodium and chloride, despite the absence of the obvious stimuli to renal salt reabsorption such as hypotension, volume depletion, low salt intake or low cardiac output [35, 36]. If one suspects this diagnosis in a patient with advanced liver disease, low amounts of sodium or chloride in the urine would support hepato-renal syndrome, while large amounts should cast doubt on the diagnosis.

Urine inappropriately low in sodium and chloride in the absence of the normal stimuli to salt reabsorption may also be seen in certain other causes of renal failure (Table 6.3). Unfortunately, urine sodium and chloride concentrations have been studied in only a few of these cases, so that absence of salt poor urine does not exclude these conditions. For the most part, the reason for the low urinary salt content in these different situations is not completely understood [49].

Inappropriately High Urine Salt Content. Assessment of renal salt avidity is commonly employed *to distinguish ischemic acute tubular necrosis from prerenal azotemia* in patients with hypotension and acute renal failure. In these cases, the appropriate renal response to reduced blood pressure would be increased tubular reabsorption of salt as seen in prerenal azotemia. In contrast, in acute tubular

Table 6.3. Causes of renal failure with inappropriately low urine salt content

---

Early urinary obstruction [37]
Vasomotor reactions
    Captopril [38]
    NSAIDs [39]
    Cyclosporin A [40, 41]
    Contrast media [42]
Atheroembolic renal disease [43]
Bilateral renal artery stenosis [44]
Acute glomerulonephritis [45, 46]
Acute interstitial nephritis [47]
Transplant rejection [48]

---

necrosis the damaged tubules are usually unable to reabsorb sodium and chloride normally and urine salt content is high. Therefore, a determination of renal salt avidity helps distinguish these two conditions [45, 46].

Unfortunately, the result has little influence on patient management, since in either condition the cornerstone of therapy is the prompt restoration of normal hemodynamics. Moreover, regardless of renal avidity for salt, the diagnosis of prerenal azotemia will depend on whether one obtains recovery of renal function in the hours to one day that follow correction of hypotension. The role of urine tests of renal salt avidity in this situation is further limited by the finding of low urinary salt content in some patients with acute tubular necrosis [50–56], and high content in some patients with prerenal azotemia. In these latter cases, the kidneys' ability to conserve sodium and chloride may be impaired by adrenal insufficiency, diuretics or renal parenchymal disease [55]. In fact, urinary salt loss may have contributed to the volume depleted state [57].

Subclinical Hypovolemia. Another circumstance where tests of tubular reabsorption of salt may be employed is in the occasional patient with prerenal azotemia associated with subtle volume depletion; the patient may have little or nothing in the history or physical examination to alert the physician to the reduced state of renal perfusion. These individuals typically have chronic renal insufficiency and have an acute worsening of azotemia due to an unrecognized acute insult such as unreported copious diarrhea. Laboratory studies showing increased renal sodium avidity may be the only clue

to the diagnosis [57–59]. Therefore, patients with *acute-on-chronic renal insufficiency* should have studies done of urine sodium and chloride content. The failure to find urine poor in salt does not exclude prerenal azotemia, however, since in many cases of chronic renal disease the tubules may be unable to reabsorb salt efficiently [55, 57].

FENa. The traditional criterion for increased renal salt avidity is a urinary sodium concentration below 20 mEq/L, while the absence of avidity is indicated by concentrations above 40 mEq/L; values from 20 to 40 mEq/L are indeterminate [45, 46]. Unfortunately, the urine sodium concentration depends not only on the efficiency of tubular reabsorption of sodium, but also on the extent of water reabsorption (urine concentration) in the distal nephron. In attempt to eliminate this confounding effect and to look at tubular salt reabsorption by itself, the renal failure index or even more commonly the fractional excretion of sodium (FENa) is determined by measuring creatinine and sodium concentrations in the serum and in a simultaneously collected urine sample:

$$FENa(\%) = \frac{\text{urine sodium (mEq/L)} \times \text{Scr (mg/dl)}^* \times 100}{\text{serum sodium (mEq/L)} \times \text{urine creatinine (mg/dl)}^*}$$

    * serum and urine creatinine may also be measured in μmol/L.

The presence of sodium avidity is indicated by a FENa below 1% and the lack of avidity by values above 1% [45, 46].

Urine Chloride Content. The physician should be aware of two situations where the salt avid patient may factitiously or transiently excrete high amounts of urinary sodium. First, one may have a natriuresis caused by hyperglycemia, mannitol therapy or diuretics.[1] Second, augmented sodium excretion may accompany high urinary anion content (1) in patients given contrast medium or high doses of penicillin analogs; (2) in uncontrolled diabetics with large amounts of ketoacids in the urine; or (3) in individuals excreting large amounts of bicarbonate, e.g. because of vomiting or resolving metabolic alkalosis [60]. When an increase in urinary sodium is caused by high anion excretion, a urinary chloride content less than 20 mEq/L or a fractional excretion of chloride (FECl) less than 1% is an equally specific and a more sensitive indicator of prerenal azotemia than is urine sodium concentration [55]. It is, therefore, recommended that urine chloride concentration or FECl always be measured, in addition to sodium concentrations, when looking for evidence of renal salt avidity [55, 60].

Renal sonogram
Ultrasonography is the preferred imaging technique in most cases where one wants to screen for gross abnormalities in renal size and structure. It is safe, accurate and if necessary, can be done at the bedside.

Obstruction. When urinary tract obstruction is suggested by the patient's initial evaluation, renal ultrasonography should be ordered for confirmation. This method will detect hydronephrosis in 90–100% of proven cases of obstruction (Figure 6.1) [61–63].

An even more important role of ultrasonography is to *exclude* obstruction, which may occur and impair renal function in occasional patients without any tell-tale signs or symptoms. The high sensitivity and freedom from morbidity of this method more than compensate for the high incidence (8–26%) of *false positive results* (usually grade I hydronephrosis) [61–63]. These may be caused by failure to empty the bladder, high urine flow, large normal calyces, post obstructive dilata-

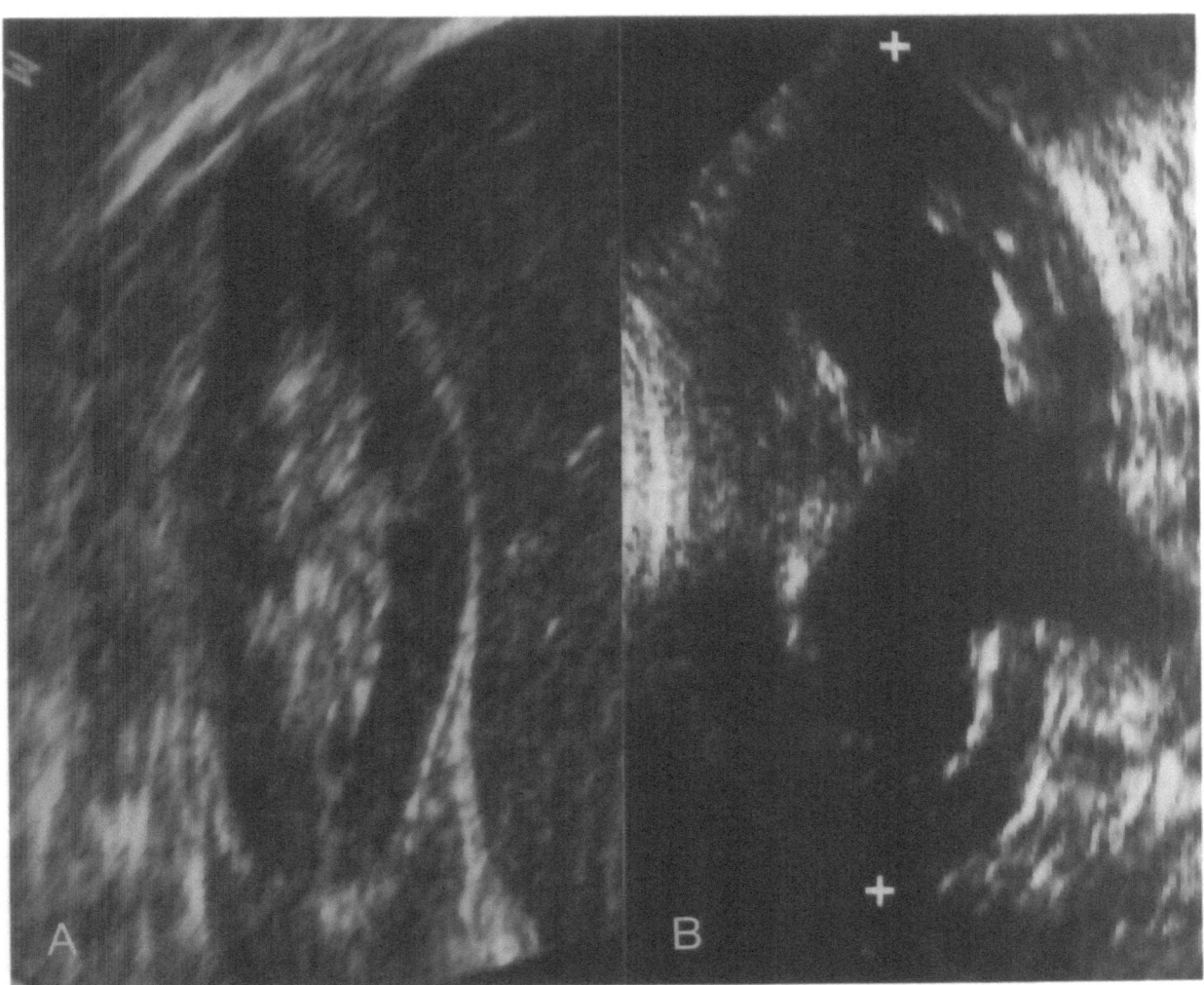

Fig. 6.1. (A) Normal sonogram. (B) Sonogram of a hydronephritic kidney showing dilated calyces.

tion, papillary necrosis, high grade vesicoureteral reflux, calyceal diverticula, peripelvic and other cysts, renal tuberculosis with cavity formation, an extra-renal pelvis or blood vessels [64]. If dilatation is due to the first two causes, a second sonogram may be negative, showing their transient nature. Blood vessels that mimic obstruction may now be detected by Doppler color flow ultrasonography [65]. Recognition of other false positives may require intravenous or retrograde urography.

Other situations where ultrasonography may be inadequate are when one or both kidneys are not clearly visualized, or collecting system dilatation is obscured by cysts or staghorn calculi [61]. In either case, intravenous or retrograde pyelography will be necessary to diagnose urinary tract obstruction.

Atrophy, Cysts and Tumors. The renal length can also be determined from the sonogram. If renal length is less than 8 cm on the right side and 8.8 cm on the left, it indicates shrunken kidneys due to chronic renal disease [66].

> Alternatively, one may multiply the height of the second lumbar vertebrae seen on X-ray by 2.8 to get a lower limit of normal of the renal length by ultrasound [67]. Criteria for normal renal length in children have also been published [68].

In some patients with chronic atrophy of renal parenchyma, a proliferation of renal sinus fat replaces the lost renal bulk and conserves the overall kidney size. This *renal sinus lipomatosis* can be seen on ultrasound as an expanded central renal sinus complex with high intensity echoes associated with thinning of the renal parenchymal [69–71]. Other information important in the diagnosis of renal failure may be obtained from the sonogram including cystic disease, massive tumor replacement of renal tissue, enlarged kidneys, or the absence or atrophy of a kidney [72]. The finding of a single kidney raises suspicion of renal failure caused by a unilateral process like obstruction, renal artery stenosis or renal embolism. Kidneys may be enlarged due to inflammation in glomerulonephritis or interstitial nephritis, or due to infiltration by amyloid, lymphoma or leukemia.

Intravenous pyelogram (IVP)
The IVP was formerly used in the evaluation of most patients with renal failure to show if two

kidneys were present, if they were of normal size, if they had any function, and if they were obstructed (Figure 6.2). The last 20 years has seen the recognition of contrast medium-induced renal failure caused by IVPs and the introduction of sonography, which needs no preparation of the patient, and can safely provide the information needed about the anatomy of the kidneys. Consequently, the IVP is now used in only special situations (see below), when it entails little added risk and provides more information than ultrasonography.

Nephrotoxic Reaction to Contrast Agents. The risk of a nephrotoxic reaction to contrast media used in IVP's increases with the severity of underlying renal impairment and with the presence of diabetes mellitus, such that with baseline Scr between 1.5 to 2.0 mg/dl (133 to 177 μmol/L) the incidence of an acute worsening of azotemia is 3% in non-diabetics and 50–58% in diabetics. With baseline Scr greater than 4.5 mg/dl (398 μmol/L), the incidence is 31% and over 90%, respectively. These figures compare to an incidence of 6% or less in both groups with baseline Scr of 1.4 mg/dl (124 μmol/L) or less [73–76]. The risk of nephrotoxicity from the new non-ionic low osmolarity contrast agents such as iohexol or iopamidol is probably less than with the older ionic agents [77, 78].

The *severity* of the nephrotoxic reaction may also increase with the degree of underlying renal impairment [79], and several authors have described permanent renal failure following IVP's, when the baseline Scr was 4.5 mg/dl (398 μmol/L) or greater, especially in diabetics [73, 74, 80, 81].

Looking at the other side of the coin, IVP's are relatively safe in non-diabetic individuals with baseline Scr of 4.5 mg/dl (398 μmol/L) or less. In this population nephrotoxic reactions may have an occurrence as low as 3% [73], are transient, lasting less than two weeks in most cases, and rarely are severe enough to require dialysis [73, 75, 79, 81, 82]. Furthermore, youth may provide added safety in that reactions are rarely, if ever, seen in non-diabetic individuals younger than 30 years [73, 79, 81, 82].

Poor Visualization. An additional problem of the IVP is inadequate visualization due to poor excretion of the contrast medium by the impaired kidneys. When the baseline Scr is 8 mg/dl (708

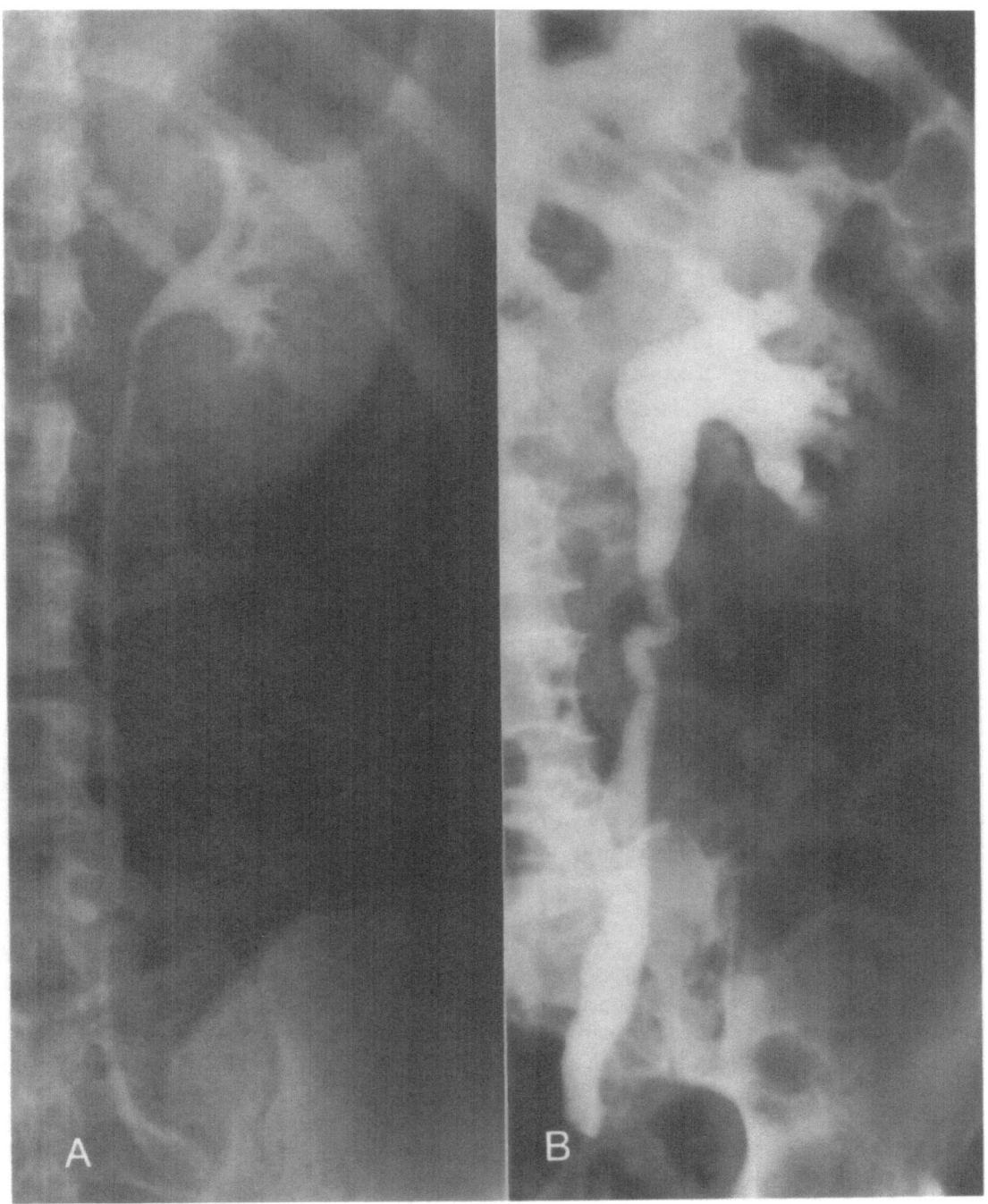

Fig. 6.2. (A) Normal IVP. (B) IVP showing hydronephrosis and hydroureter.

μmol/L) or more, only 19% of studies are satisfactory. On the other hand with Scr less than 3.9 mg/dl (343 μmol/L), 91% of IVP's are adequate [83]. If opacification of the renal structures is not satisfactory with the routine technique, nephrotomograms should be done.

Indications. The IVP has certain advantages over

renal ultrasonography in that it may demonstrate poor function of one kidney as compared to the other kidney, shows the location of any obstruction, produces a clearer image of the pelvocalyceal structures, rarely gives false positive readings for urinary obstruction, and may visualize kidneys inadequately seen by ultrasonography [61].

When an azotemic patient has a low risk for a nephrotoxic reaction to contrast medium and has *unilateral renal colic or pain* suspected to be of renal origin, an IVP is the imaging modality of choice. The renal sonogram often fails to show dilatation during the first day or two of obstruction by a stone [84], while an IVP will diagnose and identify the level of urinary obstruction. The IVP will also recognize papillary necrosis in patients with obstruction due to a sloughed papilla. If the renal pain is caused by acute pyelonephritis, renal vein thrombosis or an embolism to the kidney, unilateral poor function will be seen.

If ultrasonography inadequately visualizes the kidneys, an IVP may be indicated. The possibility of analgesic nephropathy comes up when patients have chronic renal failure and analgesic abuse. The tell-tale papillary necrosis is rarely seen by ultrasound, and usually requires an IVP for visualization. In patients with obstruction detected by ultrasound and with a low risk for contrast nephrotoxicity, one may order an IVP to confirm and localize the obstruction.

Pyelography Performed with Other Contrast Studies. Patients who are having angiography or a computed tomography with contrast enhancement for evaluation of an extrarenal problem will usually excrete enough contrast agent to get an adequate view of the kidneys and collecting system. Therefore, X-ray films of the urinary tract taken at the end of the contrast study while the contrast media is still present will provide the needed anatomical information and make ultrasonography unnecessary.

Renal Radionuclide Imaging

Technetium-99m Scan. The physician may wish to document unilateral loss of renal function in patients with azotemia caused by unilateral processes such as renal artery stenosis, renal embolism, or acute pyelonephritis. The radioagent of choice is 99 mTc mercaptoacetyltriglycine (MAG3). Radionuclide scanning is preferable to the IVP for this purpose because it has no risk of hypersensitivity or nephrotoxic contrast medium reactions. In a patient suspected of having renal artery embolism, a technetium-99m glucoheptonate or dimercaptosuccinate iron ascorbate (DMSA) scan showing unilateral poor or absent function can be particularly useful in supporting the diagnosis [85].

Gallium Citrate Scan. This is used to detect inflammatory or neoplastic tissue. It was noted by Linton et al. that the kidneys of patients with acute interstitial nephritis due to a variety of medications have intense uptake of gallium [86]. Although these authors considered a positive gallium scan to be evidence for this diagnosis, experience with the study is limited. In one report the sensitivity was only 58% [87], and others have noted moderate to marked uptake in cases with pyelonephritis, crescentic glomerulonephritis, minimal change disease and other conditions [86, 88–92].

Arteriography or Venography

Polyarteritis Nodosa. Abdominal aortography and selective renal, celiac and mesenteric angiography, can be instrumental in the diagnosis of vasculitis [1]. Typically in polyarteritis nodosa multiple small aneurysms, occlusions and stenoses of medium-sized arteries are seen in one or more of the abdominal viscera, and the nephrogram phase of the study often demonstrates renal infarcts. Although these and similar changes may occur in other vasculitides and in some instances of disseminated lupus erythematosus, the specific diagnosis is usually apparent when the overall clinical picture is considered. Negative arteriograms are sometimes seen in polyarteritis nodosa and do not, therefore, exclude the diagnosis [1].

Renal Artery Stenosis and Embolism. Renal arteriography is used to demonstrate renal artery stenosis, which if bilateral and severe enough, can lead to renal functional impairment. In patients with renal embolism the clinical findings and the results of radionuclide scanning may be convincing enough to satisfy the physician as to the diagnosis. In other cases, however, one may wish to demonstrate occlusion of the renal artery or its branches with renal angiography.

Renal Vein Thrombosis. The thrombosis is usually incomplete and unilateral, and causes renal failure only occasionally in infants and rarely in adults. Although the IVP may support the diagnosis by showing ureteral notching caused by enlarged collateral veins, renal and vena cava venography are usually necessary to confirm the diagnosis.

Computed tomography and magnetic resonance imaging

These imaging techniques are rarely useful in the diagnosis of renal failure. However, acute renal cortical necrosis [93] or renal infarction [94] can be detected by computed tomography. Spiral CT angiography [95, 96] and magnetic resonance angiography [97] are being evaluated as methods to diagnose renal artery stenosis.

Renal biopsy

A renal biopsy usually reveals the etiology of the renal failure in undiagnosed cases with intrinsic renal disease [98, 99]. When the etiology is already known, a biopsy may give the histologic stage of the disease and thereby indicate if the lesion is amenable to treatment.

Percutaneous renal biopsies are performed under local anesthesia usually with sonography or computed tomography to locate the lower pole of the kidney. Bleeding is the main complication and causes gross hematuria, perirenal hematoma, and blood loss requiring transfusion in a few percent of patients. Nephrectomy or selective embolization to stop hemorrhage is necessary in about 0.1% and deaths from bleeding occur in less than 0.1% of cases [100]. Hypertension and renal failure seem to increase the risk of complications [100]. The risks are a little less with open (surgical) renal biopsies [101]. Due to the seriousness of these complications, renal biopsies are only to be performed when the result may alter the therapy and when there are no contraindications. Before doing a renal biopsy, one must screen for bleeding dyscrasias and correct any abnormality that is found.

CONCLUSIONS

Patients with undiagnosed azotemia after the initial laboratory evaluation require additional investigation. This chapter discusses the most commonly used tests and their interpretation. These tests are listed on Table 6.4 with their indications.

NOTES

1. Obviously, urine samples for assessment of renal avidity ideally should be collected before or well after the use of a diuretic. However, if the patient is refractory to diuretics, determination of salt avidity after diuretic administration may have value. A test showing low urine salt content would be reliable, while a test showing high salt content would have to be repeated after the diuretic wears off.

Table 6.4. Summary of additional laboratory tests

Extrarenal test	Indication
CBC, chest Xray, stool guaiac, liver function tests, serum glucose, calcium, phosphorus and uric acid	All undiagnosed patients
Urine protein: creatinine, sulfosalicylic acid test	No proteinuria, over age 50
Skin/throat culture, C', ASLO titer, etc.	Impetigo, sore throat
Anti-GBM antibodies, ANCA	Lower respiratory symptoms
Sinus X-rays, ENT evaluation	Upper respiratory symptoms
ANA, C', ESR, ANCA, rheumatoid factor, cryoglobulin, arteriography, biopsy of affected tissue	Constitutional/multiorgan symptoms, hematuria and proteinuria
Protein & immunofixation electrophoresis	Proteinuria, over age 50
ANCA, C' studies (C3, C4, CH50)	Hematuria & proteinuria

Renal tests	Indication
24 hour urine protein, urine protein: creatinine	Proteinuria
Urine Na, Cl, FENa, FECl	? Hepatorenal syndrome, prerenal azotemia, ATN, hypovolemia
Renal sonogram	All undiagnosed patients
Intravenous pyelography	Renal colic, address ? raised by sonogram
Technetium scan	? Unilateral function, ? embolism
Gallium citrate scan	? Acute interstitial nephritis
Renal arteriogram	? Polyarteritis nodosa, ? renal artery occlusion
Renal venography	? Renal vein thrombosis
Renal biopsy	Undiagnosed parenchymal disease

REFERENCES

1. Travers RL, Allison DJ, Brettle RP and Hughes GRV. Polyarteritis nodosa: a clinical and angiographic analysis of 17 cases. Sem in Arth Rheum 1979; 8:184–99.

2. Piette WW and Stone MS. A cutaneous sign of IgA-associated small dermal vessel leukocytoclastic vasculitis in adults (Henoch-Schonlein purpura). Arch Dermatol 1989; 125:53–6.

3. Gorevic PD, Kassab HJ, Levo Y, Kohn R, Meltzer M, Prose P et al. Mixed cryoglobinemia: clinical aspect and long-term follow-up of 40 patients. Am J Med 1980; 69:287–308.

4. Moorthy AV and Pringle D. Urticaria, vasculitis, hypocomplementemia and immune-complex glomerulonephritis. Arch Pathol Lab Med 1982; 106:68–70.

5. Farmer and Provost TT. Immunologic studies of skin biopsy specimens in connective tissue diseases. Human Pathol 1983; 14:316–325.

6. Kumar V, Beutner EH and Chorzelski TP. Immuno-pathology of vasculitis. In: Beutner EH, Chorzelski TP and Kumar V, editors. Immunopathology of the skin. John Wiley & Sons, Inc. New York, 1987:3rd ed, 745–54.

7. Kallenberg CGM, Leontine Mulder AH and Cohen Tervaert JW. Antineutrophil cytoplasmic antibodies: a still-growing class of autoantibodies in inflammatory disorders. Am J Med 1992; 93:675–82.

8. Gans ROB, Kuizinga MC, Goldschmeding R, Assmann K, Huysmans FTM, Gerlag PGG et al. Clinical features and outcome in patients with glomerulonephritis and antineutrophil cytoplasmic autoantibodies. Nephron 1993; 64:182–8.

9. Geffriaud-Ricouard C, Noel LH, Chauveau D, Houhou S, Grunfeld JP and Lesavre P. Clinical spectrum associated with ANCA of defined antigen specificities in 98 selected patients. Clin Nephrol 1993; 39:125–36.

10. Niles JL, Pan G, Collins AB, Shannon T, Skates S, Fienberg R et al. Antigen-specific radioimmunoassays for anti-neutrophil cytoplasmic antibodies in the diagnosis of rapidly progressive glomerulonephritis. J Am Soc Nephrol 1991; 2:27–36.

11. Buxbaum JN, Chuba JV, Hellman GC, Solomon A and Gallo GR. Monoclonal immunoglobulin deposition disease: light chain and light and heavy chain deposition diseases and their relation to light chain amyloidosis. Ann Intern Med 1990; 112:455–64.

12. Fogazzi GB, Pozzi C, Passerini P, Simonini P, Locatelli F and Ponticelli C. Utility of immunofluorescence of urine sediment for identifying patients with renal disease due to monoclonal gammopathies. Am J Kidney Dis 1991; 17:211–7.

13. Pedersen NS and Axelsen NH. Detection of M-components by an easy immunofixation procedure: comparison with agarose gel electrophoresis and classical immunoelectrophoresis. J Immunol Meth. 1979; 30:257–62.

14. Kyle RA. Bence Jones proteins. In: Pathology of immunoglobulins: diagnostic and clinical aspects. Alan R Liss, Inc., New York 1982:261–92.

15. Hebert LA, Cosio FG and Neff JC. Diagnostic significance of hypocomplementemia. Kidney Int 1991; 39:811–21.

16. Kampmann J, Siersback-Nielsen K, Kristensen M and Hansen JM. Rapid evaluation of creatinine clearance. Acta Med Scand 1974; 196:517–20.

17. Cockcroft DW and Gault MH. Prediction of creatinine clearance from serum creatinine. Nephron 1976; 16:31–41.

18. Kawakami H, Murakami T and Kajii T. Normal values for 24-h urinary protein excretion: total and low molecular weight proteins with a sex-related difference. Clin Nephrol 1990; 33:232–6.

19. Pillay VKG, Schwartz FD and Kark RM. Proteinuria in malignant hypertension. Lancet 1968; 2:1263–4.

20. Eknoyan G and Riggs SA. Renal involvement in patients with thrombotic thrombocytopenic purpura. Am J Nephrol 1986; 6:117–31.

21. Habib R. Hemolytic uremic syndrome. In: Royer P, Habib R, Mathieu H and Broyer M, editors. Pediatric nephrology. W.B. Saunders Company, Philadelphia, 1974;291–301.

22. Kaplan BS, Thomson PD and de Chadarevian J-P. The hemolytic uremic syndrome. Pediat Clin N Amer 1976; 23:761–77.

23. Kumar A and Shapiro AP. Proteinuria and nephrotic syndrome induced by renin in patients with renal artery stenosis. Arch Intern Med 1980; 140:1631–4.

24. Sato H, Saito T, Kasai Y, Abe K and Yoshinaga K. Massive proteinuria due to renal artery stenosis. Nephron 1989; 51:136–7.

25. Galpin JE, Shinaberger JH and Stanley TM. Acute interstitial nephritis due to methicillin. Am J Med 1978; 65:756–65.

26. Endreny RG, Zipin S, Chazan J and King B. Atheroembolic renal disease – Presentation and clinical course in ten patients. Am J Kidney Dis 1988; 11:A6

27. Williams HH, Wall BM and Cooke CR. Case Report: reversible nephrotic range proteinuria and renal failure in atheroembolic renal disease. Am J Med Sci 1990; 299:58–61.

28. Lessman RK, Johnson SF, Coburn JW and Kaufman JJ. Renal artery embolism: clinical features and long term follow-up of 17 cases. Ann Intern Med 1978; 89:477–82.

29. Schwab SJ, Christensen RL, Dougherty K and Klahr S. Quantitation of proteinuria by the use of protein-to-creatinine ratios in single urine samples. Arch Intern Med 1987;147:943–4.

30. Baumelou A, Colin B, Thiollieres JM, Percheron F and Legrain M. Quantification de la protéinurie par la mesure du rapport protéine sur créatinine. La Presse Med 1987;16:343–5.

31. Lemann J Jr. and Doumas BT. Proteinuria in health and disease assessed by measuring the urinary protein/creatinine ratio. Clin Chem 1987; 33:297–9.

32. Shaw AB, Risdon P and Lewis-Jackson JD. Protein creatinine index and Albustix in assessment of proteinuria. BMJ 1983; 287:929–32.

33. Ginsberg JM, Chang BS, Matarese R and Garella S. Use of single voided urine samples to estimate quantitative proteinuria. N Engl J Med 1983; 309:1543–6.

34. Kristal B, Shasha SM, Labin L and Cohen A. Estimation of quantitative proteinuria by using the protein-creatinine ratio in random urine samples. Am J Nephrol 1988; 8:198–203.

35. Linas SL, Schaefer JW, Moore EE, Good JT Jr. and Gian-siracusa R. Peritoneovenous shunt in the management of the hepatorenal syndrome. Kidney Int 1986; 30:736–40.

36. Levenson DJ, Skorecki KL, Newell GC and Norins RG. Acute renal failure with hepatobiliary disease. In: Brenner BM and Lazarus M, editors. Acute renal failure. Churchill Livingston Inc., 1988;535–81.

37. Hoffman LM and Suki WN. Obstructive uropathy mimicking volume depletion. JAMA 1976; 236:2096–7.

38. Textor SC, Biscardi A, Bravo EL, Tarazi RC and Fouad FM. Acute renal failure during converting enzyme inhibition in patients with renal artery stenosis. Abstracts American Soc Nephrol 1982:45.

39. Blackshear JL, Davidman M and Stillman T. Identification of risk for renal insufficiency from nonsteroid anti-inflammatory drugs. Arch Intern Med 1983; 143:1130–4.

40. Myers BD. Cyclosporine nephrotoxicity. Kidney Int. 1986; 30:964–74.

41. Greenberg A, Egel J, Thompson M, Bahnson H, Griffith B, Hardesty R et al. Renal failure in heart transplant patients receiving cyclosporin A. Clin Res 1983; 31:429A.

42. Fang LST, Sirota RA, Ebert TH and Lichtenstein NS. Low fractional excretion of sodium with contrast media-induced acute renal failure. Arch Intern Med 1980; 140:531–3.

43. Case Records of the Massachusetts General Hospital (Case 30-1986). N Engl J Med 1986; 315:308–315.

44. Besarab A, Brown RS, Rubin NT, Salzman E, Wirthlin L, Steinman T et al. Reversible renal failure following bilateral renal artery occlusive disease: Clinical features, pathology, and the role of surgical revascularization. JAMA 1976; 235:2838–41.

45. Miller TR, Anderson RJ, Linas SL, Henrich WL, Berns AS, Gabow PA et al. Urinary diagnostic indices in acute renal failure. Ann Intern Med 1978; 89:47–50.

46. Espinal CH and Gregory AW. Differential diagnosis of acute renal failure. Clin Nephrol 1980; 13:73–7.

47. Case Records of the Massachusetts General Hospital. Case 42-1983 N Engl J Med 1983; 309:970–8.

48. Hong CD, Kapoor BS and First MR. Fractional excretion of sodium after renal transplantation. Kidney Int 1979; 16:167–78.

49. Steiner RW. Interpreting the fractional excretion of sodium. Am J Med 1984; 77:699–702.

50. Vaz AJ. Low fractional excretion of urine sodium in acute renal failure due to sepsis. Arch Intern Med 1983; 143:738–9.

51. Diamond JR and Yoburn DC. Nonoliguric acute renal failure with a low fractional excretion of sodium. Ann Intern Med 1982; 96:597–600.

52. Planas M, Wachtel T, Frank H and Henderson LW. Characterization of acute renal failure in the burned patient. Arch Intern Med 1982; 142:2087–91.

53. Corwin HL, Schreiber MJ and Fang LST. Low fractional excretion of sodium. Occurrence with hemoglobinuric- and myoglobinuria-induced acute renal failure. Arch Intern Med 1984; 144:981–2.

54. Steiner RW. Low fractional excretion of sodium in myoglobinuric renal failure. Arch Intern Med 1982; 142:1216–7.

55. Anderson RJ, PA Gabow and Gross PA. Urinary chloride concentration in acute renal failure. Min Electrolyte Metabl 1984; 10:93–7.

56. Brosius FC and Lau K. Low fractional excretion of sodium in acute renal failure: role of timing of the test and ischemia. Am J Nephrol 1986; 6:450.

57. Polak A. Sodium depletion in chronic renal failure. J Roy Coll Phycns Lond 1971; 5:333–43.

58. Coleman AJ, Areas M, Carter NW, Rector FC and Seldin DW. The mechanism of salt wastage in chronic renal failure. J Clin Invest 1966; 45:1116–24.

59. Nickel JF, Blowrance P, Leifer E and Bradley SE. Renal function, electrolyte excretion and body fluids in patients with chronic renal insufficiency before and after sodium deprivation. J Clin Invest 1953; 32:68–79.

60. Sherman RA and Eisinger RP. Urinary sodium and chloride during renal salt retention. Am J Kidney Dis 1983; 3:121–3.

61. Webb JAW, Reznek RH, White FE, Cattell WR, Fry IK and Baker LRI. Can ultrasound and computed tomography replace high-dose urography in patients with impaired renal function? Quart J Med 1984; 53:411–25.

62. Ellenbogen PH, Scheible FW, Talner LB and Leopold GR. Sensitivity of grey scale ultrasound in detecting urinary tract obstruction. Am J Roentgenol 1978; 130:731–3.

63. Lee JKT, Baron RL, Melson GL, McClennan BL and Weyman PJ. Can real-time ultrasonography replace static B-scanning in the diagnosis of renal obstruction? Radiology 1981; 139:161–5.

64. Amis ES, Cronin JJ, Pfister RC and Yoder IC. Ultrasonic inaccuracies in diagnosing renal obstruction. Urology 1982; 19:101–5.

65. Scola FH, Cronan JJ and Schepps B. Grade I hydronephrosis: Pulsed Doppler US evaluation. Radiology 1989; 171:519–20.

66. Brandt TD, Neiman HL, Dragowski MJ, Bulawa W and Claykamp G. Ultrasound assessment of normal renal dimensions. J Ultrasound Med 1982; 1:49–52.

67. Dhar SK, Chandrasekhar H and Smith EC. Renosonogram in diagnosis of renal failure. Clin Nephrol 1977; 7:15–20.

68. Rosenbaum DM, Korngold E and Teele RL. Sonographic assessment of renal length in normal children. AJR 1983; 142:467–9.

69. Olsson O and Weiland P-O. Renal fibrolipomatosis. Acta Radiol (Diagn) 1963; 1:1061–70.

70. Subramanyam BR, Bosniak MA, Horii SC, Megibow AJ and Balthazar EJ. Replacement lipomatosis of the kidney: diagnosis by computed tomography and sonography. Radiology 1983; 148:791–92.

71. Davidson AJ. Renal sinus abnormalities. In: Radiology of the kidney. WB Saunders Company, Philadelphia 1985:510–17.

72. Koenigsberg M. Ultrasonography of the urinary tract. Chapter 16. In: Elkin M, editor. Radiology of the urinary system. Little, Brown and Company, Boston, 1980; 1190–259.

73. Van Zee BE, Hoy WE, Talley TE and Jaenike JR. Renal injury associated with intravenous pyelography in nondiabetic and diabetic patients. Ann Intern Med 1978; 89:51–4.

74. Harkonen S and Kjellstrand CM. Intravenous pyelography in nonuremic diabetic patients. Nephron 1979; 24:268–70.

75. Shafi T, Chou S-Y, Porush JG and Shapiro WB. Infusion intravenous pyelography and renal function. Effect in patients with chronic renal insufficiency. Arch Intern Med 1978; 138:1218–21.

76. Parfrey PS, Griffiths SM, Brendan RN, Barrett J, Paul MD, Genge M et al. Contrast material-induced renal failure in patients with diabetes mellitus, renal insufficiency, or both. N Engl J Med 1989; 320:143–9.

77. Barrett BJ and Carlisle EJ. Metaanalysis of the relative nephrotoxicity of high- and low-osmolality iodinated contrast media. Radiology 1993; 188:171–8.

78. Lautin EM, Freeman NJ, Schoenfeld AH, Bakal CW, Haramiti N, Friedman AC et al. Radiocontrast-associated renal dysfunction: A comparison of lower-osmolality and conventional high-osmolality contrast media. AJR 1991; 157:59–65.

79. Teruel JL, Marcen R, Onaindia JM, Serrano A, Quereda C and Ortuno J. Renal function impairment caused by intravenous urography. A prospective study. Arch Intern Med 1981; 141:1271–4.

80. Diaz-Buxo JA, Wagoner RD, Hatterly RR and Palumbo PJ. Acute renal failure after excretory urography in diabetic patients. Ann Intern Med 1975; 83:155–8.

81. Anzari Z and Baldwin DS. Acute renal failure due to radiocontrast agents. Nephron 1975; 17:28–40.

82. Carvalho A, Rakowski TA, Argy WP and Schreiner GE. Acute renal failure following drip infusion pyelography. Am J Med 1978; 65:38–45.

83. Ensor RD, Anderson EE and Robinson RR. Drip infusion urography in patients with renal disease. J Urol 1970; 103:267–71.

84. Platt JF, Rubin JM and Ellis JH. Acute renal obstruction: evaluation with intrarenal duplex Doppler and conventional US. Radiology 1993; 186:685–8.

85. Lessman RK, Johnson SF, Coburn JW and Kaufman JJ. Renal artery embolism: clinical features and long term follow-up of 17 cases. Ann Intern Med 1978; 89:477–82.

86. Linton AL, Richmond JM, Clark WF, Lindsay RM, Driedger AA, and Lamki LM. Gallium 67 scintigraphy in the diagnosis of acute renal disease. Clin Nephrol 1985; 24:84–7.

87. Graham GD, Lundy MM and Moreno AJ. Failure of gallium-67 scintigraphy to identify reliably noninfectious interstitial nephritis: Concise communication. J Nucl Med 1983; 24:568–70.

88. Bakir AA, Lopez-Majano V, Hryhorczuk DO, Rhee HL and Dunea G. Appraisal of lupus nephritis by renal imaging with gallium 67. Am J Med 1985; 79:175–82.

89. Bakir AA, Lopez-Majano V, Levy PS, Rhee HL and Dunea G. Gallium 67 scintigraphy in glomerular disease. Am J Kidney Dis 1988; 12:481–6.

90. Fawwaz RA and Johnson PM. Renal localization of radiogallium – a retrospective study. J Nucl Med 1977; 18:595.

91. Golper TA, Houghton DC, Specht HD and Porter GA. The diagnostic value of gallium – 67 scans in various nephropathies. Am Soc Nephrol, Abstracts, 1984:41.

92. Linton AL, Clark WF, Driedger AA, Turnbull I and Lindsay RM. Acute interstitial nephritis due to drugs. Review of the literature with a report of nine cases. Ann Intern Med 1980; 93:735–41.

93. Goergen TG, Lindstrom RR, Tan H and Lilley JJ. CT appearance of acute renal cortical necrosis. AJR 1981; 137:176–7.

94. Choyke PL and Pollack HM. The role of MRI in diseases of the kidney. Radiol Clin N Amer 1988; 26:617–31.

95. Galanski M, Prokop M, Chavan A, Schaefer CM, Jandeleit K and Nischelsky JE. Renal arterial stenoses: spiral CT angiography. Radiology 1993; 189:185–92.

96. Rubin GD, Dake MD, Napel S, Jeffrey RB Jr., McDonnell CH, Sommer FG et al. Spiral CT of renal artery stenosis: comparison of three-dimensional rendering techniques. Radiology 1994; 190:181–9.

97. Postma CT, Hartog O, Rosenbusch G and Thien T. Magnetic resonance angiography in the diagnosis of renal artery stenosis. J Hypertension 1993; 11:S204–5.

98. Mustonen J, Pasternack A, Helin H, Pystynen S and Tuominen T. Renal biopsy in acute renal failure. Am J Nephrol 1984; 4:27–31.

99. Duhoux P, Kourilsky O, Sraer JD and Richet G. Les insuffisances rénales aigues nécessitant un traitement étiopathogenique (utilité de la biopsie rénale précoce). In: Kuss R and Legrain M, editors. Séminaire néphro-urologie: la Pitiée Salpêtrière. Mason, Paris, 1981; 226–240.

100. Gault MH and Muehrcke RC. Renal biopsy: current views and controversies. Nephron 1983; 34:1–34.

101. Nomoto Y, Tomino Y, Endoh M, Suga T, Miura M, Nomoto H et al. Modified open renal biopsy: results in 934 patients. Nephron 1987; 45:224–8.

PART THREE

The various causes of renal failure and their diagnoses

Part II of this book was a discussion of the first diagnostic step, *gathering basic information* about the patient. In the second diagnostic step, *syndrome recognition*, the physician looks at the clinical picture and recognizes the condition responsible for the renal failure. This requires an adequate fund of information about the disorders that produce renal failure. These are now described in Part III.

False renal failure and chronic renal failure are discussed first (Chapter 7), since they are easy to identify, and require little further investigation. Failure to recognize these conditions can lead to invasive, costly and useless tests.

Next, we turn to the causes of acute and subacute renal failure. Prerenal and postrenal conditions (Chapters 8 and 9) should be distinguished from parenchymal diseases early on. Prerenal conditions (low perfusion states) and postrenal conditions (states that impede urine outflow) are common, readily recognized, and are often easy to treat.

Finally, in Chapters 10 to 13, we discuss parenchymal renal disorders: vascular, glomerular, tubular and interstitial diseases. *Confirmation of the diagnosis*, the third diagnostic step, is also described here in Part III for each of the various conditions discussed.

7. False renal failure and chronic renal failure

J. GARY ABUELO

FALSE RENAL FAILURE

False renal failure is an increase in Scr without a fall in GFR due to one of the etiologies listed in Table 7.1. (See the section, *Misleading Elevation in Scr*, in Chapter 5.) The physician needs to consider this diagnosis when the Scr increases without a change in BUN or when he recognizes one of the conditions on Table 7.1. For confirmation, one should stop the suspected drug or in the case of chemical interference, measure Scr with another method. With muscular individuals, a creatinine clearance should be performed.

CHRONIC RENAL FAILURE

Definition

Chronic renal failure is persistent azotemia caused either by gradual renal parenchymal damage or by tissue loss from a short-lived process, such as a poststreptococcal glomerulonephritis. One usually sees a slow progressive loss of GFR over years, eventuating in uremia. This is due to continued activity of the underlying disease, and to a poorly understood sclerosing process that occurs even if the original disease runs its course and leaves enough nephrons to sustain life [1, 2]. Chronic renal failure is generally irreversible, although exceptions occur, as discussed below.

Causes

Table 7.2 lists the etiologies of chronic renal failure [3–5]. In general, diabetic nephropathy, nephrosclerosis due to hypertension, and chronic glomerulonephritis each account for 20–30% of cases, while the next most common causes, polycystic kidney disease and obstructive

Table 7.1. Causes of false renal failure*

Increased creatinine load
    Large meal well cooked meat
    Greatly increased muscle mass
Impaired tubular secretion of creatinine
    Salicylate
    Cimetidine
    Trimethoprim
Positive interference with creatinine measurement
    Jaffe reaction
        Drugs
            Cefoxitin
            Acetohexamide
            Methyldopa
        Acetone and acetoacetic acid
            Diabetic, alcoholic or starvation ketosis
            Ingestion of isopropyl alcohol
            Inhalation of acetylene
    Creatinine imidohydrolase method[†] (5-flucytosine)

---

* For references see Chapter 5 – *Misleading Elevation in Scr*.
† *Ektachem method (Eastman Kodak Company, Rochester, NY).*

nephropathy, each are found in less than 5% of cases.

> Most patients with chronic glomerulonephritis have not had a renal biopsy to define the pathologic lesion; among those who have had a biopsy, IgA nephropathy, focal segmental glomerulosclerosis and crescentic glomerulonephritis are the most common forms of chronic glomerulonephritis [4, 5].

Sometimes the cause of chronic renal failure may be evident from a previous renal biopsy or might be surmised from a history of an underlying disease like severe longstanding hypertension or diabetes mellitus. In many cases an etiology is never determined, since renal biopsies are rarely performed be-

J.G. Abuelo (ed.), Renal Failure, 49–53.

Table 7.2. Causes of chronic renal failure

Glomerular diseases	Vascular diseases
Primary*	Hypertensive vascular disease*
Chronic glomerulonephritis (indeterminate type)	Benign arteriolar nephrosclerosis
IgA nephropathy	Malignant arteriolar nephrosclerosis
Focal segmental glomerulosclerosis	Atheroembolic disease
Idiopathic crescentic glomerulonephritis	Bilateral renal artery stenosis
Membranous glomerulonephritis	Hemolytic uremic syndrome
Membranoproliferative glomerulonephritis	Acute cortical necrosis
Secondary	*Tubulointerstitial diseases*
Diabetic nephropathy*	Polycystic kidney disease/other cystic diseases
Amyloidosis	Myeloma kidney
Lupus nephritis	Obstructive uropathy
Hereditary nephritis	Reflux nephropathy (chronic pyelonephritis)
Heroin nephropathy	Chronic calcium nephropathy
HIV-associated nephropathy	Oxalate nephropathy
Goodpasture's syndrome	Lead nephropathy
Light chain deposition disease	Balkan nephropathy
Vasculitides	Drug induced interstitial nephritis
Polyarteritis nodosa	Analgesic nephropathy
Wegener's granulomatosis	Cis-platinum nephropathy
Henoch-Schonlein purpura	Nitrosourea nephropathy
Essential mixed cryoglobulinemia	Lithium nephropathy (?)

* 20–30% of patients.

cause of the low likelihood of finding a reversible lesion.

Clinical picture

Chronic renal failure is usually asymptomatic initially and is recognized by a slowly rising Scr recorded over many years. Uremic symptoms like itching or anorexia and manifestations of volume overload like hypertension, pulmonary or peripheral edema usually appear as renal failure approaches end-stage. Proteinuria varies from none to massive amounts, and depends on the underlying etiology with glomerular diseases generally causing the most protein excretion. The degree of hematuria also varies widely.

An elevated Scr is often the first sign that something is wrong with the kidneys. Indeed, an evaluation for an apparently minor complaint of tiredness or poor appetite may show a Scr over 10 or even 20 mg/dl (1770 μmol/L)! In some cases, the chronicity of the process is supported by the presence of long-standing nocturia (loss of concentrating ability), anemia, edema, uremic symptoms, or by short stature in children and young adults. On the other hand, a normal hemoglobin concentration is uncommon in severe chronic renal failure (Scr greater than 6 mg/dl or 530 μmol/L) and would suggest acute renal failure.

Diagnosis

In evaluating patients with azotemia the first step is to decide whether it is acute (often reversible) or chronic (usually irreversible). The most reliable means is to review old values of Scr. Although an acute process may be suspected initially, a stable Scr over several weeks would suggest that the renal insufficiency is chronic. However, a stable or slowly rising Scr for at least three months is necessary to exclude acute or subacute disease and diagnose chronic renal failure. If previous Scr levels are not available, finding atrophic kidneys by ultrasonography or by X-ray also confirms chronic renal failure, as does renal osteodystrophy detected by roentgenologic bone survey. However, the absence of small kidneys and osteodystrophy does not exclude chronic renal failure. Therefore, patients with normal kidney size and a recently discovered stable elevation in Scr can present a difficult decision about how extensive an evaluation for acute renal failure to perform. For example, if the patient is otherwise healthy and has nothing to suggest chronic renal failure other than the stable elevated Scr, the patient is assumed to have acute renal failure and an aggressive investigation as outlined in subsequent chapters is appropriate. On the other hand, if the patient with normal kidney size and a stable elevation of Scr is elderly, severely debilitated, and has longstanding hypertension, one tends to limit the evaluation of azotemia, and to assume that it is due to chronic renal failure caused by (benign arteriolar) nephrosclerosis. One should just measure Scr periodically and only investigate further if a rapid rise is noted.

In deciding how much of an evaluation to carry out, the physician must consider the likelihood of a treatable etiology, the risk, pain and expense of the tests involved, the quality of life and the desires of the patient.

Renal Sonogram. *Ultrasonography of the kidneys should be carried out in all patients with suspected or confirmed chronic renal failure. If one cannot distinguish acute from chronic azotemia, the finding of small kidneys or normal size kidneys with parenchymal atrophy supplanted by replacement lipomatosis [6–8] confirms the chronic nature of the renal disease. The ultrasound may also indicate the cause of chronic renal failure by detecting polycystic kidneys, signs of analgesic nephropathy, an atrophic kidney due to renovascular disease, or a dilated collecting system due to obstruction.*

Roentgenologic Bone Survey. *Perhaps 10–30% of patients with end stage renal disease show X-ray changes of renal osteodystrophy, typically erosion of the terminal phalanges on plain films of the hands [4, 9]. These cases almost always have an increased serum alkaline phosphatase concentration. Although uncommon, the finding of osteodystrophy will confirm that the renal failure is longstanding. Therefore, if the serum alkaline phosphatase level is high and chronic renal failure is suspected, X-rays of the hands should be obtained.*

Treatable Causes. *A diagnosis of chronic renal failure usually means that a progressive loss of GFR is unavoidable. Further diagnostic studies should be limited and a renal biopsy is rarely indicated. Nevertheless, there are several causes of chronic renal failure that should be carefully excluded, since their treatment may stabilize or reverse the loss of GFR.*

Severe hypertension may be a clue to the cause of chronic renal failure. Renal artery stenosis *can lead to gradually declining renal function, which may be im-* proved by relief of the renal artery stenosis with surgery or angioplasty, even in the face of total renal arterial occlusion [10] (see Chapter 10, Vascular Causes of Renal Failure). One should suspect renal artery stenosis in older hypertensive patients with generalized atherosclerosis, worsening hypertension, and asymmetric renal size [11], and should consider performing arteriography.

Many reversible etiologies produce interstitial or tubular damage. Chronic urinary tract obstruction *is one such disorder; fortunately, it is easily recognized on ultrasonography, and renal failure may improve with relief of obstruction, if parenchymal atrophy has not occurred (see Chapter 9, Postrenal Renal Failure).* Analgesic nephropathy *is a combination of chronic interstitial nephritis and papillary necrosis formerly observed in individuals abusing phenacetin over many years. Now that phenacetin has been removed from most markets, a similar condition occasionally without papillary necrosis is being observed with prolonged use of acetaminophen and nonsteroidal anti-inflammatory drugs [12–16]. It should be suspected in patients with chronic backache, arthritic pain or headaches. Analgesic nephropathy is usually diagnosed by showing papillary necrosis on intravenous or retrograde pyelography. However, renal tomography alone is a sensitive screening test [16], and should be ordered in patient's with longstanding analgesic use. Renal function may improve or stabilize with discontinuation of the analgesic abuse.* Chronic hypercalcemia *of many causes produces nephrocalcinosis and interstitial nephritis. A serum calcium concentration should be measured, since improvement of renal insufficiency due to hypercalcemia may be observed after normalization of the serum calcium [17–19] (see Chapter 10, section on Vasomotor Disturbances).*

Patients older than 40 years with normal kidney size and proteinuria should be tested for multiple myeloma *or* light chain deposition disease *with urine and serum protein and immunofixation electrophoresis, since monoclonal gammopathies may present with chronic renal insufficiency, and chemotherapy may occasionally lead to partial recovery of renal function [20–22] (see Chapter 11, section on Nephrotic Diseases, and Chapter 12, section on Tubular Obstruction).*

Acute Fall in Renal Function. Patients with pre-existing chronic renal failure are at higher risk for acute renal insufficiency than are patients with normal renal function [23, 24], especially in the post-operative setting [25, 26]. In fact, at some time up to a quarter of patients with chronic renal impairment experience "acute-on-chronic" renal failure, usually due to volume depletion, aggressive treatment of hypertension, urinary obstruction or infection [27, 28, 29].

It is important to detect "acute-on-chronic" renal failure since the acute component is usually reversible with appropriate treatment. Typically, the Scr rises more rapidly than expected for simple progression of chronic disease. To get an idea of the expected rise in Scr, one may plot the reciprocal of the previous Scr values (1/Scr) versus time on graph paper and draw the best fitting straight line through the points. This line will show the predicted Scr with which one may compare the current values [30] (Figure 7.1). Another clue to acute-on-chronic renal failure is a BUN to Scr ratio greater than 20 : 1 (0.08 in SI units), since such ratios are rare in uncomplicated chronic renal failure [4, 31].

If one detects or suspects an unusually rapid fall in GFR, one must look for a treatable cause, especially one of the etiologies mentioned above. In patients with pyuria (more than 3–5 white blood cells per high power field) a urine culture should be done and any infection should be treated [29].

CONCLUSION

Chronic renal failure as a cause of azotemia is diagnosed by any one of the following:
(1) a progressive increase in Scr;
(2) an elevated Scr that is stable for three months or more;

(3) atrophic renal parenchyma by X-ray or sonography;
(4) renal osteodystrophy on skeletal survey.

Hypercalcemia and obstruction need to be excluded with a serum calcium determination and renal sonography, respectively. Clinical clues to other treatable causes are indicated on Table 7.3.

REFERENCES

1. Maschio G, Oldrizzi L and, Rugiu C. Is there a "point of no return" in progressive renal disease? Am Soc Nephrol 1991; 2:832–40.
2. Klahr S, Schreiner G and, Ichikawa I. Mechanisms of disease. N Engl J Med 1988; 318:1657–66.
3. U.S. Renal Data System, USRDS 1993 Annual Data Report, The National Institutes of Health, National Institute of Diabetes and Digestive and Kidney Diseases, Bethesda, MD, March 1993, p 24.
4. Malangone JM, Abuelo JG, Pezzullo JC, Lund K and McGloin CA. Clinical and laboratory features of patients with chronic renal disease at the start of dialysis. Clin Nephrol 1989; 31:77–87.
5. Simon P, Ang KS, Cam G and Ramee MP. La glomerulonephrite a depots d'immunoglobulines A est une des causes les plus frequentes d'insuffisance renale terminale. Enquete epidemiologique. La Presse Med 1988; 17:121.
6. Davidson AJ. Renal sinus abnormalities. In: Radiology of the kidney. WB Saunders Company, Philadelphia 1985:510–7.
7. Olsson O and Weiland P-O. Renal fibrolipomatosis. Acta Radiol (Diagn) 1963; 1:1061–70.

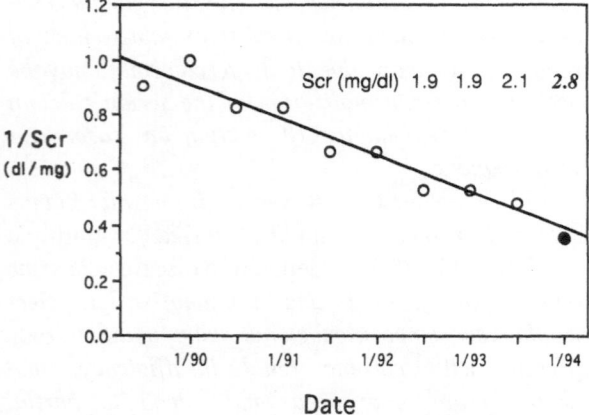

Fig. 7.1. A patient with chronic renal failure has had a Scr in the area of 2.0 mg/dl for the past year. A Scr of 2.8 mg/dl is obtained at a routine visit. Does this indicate acute-on-chronic renal failure? The plot of 1/Scr shows that the 2.8 mg/dl measurement is not very different from the predicted value – about 2.5 mg/dl, and suggests that no acute process has occurred.

Table 7.3. Clinical clues to treatable causes of chronic renal failure

Condition	Clues
Renal artery stenosis	Generalized atherosclerosis, abdominal bruits, symmetric kidneys, severe hypertension
Obstruction	Bladder symptoms, prostatic hypertrophy, gross hematuria, abdominal or flank pain, pelvic or urologic malignancy
Analgesic nephropathy	Acetaminophen, NSAID's, chronic headache, backache or joint pains
Myeloma kidney/light chain deposition disease	Proteinuria, bone pain, anemia, age over 40, frequent infections, hypercalcemia
Acute-on-chronic renal failure	Unexpected "jump" in Scr, recent volume loss, BUN/Scr > 20 : 1 (0.08 in SI units)

8. Subramanyam BR, Bosniak MA, Horii SC, Megibow AJ, and Balthazar EJ. Replacement lipomatosis of the kidney: Diagnosis by computed tomography and sonography. Radiology 1983; 148:791–2.
9. Hutchinson AJ, Whitehouse RW, Boulton HF, Adams JE, Mawer EB, Freemont TJ, et al. Correlation of bone histology with parathyroid hormone, vitamin D3, and radiology in end-stage renal disease. Kidney Int 1993; 44:1071–7.
10. Jacobson HR. Ischemic renal disease: An overlooked clinical entity? Kidney Int 1988; 34:729–43.
11. Novick AC, Textor SC, Bodie B and Khauli RB. Revascularization to preserve renal function in patients with atherosclerotic renovascular disease. Urol Clin NA 1984; 11:477–90.
12. Adams DH, Michael J, Bacon PA, Howie AJ, McConckey B and Adu D. Non-steroidal anti-inflammatory drugs and renal failure. Lancet 1986; i:57–60.
13. Segasothy M, Kong Chiew Tong B, Kamal A, Murad Z, Suleiman AB. Analgesic nephropathy associated with paracetamol. Aust NZ J Med 1984; 14:23–6.
14. Krikler DM. Paracetamol and the kidney. BMJ 1967; 2:615–6.
15. Schwarz A, Keller F, Kunzendorf U, Kuhn-Freitag G, Heinemeyer G, Pommer W, et al. Characteristics and clinical course of hemodialysis patients with analgesic-associated nephropathy. Clin Nephrol 1988; 29:299–306.
16. De Broe ME and Elseviers MM. Analgesic nephropathy – Still a problem? Nephron 1993; 64:505–13.
17. Orwoll ES. The milk-alkali syndrome: current concepts. Ann Intern Med 1982; 97-242–8.
18. Agus ZS, Goldfarb S and Wasserstein A. Disorders of calcium and phosphate balance. In: The Kidney 2nd edition, Brenner BM, Rector FC, Jr., WB Saunders, Philadelphia 1981: 940–1022.
19. Schuman CA and Jones HW, III. The "milk-alkali" sydrome: Two case reports with discussion of pathogenesis. Quart J Med 1985; 55:119–26.
20. Emmett M, Bengfort L, Warren E, Hull A and Dallas Neph Assocs: Recovery from end stage renal disease. Am Soc Nephrol Abstracts 1979: 116A.
21. Brown WW, Hebert LE, Piering WF, Psciotta AV, Lemann J and Garancis JC. Reversal of chronic end-stage renal failure due to myeloma kidney. Ann Intern Med 1979; 90:793–4.
22. Heilman RL, Holley K, Offord K, Velosa J and Kyle R. Apparent renal response to melphalan and prednisone (MP) in light chain deposition disease (LCDD). Kidney Int 1989; 35:209.
23. Hou SH, Bushinsky DA, Wish JB, Cohen JJ and Harrington JT. Hospital-acquired renal insufficiency: a prospective study. Am J Med 1983; 74:243–8.
24. Rasmussen HH and Ibels LS. Acute renal failure. Multivariate analysis of causes and risk factors. Am J Med 1982; 73:211–8.
25. Abel RM, Buckley MJ, Austen WG, Barnett GO, Beck CH and Fischer JE. Etiology, incidence and prognosis of renal failure following cardiac operations. Results of a prospective analysis of 500 consecutive patients. J Thorac Cardiovasc Surg 1976; 71:323–33.
26. Tilney NL and Lazarus JM. Acute renal failure in surgical patients. Causes, clinical patterns and care. Surg Clin NA 1983; 63:357–77.
27. Maher JF, Bryan CW and Ahearn DJ. Prognosis of chronic renal failure. II. Factors affecting survival. Arch Intern Med 1975; 135:273–8.
28. Davidman M, Olson P, Kohen J, Leither T and Kjellstrand C. Iatrogenic renal disease. Arch Intern Med 1991; 151; 1809–12.
29. Ahmed Z, de la Rosa J and Levison SP. Reversible acute renal failure due to urinary tract infection in chronic renal insufficiency patients. Kidney Int 1986; 29:176.
30. Oska H, Pasternack A Luomala, M and Sirvio M. Progression of chronic renal failure. Nephron 1983; 35:31–4.
31. Morgan DB, Carver ME and Payne RB. Plasma creatinine and urea: creatinine ratio in patients with raised plasma urea. BMJ 1977; 2:929–32.

8. Prerenal renal failure

J. GARY ABUELO

Definition and causes

Prerenal renal failure or azotemia results when a disturbance in systemic hemodynamics reduces renal perfusion. The most common causes of prerenal renal failure are congestive heart failure, sepsis, and volume depletion. Specific etiologies are listed on Table 8.1.

Clinical picture

The typical patient with prerenal renal failure has had a recent cardiac insult or obvious volume loss and has recumbent or orthostatic hypotension. He may complain of weakness or lightheadedness when standing relieved by sitting or lying. The urine flow is usually in the oliguric range (less than

Table 8.1. Causes of prerenal renal failure

Cardiovascular causes (primary pump failure)	Blood loss
Myocardial disease	Fluid loss to the outside
Infarction	Gastrointestinal
Cardiomyopathy	Vomiting
Pericardial disease	Diarrhea
Tamponade	Fistula
Constrictive pericarditis	Drainage tubes
Pulmonary vascular obstruction	Renal
Embolism	Diuretics
Pulmonary hypertension	Primary adrenal insufficiency
Arrhythmias	Osmotic diuresis
Valvular disease	Hypercalcemia
Myxoma	Pituitary and nephrogenic diabetes insipidus
Hypocalcemia	Salt wasting nephropathies
	Dermal
Volume depletion (secondary pump failure)	Burns
Fluid loss to the third space	Sweat
Tissue damage	Dehydration 2° to ↓↓ intake
Pancreatitis	Water not available
Peritonitis	Thirst mechanism not operative
Rhabdomyolysis	
Burns	*Reduced vascular resistance*
Hypoalbuminemia	Sepsis
Malnutrition	Antihypertensive medications
Nephrosis	Overdose of barbiturates, etc.
Liver failure	Carcinoid syndrome [2]
Enteropathy	Interleukin-2 therapy [3–8]
Small or large bowel obstruction	Arteriovenous fistula
Capillary leak 2° to ovarian stimulation [1]	Coronary vasodilators
	Nitrates
	Calcium channel blockers

J.G. Abuelo (ed.), Renal Failure, 55–57.
© 1995 *Kluwer Academic Publishers.*

500 ml/day) due to low GFR and avid tubular reabsorption of salt and water. The BUN to Scr ratio is near 20 or greater (0.08 in SI units), the urine specific gravity is 1.015–1.020 or greater, the dipstick for urine protein is trace or negative, the urine sediment is normal, and urinary sodium and chloride concentrations are low. A high hematocrit may be seen in patients with fluid loss. Renal function returns promptly to normal if effective circulation is restored.

Occasional patients have *nonoliguric* prenal renal failure with urine flows as high as 3 L/day [9, 10]. In some cases the tubules are unable to concentrate appropriately for various reasons [9], while in other cases a catabolic state or excess tube feeding increases urea production, which in turn causes an osmotic diuresis [10].

Diagnosis

The physician usually can recognize the clinical picture of prerenal azotemia and may consider the diagnosis confirmed if Scr returns to normal with correction of the volume deficit and blood pressure. Unfortunately, cardiogenic and septic shock may not respond to therapy and the high BUN to Scr ratio and renal salt avidity themselves must serve as presumptive evidence.

Pitfalls. The diagnosis can be missed when the patient's blood pressure is decreased, but still in the normal range. In such cases, a circulatory disturbance, while not great enough to cause frank hypotension, can still produce prerenal renal failure, because underlying factors reduce the kidneys' autoregulatory capacity and increase susceptibility of GFR to a small fall in perfusion pressure. These factors include hypertension, renal artery stenosis, chronic renal insufficiency, diabetic arteriolosclerosis and treatment with drugs that interfere with renal autoregulation (angiotensin converting enzyme inhibitors, non-steroidal anti-inflammatory drugs) [11].

Although *hypovolemia* is responsible for many cases of prerenal azotemia, *hypervolemia* occurs in prerenal azotemia due to cardiogenic shock, and *euvolemia* is common in septic shock. (The three situations have arterial underfilling in common.) When assessing a patient's hemodynamic status, the physician should remember that all of these *volume variations* are possible.

Also, the recognition of intravascular hypovolemia is not always straightforward in cases of prerenal azotemia. In critically ill patients with *hypoalbuminemia*, the presence of edema should not be used to exclude intravascular volume depletion. Alternatively, the physician may not appreciate occult volume loss such as that due to a simple reduction in salt intake in the presence of obligatory renal salt losing. *Salt losing kidneys* can be caused by cisplatin [12] or by many

chronic renal diseases particularly tubulointerstitial, cystic and obstructive processes [13–16]. Also, renal salt loss may be due to diuretics, hypercalcemia, primary adrenal insufficiency or osmotic diuresis from hyperglycemia, mannitol or enteric tube feeding [17]. Urine tests in these cases show renal salt loss and not salt avidity.

One may encounter other misleading laboratory findings in prerenal azotemia. A rise in BUN to Scr ratio may be blunted by low dietary protein, voluminous diarrheal stools and other factors (see Urea. *Low Ratios* in Chapter 5). The expected high urine specific gravity, normal protein excretion, and normal urine sediment may be masked by underlying renal disease or other factors.

As detailed in the Pitfalls *section above, prerenal renal failure sometimes occurs without frank hypotension or without typical historical and laboratory features. This means that one must always consider this diagnosis in patients with unexplained renal failure. Orthostatic changes in blood pressure and pulse should be sought. Hypertension and signs of volume overload rule out volume depletion, but normal blood pressure and apparent euvolemia do not.*

Fluid "Challenge". *A trial of volume expansion in normotensive apparently euvolemic patients can diagnose hypovolemic prerenal azotemia. One should administer normal saline intravenously or give salt orally (NaCl tablets, bouillon, highly-salted foods) to look for improvement in BUN and Scr. An adequate salt load increases the weight by three to four kilograms over about three days, brings the blood pressure to 140/90 mmHg or produces mild volume overload. Also when a patient's hemodynamic status is uncertain, hypovolemia, low vascular resistance, and primary pump failure may be diagnosed by placing a Swan-Ganz catheter and measuring pulmonary capillary wedge pressure, peripheral resistance and cardiac output.*

Furosemide "Challenge". Some physicians give a furosemide "challenge" to oliguric patients, since a diuretic response is thought to indicate prerenal azotemia. The diagnostic value of this maneuver is doubtful as urine flow may rise regardless of the diagnosis. Also, the creation of a brisk diuresis in a volume depleted individual is hazardous.

Conclusion

Classic prerenal renal failure with its constellation of hypotension, high BUN:Scr ratio and high urine specific gravity is easily diagnosed and often responds quickly to treatment. The challenge to the

Table 8.2. Clinical clues to prerenal renal failure

Recent volume loss	Blood pressure < usual level
Recent cardiac insult	BUN/Scr > 20 : 1 (<0.08 SI)
Fever or other signs of sepsis	Urine specific gravity > 1.020
Orthostatic symptoms	Albumin <3 g/dL without edema

physician is to recognize this condition when hypotension or other hallmarks are absent. Clinical clues to prerenal renal failure are listed on Table 8.2.

REFERENCES

1. Golan A, Ron-El R, Herman A, Soffer Y, Weinraub Z and Caspi E. Ovarian hyperstimulation syndrome: an update review. Obstet and Gynecol Survey 1989; 44:430–40.
2. Couttenye MM, Verpooten GA, Daelemans RA and DeBroe ME. Functional acute renal failure in a patient with carcinoid syndrome. Nephron 1987; 47:131–3.
3. Kozeny GA, Nicolas JD, Creekmore S, Sticklin L, Hano JE and Fisher RI. Effects of interleukin-2 immunotherapy on renal function. J Clin Oncol 1988; 6:1170–6.
4. Belldegrun A, Webb DE, Austin III HA, Steinberg SM, White DE, Linehan WM et al. Effects of interleukin-2 on renal function in patients receiving immunotherapy for advanced cancer. Ann Intern Med 1987; 106:817–22.
5. Christiansen NP, Skubitz KM, Nath K, Ochoa A and Kennedy BJ. Nephrotoxicity of continuous intravenous infusion of recombinant interleukin-2. Am J Med 1988; 84:1072–5.
6. Webb DE, Austin HA III, Belldegrun A, Vaughan E, Linehan WM and Rosenberg SA. Metabolic and renal effects of interleukin-2 immunotherapy for metastatic cancer. Clin Nephrol 1988; 30:141–5.
7. Textor SC, Margolin K, Blayney D, Carlson J and Doroshow J. Renal, volume, and hormonal changes during therapeutic administration of recombinant interleukin-2 in man. Am J Med 1987; 83:1055–61.
8. Rosenberg SA, Packard BS, Aebersold PM, Solomon D, Topalian SL, Toy ST et al. Use of tumor-infiltrating lymphocytes and interleukin-2 in the immunotherapy of patients with metastatic melanoma. N Engl J Med 1988; 319:1676–80.
9. Miller PD, Krebs RA, Neal BJ and McIntyre DO. Polyuric prerenal failure. Arch Intern Med 1980; 140:907–9.
10. Kamm DE, Spital A and Sterns R. Non-oliguric prerenal azotemia. Kidney Int. 1983; 23:127.
11. Badr KF and Ichikawa I. Prerenal failure: a deleterious shift from renal compensation to decompensation. N Engl J Med 1988; 319:623–9.
12. Hutchison FN, Perez EA, Gandara DR, Lawrence HJ and Kaysen GA. Renal salt wasting in patients treated with cisplatin. Ann Intern Med 1988; 108:21–5.
13. Conte G, Dal Canton A, Marcuccio F, Stanziale P and Andreucci VE. Polyuric prerenal failure after reduction from high to normal dietary intake of sodium. Arch Intern Med 1986; 146:1814–7.
14. Morgan DB, Ball SR, Thomas TH and Lee MR. Sodium losing renal disease: two cases of a review of the literature. Quart J Med 1978; N.S. 47:21–34.
15. Peer G, Wigler I and Aviram A. Prolonged volume depletion imitating end-stage renal failure. Am J Med Sci 1987; 30:214–7.
16. Uribarri J, Oh MS and Carroll HJ. Salt-losing nephropathy. Am J Nephrol 1983; 3:193–8.
17. Cataldi-Betcher EL, Seltzer MH, Slocum BA and Jones KW. Complications occurring during enteral nutrition support: a prospective study. J Parenteral and Enteral Nutrition 1983; 7:546–52.

9. Postrenal renal failure

J. GARY ABUELO

Definition

Postrenal renal failure results from a disturbance at any point in the normal passage of urine from the kidneys to the outside. Most cases involve mechanical blockage, but a neurogenic bladder or a ruptured bladder with intraperitoneal extravasation also disrupts urine outflow. Acutely, obstruction causes dilatation of the renal pelvis and calyces and a reversible fall in GFR; chronically progressive dilatation of the collecting system and parenchymal atrophy lead to massive hydronephrosis and irreversible renal failure.

Pathophysiology

Complete obstruction of the bladder outlet, both ureters or the ureter from a single functioning kidney produces total cessation of function with anuria. Partial obstruction often reduces GFR and urine flow, but can also reduce GFR and *increase urine flow* due to interference with urine concentration. Complete obstruction of one of two functioning kidneys should acutely halve the GFR and double the Scr, e.g. from 1 to 2 mg/dl (88 to 176 μmol/L). With underlying chronic renal failure the rise in Scr with unilateral obstruction may be more significant, e.g. doubling after the obstruction from 4 to 8 mg/dl (354 to 708 μmol/L). In the first example, compensatory hypertrophy of the unobstructed normal kidney will return GFR and Scr close to normal. With chronic renal failure, however, compensatory hypertrophy is minimal.

Causes

The causes of postrenal renal failure are many and appear in Table 9.1. Obstruction in women occurs most often in the middle years of life, and is due to stones and pelvic malignancies. Stones are responsible for most cases in men before age 60; afterwards prostatic cancer and hypertrophy are the leading causes. Congenital ureteropelvic junction obstruction is the most common cause of hydronephrosis in young children and is also seen in adults.

Clinical picture

In typical cases of postrenal renal failure the initial evaluation gives a clue to the diagnosis.

On history the patient may have active manifestations of urologic disease like bladder symptoms, gross hematuria, signs of urinary infection or pain from the urinary tract (see *Other Renal or Urologic Symptoms* in Chapter 3). As mentioned above, urine output may be increased, reduced or absent. The setting may suggest a higher *risk* of urologic disease or obstruction. The risk is increased by old age in men, a solitary kidney, anticholinergic drugs, diabetes mellitus, previous urologic disease, and surgery, malignancy or other disorder of the periurinary structures.

The physical examination may show a palpable hydronephrotic kidney, distended bladder or a pelvic or prostatic mass. However, when benign prostatic hypertrophy of the subcervical lobe produces postrenal renal failure, the prostate may be of normal size and consistency on rectal examination.

The urinalysis reveals an isotonic specific gravity ($\sim$1.010), negative to trace protein, occasionally increased red cells, and if infection is present, pyuria and bacteria.

Renal salt avidity and high BUN to Scr ratio are occasionally present [36–39], but renal salt losing with volume depletion may also be seen [40]. Defects in distal tubular potassium and acid secretion may produce hyperkalemia or metabolic acidosis out of proportion to the severity of renal failure [41].

J.G. Abuelo (ed.), Renal Failure, 59–63.
© 1995 *Kluwer Academic Publishers.*

Table 9.1. Causes of postrenal renal failure

Ureteropelvic junction
Stricture [1]
Fibrous band
Aberrant vessel

Ureter [2]
Trauma
    Edema after retrograde catheter [3]
    Surgical ligation or other injury [4]
    Stricture after instrumentation
Congenital
    Ureterocele
    Severe vesicoureteral reflux
    Ectopic location of ureter
    Ectopic kidney
    Bladder diverticula
    Stricture
Intraluminal objects
    Stone*
    Sloughed papilla
        Sickle cell anemia and trait
        Diabetes mellitus
        Nonsteroidal anti-inflammatory drugs
        Pyelonephritis
    Blood clots
        Bleeding diathesis [5]
        Aminocaproic acid [6]
    Fungus balls [7, 8]
Inflammatory process
    Retroperitoneal fibrosis
        Idiopathic
        Bromocriptine [9]
        Methysergide [10]
        Dihydroergotamine [11]
        Aortic aneurysm with perianeurysmal fibrosis [12]
        Post aortoiliac [13] or other surgery
        Crohn's disease, diverticulitis, appendicitis or other
            contiguous inflammatory processes [14]
    Retroperitoneal or pelvic abscess
    Retroperitoneal bleeding [15]
    Urinoma (post trauma)
    Tuberculosis [16]
    Vasculitis [17–19]
    Schistosomiasis [20]
    Sarcoidosis and other granulomatous disease
Uterine process
    Pregnancy [21–23]
    Prolapse [24]
    Endometriosis [25, 26]

Tumors
    Urinary neoplasms
        Carcinoma of ureter, bladder or prostate
        Polyps
        Sarcoma and other rare tumors
    Extraurinary neoplasms
        Carcinoma of cervix or ovary*
        Retroperitoneal lymphoma
        Breast or other retroperitoneal metastatic malignancy
Amyloidosis [27, 28]
Iliac artery aneurysm
Idiopathic post-ileal conduit [29]
Submucosal bleeding (warfarin) [30]

Bladder
Neurogenic bladder
    Meningomyelocele and other congenital defects
    Diabetes mellitus [31]
    Spinal cord lesions
        Trauma
        Tumor
        Abscess
        Tabes dorsalis
    Herpes and other viral infections [32, 33]
    Narcotics
    Drugs with anticholinergic activity
        Antihistamines
        Phenothiazines
        Disopyramide phosphate
    Multiple sclerosis
Rupture due to trauma [34]
Chronic (lupus) interstitial cystitis [35]

Urethra
Benign prostatic hypertrophy*
Neoplasms
    Prostate
    Bladder
    Other tumors
Intraluminal object
    Stone
    Foreign body
    Obstructed indwelling catheter
Congenital
    Posterior urethral valves
    Anomalous location
    Urethral diverticula
Post infectious or traumatic stricture
Meatal stenosis
Phimosis

* Most common causes.

Diagnosis

Urethral Catheter. *A urethral catheter should be inserted in patients with acute urinary retention or other urinary symptoms, as well as in elderly men with undiagnosed renal failure. If possible the patient should void just before catheterization. A postvoid residual urine volume of up to 100 to 150 ml excludes impaired bladder outflow as a cause of renal failure, and the catheter should be removed. If the postvoid residual urine volume is 150 to 400 ml, the catheter should be left in for 24 to 48 hours to look for an improvement of Scr; however, impairment of bladder outflow severe enough to produce renal failure usually leads to residual urine volumes of 400 ml or more. Drainage of a large amount of urine from the bladder followed by a fall in Scr confirms the postrenal azotemia. Relief of obstruction may also lead to a continuous diuresis of 3 L/day or more, but in chronic obstruction, recovery of renal function may occur without such a diuresis [42]. A large bladder volume without a subsequent fall in Scr indicates that permanent damage from bladder outlet obstruction has occurred and improvement, if any, will be slow and incomplete. It may also reflect concurrent ureteral obstruction.*

Imaging of the Urinary Tract. *Patients suspected of postrenal azotemia should have a renal sonogram. It will show hydronephrosis in virtually all patients with urinary obstruction, although dilatation may only be minimal (Grade I hydronephrosis) [43, 44]. Alternatively, in patients with acute renal colic, if not contraindicated (see section on* Intravenous Pyelogram, *Chapter 6), an IVP should be ordered to look for obstruction behind a stone or sloughed papilla. If the diagnosis remains in doubt or further definition of the lesion is needed, cystoscopy with retrograde pyelography or in sicker patients, percutaneous nephrostomy with antegrade pyelography is indicated [45]. A urologist should be consulted at this point for guidance in further diagnosis and management of obstructed patients.*

Since a renal sonogram ought to be done in all undiagnosed cases of renal failure, postrenal renal failure should be detected even in patients with no clinical indications of an obstruction [46].

A renal sonogram or IVP is not always adequate to diagnose urinary obstruction. With minimal hydronephrosis, residual hydronephrosis and hydronephrosis of pregnancy, one may be unsure of the clinical significance of urinary tract dilatation. *Moreover, rare obstructed patients have no hydronephrosis at all!*

Minimal or no Hydronephrosis. *Rarely obstruction causing renal failure produces little or no dilatation. This can occur early after obstruction before much distention takes place [44, 47, 48] or when retroperitoneal fibrosis or tumor encases the ureter and renal pelvis [45]. The diagnosis of postrenal renal failure may be missed in these patients, because no hydronephrosis has developed or the slight dilatation is erroneously thought to be inadequate to explain the degree of renal failure [43, 45]. Within the first 24 hours of acute obstruction by calculi a third of patients have no hydronephrosis detected on ultrasound, but mild ureteral dilatation and the point of obstruction will be seen on IVP [47]. Therefore, the IVP is a better test than sonography in most patients with acute renal colic.*

Residual Hydronephrosis of Questionable Significance. *Relief of longstanding urinary obstruction may improve GFR, but bring about little or no improvement in chronic dilatation of the urinary tract. If a new obstructing lesion causes a rise in Scr, the residual hydronephrosis can interfere with detection of the new obstruction. While a clear increase in dilatation points to urinary tract blockage, a significant obstruction may produce no change in dilatation.*

Hydronephrosis of Pregnancy. *Postrenal renal failure may be produced by the gravid uterus, especially one overdistended by polyhydramnios or multiple gestations [21, 23, 49]. It can be difficult to recognize in pregnant women who normally develop up to Grade II hydronephrosis without loss of renal function [50–52]. The mechanism of this physiologic dilatation is not known. If the initial evaluation suggests postrenal azotemia or if the dilatation on ultrasound is more than that anticipated for the stage of pregnancy [50–52], the diagnosis of a pathologic blockage may be confirmed by a fall in Scr following relief of the obstruction. Delivery or placement of a ureteral catheter or percutaneous nephrostomy tube should be carried out [21–23]. Alternatively, in women with polyhydramnios, amniotomy may decompress the ureters [23].*

Several procedures may be useful in assessing the significance of dilatation in these three situations. Diuretic renography *may be carried out by combining a technetium scan with furosemide. The half time or time for half the tracer to exit the collecting system is normally less than 15 min, and is over 20 min in clear-cut obstruction. Unfortunately, many patients fall in the indeterminate range of 15 to 20 min [53]. Alternatively, one may do a functional study, the* Whitaker test, *in which fluid is infused into the renal pelvis through a percutaneous needle at high flow and the hydrostatic pressure response is* monitored [54]. High pressure indicates obstruction. Inaccurate results occur with both these tests, leading some to question their value [55–57]. If urinary obstruction cannot be ruled out, retrograde or antegrade pyelography and a trial of urinary drainage should be considered. Obviously, a urologist should be involved in the evaluation of these difficult cases.

Conclusion

Most patients with postrenal renal failure give a history suggestive of an obstructive process in the urinary tract. The most common clues to problems of urine outflow are given on Table 9.2. The diagnosis of impaired bladder emptying is confirmed by urethral catheterization, while upper tract lesions are easily documented by renal sonography. Even cases with asymptomatic obstruction should not be missed, since the evaluation of undiagnosed renal failure includes renal sonography.

Table 9.2. Clinical clues to postrenal renal failure

Bladder symptoms	Anticholinergic drugs
Old age in men	History of pelvic or urologic malignancy
Solitary kidney	Prostatic hypertrophy
Urinary tract pain	Gross hematuria

REFERENCES

1. Kerr PG, Wilson DM, Lawson PS and Dawborn JK. Bilateral pelviureteric junction obstruction causing renal failure in two elderly patients. Am J Nephrol 1989; 9:47–50.
2. Norman RW, Mack FG, Awad SA, Belitsky P, Schwarz RD and Lannon SG. Acute renal failure secondary to bilateral ureteric obstruction: review of 50 cases. Canad Med Assoc J 1982; 127:601–4.
3. Hurley RM. Acute renal failure secondary to bilateral retrograde pyelography. Clin Pediatr 1979; 18:754–6.
4. Dowling RA, Corriere JN Jr. and Sandler CM. Iatrogenic ureteral injury. J Urol 1986; 135:912–5.
5. Prentice CRM, Lindsay RM, Barr RD, Forbes CD, Kennedy AC, McNicol GP et al. Renal complications in haemophilia and Christmas disease. Quart J Med 1971; 40:47–61.
6. Pitts TO, Spero JA, Bontempo FA and Greenberg A. Acute renal failure due to high-grade obstruction following therapy with e-aminocaproic acid. Am J Kidney Dis 1986; 8:441–4.
7. Domart Y, Delmas V, Cornus F, Bouchama A, Chastre J and Gibert C. Obstruction des voies urinaires par des bezoars candidosiques, ou "fungus balls". La Presse Med 1986; 15:153–6.
8. Bartone FF, Hurwitz RS, Rojas EL, Steinberg E and Franceschini R. The role of percutaneous nephrostomy in the management of obstructing candidiasis of the urinary tract in infants. J Urol 1988; 140:338–41.
9. Bowler JV, Ormerod IE and Legg NJ. Retroperitoneal fibrosis and bromocriptine. Lancet 1986; 2:466.
10. Graham JR, Suby JI, LeCompte PR and Sandowsky NL. Fibrotic disorders associated with methysergide therapy for headache. N Engl J Med 1966; 274:359–368.
11. Malaquin F, Urban T, Ostinelli J, Ghedira H and Lacronique J. Pleural and retroperitoneal fibrosis from dihydroergotamine. N Engl J Med 1989; 321:1760.
12. Rault R, Kapoor W and Kam W. Perianeurysmal fibrosis and ureteric obstruction: case report and review of literature. Clin Nephrol 1982; 18:159–62.
13. Schubart P, Fortner G, Cummings D, Reed D, Thiele BL, Bandyk DF et al. The significance of hydronephrosis after aortofemoral reconstruction. Arch Surg 1985; 120:377–81.
14. Wagenknecht LV and Hardy JC. Value of various treatments for retroperitoneal fibrosis. Eur Urol 1981; 7:193–200.
15. Weinberg MS, Quigg R and Krane RL. Retroperitoneal bleeding: hidden culprit of acute renal failure. Urology 1983; 21:291–4.
16. Lazarus L and Peraino RA. Reversible uremia due to bilateral ureteral obstruction from tuberculosis. Am J Nephrol 1984; 4:322–7.
17. Rich LM and Piering WF. Ureteral stenosis due to recurrent Wegener's granulomatosis after kidney transplantation. J Am Soc Nephrol 1994; 4:1516–21.
18. Smet M-H, Marchal G, Oyen R and Breysem L. Stenosing hemorrhagic ureteritis in a child with Henoch-Schonlein purpura: CT appearance. J Comp Assist Tomog 1991; 15:326–8.
19. Lie JT. Retroperitoneal polyarteritis nodosa presenting as ureteral obstruction. J Rheumatol 1992; 19:1628–31.
20. El-Said W. Obstructive uropathy as a cause of renal failure among dialysis patients. Kidney Int. 1984; 26:557 (abstract).
21. Lowes JJ, Mackenzie JC, Abrams PH and Gingell JC. Acute renal failure and acute hydronephrosis in pregnancy: use of the double-J stent. J Royal Soc Med 1987; 80:524–5.
22. Eckford SD and Gingell JC. Ureteric obstruction in pregnancy – diagnosis and management. Brit J Obstet and Gynecol 1991; 98:1137–40.
23. Brandes JC and Fritsche C. Obstructive acute renal failure by a gravid uterus: a case report and review. Am J Kidney Dis 1991; 18:398–401.
24. Churchill DN, Afridi S, Dow D and McManamon P. Uterine prolapse and renal dysfunction. J Urol 1980; 124:899–900.
25. Kane C and Drouin P. Obstructive uropathy associated with endometriosis. Am J Obstet and Gynecol 1985; 151:207–11.
26. Slutsky JN and Callahan D. Endometriosis of the ureter can present as renal failure: a case report and review of endometriosis affecting the ureters. J Urol 1983; 130:336–7.

27. Weinrauch LA, Desautels RE, Christlieb AR, Kaldany A and D'Elia JA. Amyloid deposition in serosal membranes. Arch Intern Med 1984; 144:630–2.

28. Rao KV, Kjellsen D and Wolseth D. Renal failure due to bilateral obstructive amyloidosis of the urinary tract. Arch Pathol Lab Med 1979; 103:540–2.

29. Neal DE. Complications of ileal conduit diversion in adults with cancer followed up for at least five years. BMJ 1985; 290:1695–7.

30. Kolko A, Kiselman R, Russ G, Bacques O and Kleinknecht D. Acute renal failure due to bilateral ureteral hematomas complicating anticoagulant therapy. Nephron 1993; 65:165–6.

31. Kahan M, Goldberg PD and Mandel EE. Neurogenic vesical dysfunction and diabetes mellitus. NY State J Med 1970; 70:2448–55.

32. Michaelson RA, Benson GS and Friedman HM. Urinary retention as the presenting symptom of acquired cytomegalovirus infection. Am J Med 1983; 74:526–8.

33. Oates JK and Greenhouse PRDH. Retention of urine in anogenital herpetic infection. Lancet 1978; 1:691.

34. Dees A, Kluchert SA and van Vliet AC. Pseudo-renal failure associated with internal leakage of urine. Neth J Med 1990; 37:197–201.

35. Meulders Q, Michel C, Marteau P, Grange JD, Mougenot B, Ronco P et al. Association of chronic interstitial cystitis, protein-losing enteropathy and paralytic ileus with seronegative systemic lupus erythematosus: case report and review of the literature. Clin Nephrol 1992; 37:239–44.

36. Espinal CH and Gregory AW. Differential diagnosis of acute renal failure. Clin Nephrol 1980; 13:73–7.

37. Miller TR, Anderson RJ, Linas SL, Henrich WL, Berns AS, Gabow PA et al. Urinary diagnostic indices in acute renal failure. Ann Intern Med 1978; 89:47–50.

38. Hoffman LM and Suki WN. Obstructive uropathy mimicking volume depletion. JAMA 1976; 236:2096–7.

39. Marshall S. Urea-creatinine ratio in obstructive uropathy and renal hypertension. JAMA 1964; 190:719–20.

40. Morgan DB, Ball SR, Thomas TH and Lee MR. Sodium losing renal disease: two cases and a review of the literature. Quart J Med 1978; 47:21–34.

41. Batlle DC, Arruda JAL and Kurtzman NA. Hyperkalemic distal renal tubular acidosis associated with obstructive uropathy. N Engl J Med 1981; 304:373–80.

42. Bishop MC. Diuresis and renal functional recovery in chronic retention. Br J Urol 1985; 57: 1–5.

43. Kamholtz RG, Cronan JJ and Dorfman GS. Ultrasound, obstruction, and the minimally dilated collecting system. Radiology 1989; 170:51–3.

44. Cronan JJ. Contemporary concepts for imaging urinary tract obstruction. Urol Radiol 1992; 14:8–12.

45. Spital A, Valvo JR and Segal AJ. Nondilated obstructive uropathy. Urology 1988; 31:478–82.

46. WW Ritchie, CW Vick, SK Glocheski and Cook DE. Evaluation of azotemic patients: diagnostic yield of initial US examination. Radiology 1988; 167:245–7.

47. Platt JF, Rubin JM and Ellis JH. Acute renal obstruction: evaluation with intrarenal duplex doppler and conventional US. Radiology 1993; 186:685–8.

48. Haddad MC, Sharif HS, Shahed MS, Mutaiery MA, Samihan AM, Sammak BM et al. Renal colic: diagnosis and outcome. Radiology 1992; 184:83–8.

49. Hamilton DV, Kelly MB and Pryor JS. Polyhydramnios and acute renal failure. Postgrad Med J 1980; 56:798–9.

50. Muller-Suur R and Tyden O. Evaluation of hydronephrosis in pregnancy using ultrasound and renography. Scand J Urol Nephrol 1985; 19:267–73.

51. Peake SL, Roxburgh HB and Langlois S Le P. Ultrasonic assessment of hydronephrosis of pregnancy. Radiology 1983; 146:167–70.

52. Cietak KA and Newton JR. Serial qualitative maternal nephrosonography in pregnancy. Brit J Radiol 1985; 58:399–404.

53. Kass EJ and Fink-Bennett D. Contemporary techniques for the radioisotopic evaluation of the dilated urinary tract. Urol Clin N Amer 1990; 17:273–89.

54. Witherow RO'N and Whitaker RH. The predictive accuracy of antegrade pressure flow studies in equivocal upper tract obstruction. Br J Urol 1981; 53:496–9.

55. Poulsen EU, Frokjaer J, Taagehoj-Jensen F, Jorgensen TM, Norgaard JP, Hedegaard M et al. Diuresis renography and simultaneous renal pelvic pressure in hydronephrosis. J Urol 1987; 138:272–5.

56. Djurhuus JC, Sorensen SS, Jorgensen TM and Taagehoj-Jensen F. Predictive value of pressure flow studies for the functional outcome of reconstructive surgery for hydronephrosis. Br J Urol 1985; 57:6–9.

57. Kass EJ and Majd M. Evaluation and management of upper urinary tract obstruction in infancy and childhood. Urol Clin North Amer 1985; 12:133–41.

10. Vascular causes of renal failure

J. GARY ABUELO

DEFINITION AND CAUSES

Vascular causes of renal failure are listed on Table 10.1 and break down into three categories: *Vasomotor disturbances* refer to changes in glomerular arteriolar tone that reduce glomerular capillary pressure and as a result decrease glomerular filtration. These are functional rather than structural disorders, since the fall in renal perfusion that usually occurs is not enough to cause ischemic injury to renal tissue. *Small vessel involvement* consists of the blockage of small arteries and arterioles by cholesterol crystals, thrombi or pathological processes in the vessel wall. *Large vessel involvement* comprises the occlusion of the renal arteries and their main branches by a variety of conditions. Main renal artery lesions are included here although they do not involve intrinsic renal structures.

Table 10.1. Vascular causes of renal failure

Vasomotor disturbances
    Hepatorenal syndrome
    Hypercalcemia
    Sepsis
    Drugs and contrast media
Small vessel involvement
    Atheroembolic disease
    Scleroderma
    Malignant hypertension
    Hemolytic uremic syndrome
    Thrombotic thrombocytopenic purpura
    Acute cortical necrosis
    Benign arteriolar nephrosclerosis
    Radiation nephritis
Large vessel involvement
    Renal artery stenosis
    Renal infarction

INCIDENCE

Adults

Vascular disorders are responsible for about 5% of renal failure due to intrinsic renal disease (Chapter 2, Table 2.2). Vasomotor disturbances caused, for example, by angiotensin-converting-enzyme (ACE) inhibitors, are the most common type of vascular renal failure [1]. Of the conditions affecting small vessels, (benign arteriolar) nephrosclerosis from chronic hypertension and atheroembolic renal disease occur most frequently. Despite widespread atherosclerosis in the elderly, renal failure due to large vessel involvement is rarely observed. Both renal arteries are generally not completely blocked, and segmental, unilateral or partial occlusion usually allows enough perfusion to prevent azotemia. Also, few patients with severe enough bilateral renal artery stenosis to produce azotemia undergo the arteriography needed for diagnosis because of their frail state of health or of failure to consider the diagnosis. Thus, few of the cases that do occur are diagnosed.

Pediatric age group

With the exception of transient azotemia in infants treated with indomethacin for patent ductus arteriosus, renal failure due to vasomotor disturbance is rare in children and adolescents. In contrast, hemolytic uremic syndrome, which affects small vessels, is responsible for 25% or more of cases of acute renal failure [2–5], and renal vein thrombosis is a common cause of renal failure in infants [2, 3, 6, 7].

65

VASOMOTOR DISTURBANCES

Causes
Table 10.2 lists the vasomotor etiologies of renal failure, the most common of which are drugs and contrast media.

Definition and pathophysiology
Vasomotor disturbances impair GFR by reducing glomerular capillary pressure either through constriction of the afferent glomerular arterioles or through dilation of the efferent glomerular arterioles. The fall in renal perfusion produced by afferent arteriolar constriction is not enough to cause anoxic cell damage. Thus, renal failure of vasomotor origin is rapidly reversible if the cause is removed.

> *Afferent Glomerular Arteriolar Constriction.* Hepatorenal syndrome, hypercalcemia, sepsis and drugs such as cyclosporine A increase afferent arteriolar resistance and, thus, can interfere with the transmission of arterial pressure to the glomerular capillaries. In states of low cardiac output or low blood pressure, this may also occur with nonsteroidal anti-inflammatory drugs (NSAIDs). Ordinarily, in these low perfusion states, prostaglandins maintain glomerular capillary pressure and blood flow by dilating the afferent arterioles (Figure 10.1B). NSAIDs interfere with this homeostatic mechanism by decreasing prostaglandin production; as a result, afferent arterioles do not dilate and glomerular capillary pressure is inadequate to sustain normal GFR (Figure 10.1C).
>
> > *Efferent Glomerular Arteriolar Dilation.* Low perfusion states also stimulate the renin-angiotensin system. Angiotensin II constricts the efferent arteriole and, thereby, works together with prostaglandins to support glomerular capillary pressure (Figure 10.1B). ACE inhibitors block

Table 10.2. Vasomotor disturbances that cause renal failure

Hepatorenal syndrome [8]
Hypercalcemia [9]
Sepsis [10–12]
Drugs and contrast media
   Nonsteroidal anti-inflammatory drugs
   ACE inhibitors [13, 14]
   Nifedipine (rare) [15–17]
   Cyclosporine A [18–20]
   Contrast media [21–27]
      Diatrizoate (IVP, CT scan, angiography)
      Iothalamate (IVP, CT scan, angiography)
      Iopanoic acid (oral cholecystography)
      Low osmolarity agents (angiography)

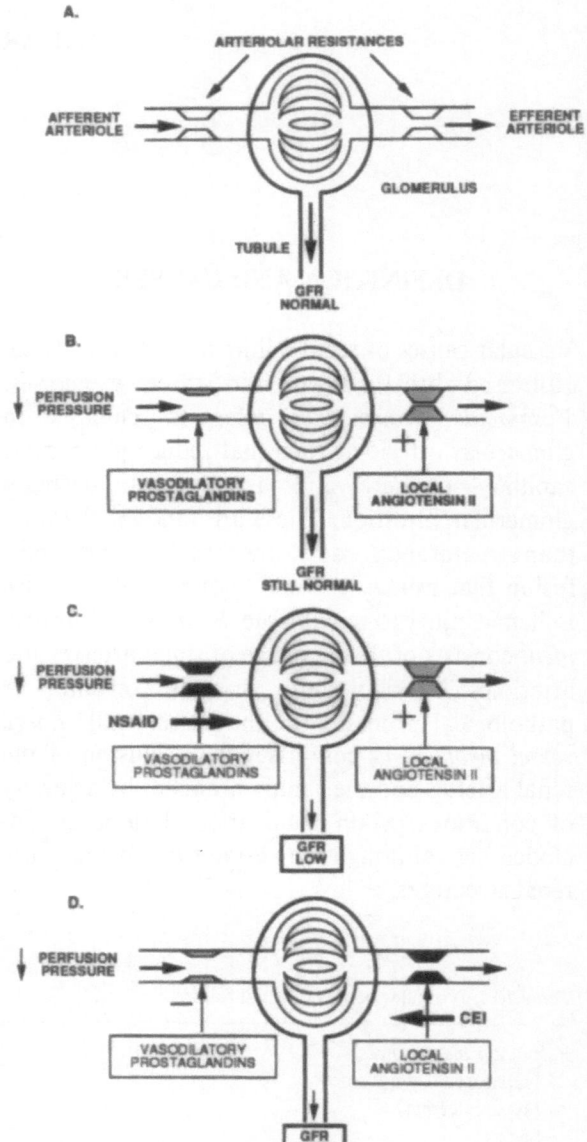

Fig. 10.1. Simplified diagram of intrarenal mechanisms for GFR autoregulation under reduced perfusion pressure, and GFR reduction by drugs. + = vasoconstriction, − = vasodilatation. (A) Normal conditions. (B) Perfusion pressure reduced within autoregulatory range. Normal glomerular capillary pressure is maintained by afferent vasodilation and efferent vasoconstriction. (C) Reduced perfusion + NSAID. Loss of vasodilatory prostaglandins increases afferent resistance. This causes glomerular capillary pressure to drop below normal and GFR to fall. (D) Reduced perfusion + angiotensin converting enzyme inhibitor (CEI). Loss of angiotensin II reduces efferent resistance. This causes glomerular capillary pressure to drop below normal and GFR to fall.

angiotensin II production, and the resulting fall in efferent arteriolar resistance reduces glomerular filtration pressure to subnormal levels (Figure 10.1D).

The mechanism of impairment of GFR with nifedipine and the various contrast agents is suspected to be vasomotor, but is not known with certainty.

Contributory factors (Figure 10.2). In most cases vasomotor disturbances reduce renal perfusion in concert with other factors that also tend to compromise circulation to the kidney. For example, NSAIDs [28–31], ACE inhibitors [13, 32, 33], contrast media [34], and hepatorenal syndrome [35–37] often produce azotemia in conjunction with renal hypoperfusion due to volume depletion or heart failure. Also, the hepatorenal syndrome, sepsis and hypercalcemia themselves usually reduce arterial blood pressure or cardiac output. Patients within hepatorenal syndrome [8, 36, 38] and sepsis [39] have a low systemic vascular resistance, while hypercalcemia induces renal salt wasting and, thereby, volume depletion. As another example of this synergy, ACE inhibitors sometimes precipitate renal failure in patients with renal artery stenosis of a solitary kidney or of both kidneys [14].

If a patient already has chronic renal insufficiency, NSAIDs [40], ACE inhibitors [33, 41, 42], contrast media and nifedipine [15, 17] are more likely to cause a reversible deterioration of renal function.

Finally, two simultaneous vasomotor disturbances in the same patient can increase the risk of renal failure. This is observed when cyclosporine A is used in conjunction with an ACE inhibitor [43] or with NSAIDs [44–46] or when patients with liver failure are septic [35, 37] or treated with NSAIDs [47].

Clinical Picture

History. Renal failure from a vasomotor disturbance occurs in various settings: severe hepatic failure, hypercalcemia, sepsis, or use of one of the agents listed in Table 10.2. The Scr usually rises within a day or so of exposure to contrast media or a vasoactive drug. Vasomotor disturbances may sometimes operate alone to cause renal failure. However, as detailed above, an acute fall in GFR is usually seen in the presence of chronic renal failure or of factors that additionally reduce renal blood flow. Such factors may be a second vasomotor disturbance or something that decreases perfusion pressure or cardiac output, such as diuretics or heart failure. Probably the best known example of this is the renal failure caused by a combination of ACE inhibitors with sodium depletion [32], congestive heart failure [13, 33] or renal artery stenosis, either bilateral or in a solitary kidney [48]. This and other reported combinations are illustrated in Figure 10.2.

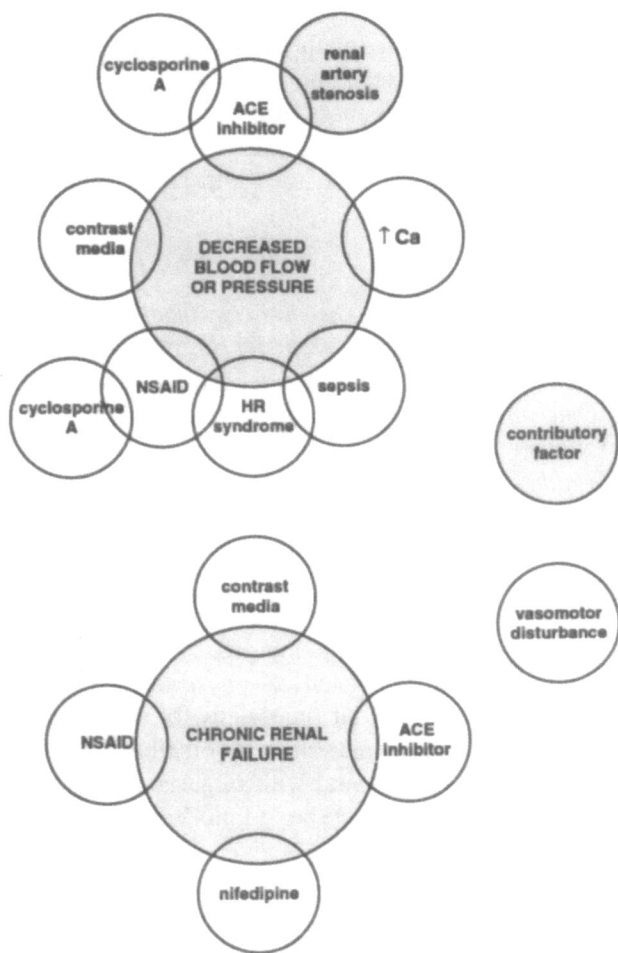

Fig. 10.2. Contributory factors and synergism in the production of renal failure by vasomotor disturbances. Schematic shows how the contributory factors like decreased blood pressure interact with the vasomotor disturbances and how certain vasomotor disturbances interact with each other. HR – hepatorenal.

Urine Tests (Figure 10.3). Vasomotor disturbances often produce renal salt avidity and urine with low sodium and chloride content (urine concentrations < 20 mEq/L; fractional excretions < 1%) [20, 31, 49–52]. In fact, it is rare to see hepatorenal syndrome in the absence of low urine salt content. Hypercalcemia is an exception because it results in renal salt-wasting [9, 53]. Also, patients with sepsis or hepatorenal syndrome tend to have a concentrated urine with a specific gravity greater than 1.015 in response to reduced effective blood volume [54–56]. However, after several days of sepsis or hepatorenal syndrome [54] renal ischemia may induce acute tubular necrosis, which blunts renal concentrating ability and salt avidity. Vasomotor disturbances do not usually cause hematuria or proteinuria, since they do not produce tissue damage and the glomerular capillary wall remains intact.

Diagnosis

General Comments. *The physician should suspect a vasomotor disturbance from the history of one or more causative factors and the characteristic urine concentration and salt content (Figure 10.3). The etiology is usually confirmed if the kidneys recover within a few days after eliminating the presumed underlying cause.*

Clinical Example. A 53-year-old woman with diabetes mellitus, gout and compensated congestive heart failure is taking digoxin, furosemide, glyburide and colchicine. A physician starts indomethacin 25 mg four times daily for acute gout. Two weeks later, while still on indomethacin, she is admitted to the hospital with oliguria and an exacerbation of congestive heart failure. Scr has risen

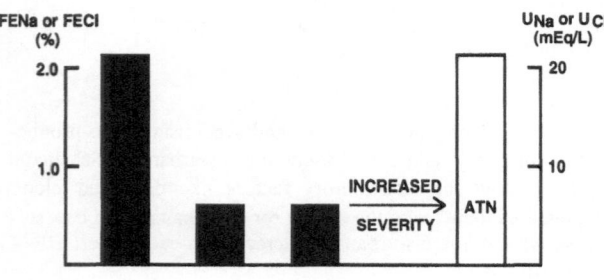

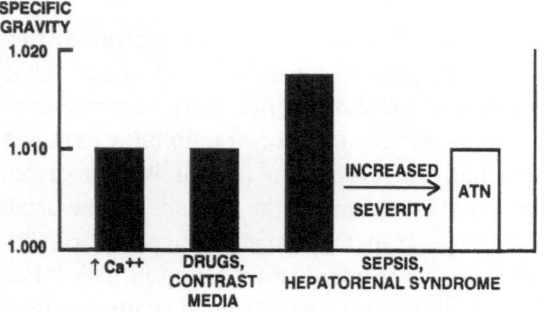

Fig. 10.3. Typical urine salt content and specific gravity seen in the vasomotor disturbances that cause renal failure. ↑ Ca++ – hypercalcemia.

from a baseline of 1.3 to 3.1 mg/dl (115 to 274 μmol/L), and the BUN from 21 to 50 mg/dl (7.5 to 17.6 μmol/L). Urine shows specific gravity 1.016, trace protein, negative sediment and U_{Na} 16 mEq/L. Suspecting that the NSAID produced vasomotor-type renal failure in the setting of poor cardiac function, the physician stops the indomethacin. Within a day there is a fall in Scr to 2.5 mg/dL (239 μmol/L) and a dramatic diuresis. Six days later, Scr and BUN return to baseline.

Some Specific Conditions-Hepatorenal Syndrome. Severe liver disease impairs renal function in this syndrome through poorly understood humoral and neural mechanisms, which vasodilate the systemic circulation and vasoconstrict the renal circulation. Despite a compensatory rise in cardiac output, blood pressure tends to fall, which contributes to poor renal perfusion [35, 37, 38].

The liver disease is generally alcoholic cirrhosis, but may involve other types of *chronic* liver disease [54, 58]. Severe acute hepatitis or other causes of fulminant *acute* liver failure can also produce hepatorenal syndrome [35, 54, 58]. Blood pressure is low normal and urine output is 500 to 1000 cc/day or less [37, 56, 57, 59]. Volume loss in the hospital due to therapeutic paracentesis, laxatives, bleeding or aggressive diuretic therapy often precedes the rise in Scr [37, 56, 57]. Renal function gradually worsens over several days to many weeks.

The diagnosis of this syndrome is based on low urine sodium or chloride content and the presence of a typical picture of chronic liver failure, portal hypertension, tense ascites, cachexia, jaundice and usually encephalopathy [37, 57, 58]. If the clinical picture suggests prerenal azotemia as an alternative or additional diagnosis, placement of a Swan-Ganz catheter (Figure 10.4) or a trial of fluid repletion is indicated. Prerenal azotemia would be suggested by typical hemodynamic readings of volume depletion and by prompt resolution with fluid repletion. In contrast, hepatorenal syndrome shows reduced systemic vascular resistance and increased cardiac output. Volume expansion produces either no effect or a slight transient improvement in urine output or renal function [36, 60].

Pitfalls. Such a seemingly favorable response in hepatorenal syndrome often kindles false hope that the patient has prerenal azotemia. Thus, patients may receive five to ten

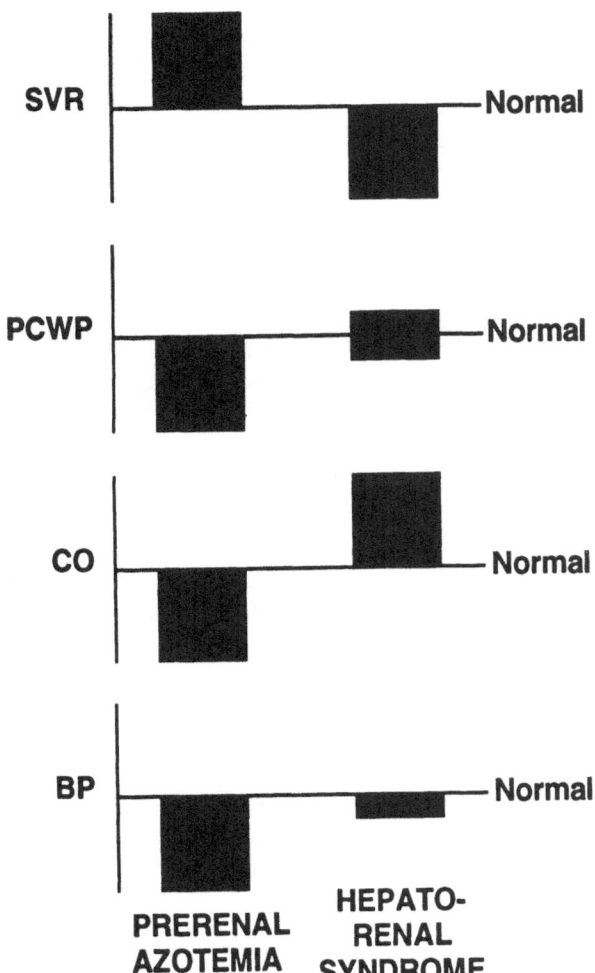

Fig. 10.4. Hemodynamic measurements in prerenal azotemia and hepatorenal syndrome. SVR – systemic vascular resistance, PCWP – pulmonary capillary wedge pressure, CO – cardiac output, BP – blood pressure.

liters of fluid and develop anasarca before it is clear that GFR has not improved significantly.

To be distinguished from hepatorenal syndrome are conditions, such as acetaminophen overdose [61], which damage both liver and kidney [35] and cases of cirrhosis complicated by urinary obstruction, acute tubular necrosis or rarely glomerulonephritis [62]. The urine findings or clinical picture usually differentiate these states from hepatorenal syndrome. Renal sonography will identify hydronephrosis.

Some Specific Conditions-Contrast Media (See Section on Intravenous Pyelogram, Chapter 6). The typical patient with a nephrotoxic reaction to contrast media has underlying renal insufficiency, is older than 40 years, receives a contrast agent during an IVP, angiography or computed tomography

and manifests acute renal insufficiency with or without oliguria within 24 hours of the procedure [22, 63–68]. Diabetes mellitus [65, 66, 69–71] and low cardiac output [34] increase the risk. Conventional high osmolality contrast media are likely more nephrotoxic than newer low osmolality contrast media [27, 72]. Oliguria, if present, usually lasts two to five days [22, 63, 66, 67] (Figure 10.5). Urine salt content is often, but not always low [51].

The diagnosis is based on the presence of risk factors, particularly chronic renal failure, and on a Scr rising within a day of the procedure and peaking within three to five days, followed by return to baseline by two to three weeks [22, 64–67]. In atypical cases, the patient may be young or have a normal baseline Scr [22, 63–69] or the renal failure may only start to improve after five to ten days or be irreversible [22, 66].

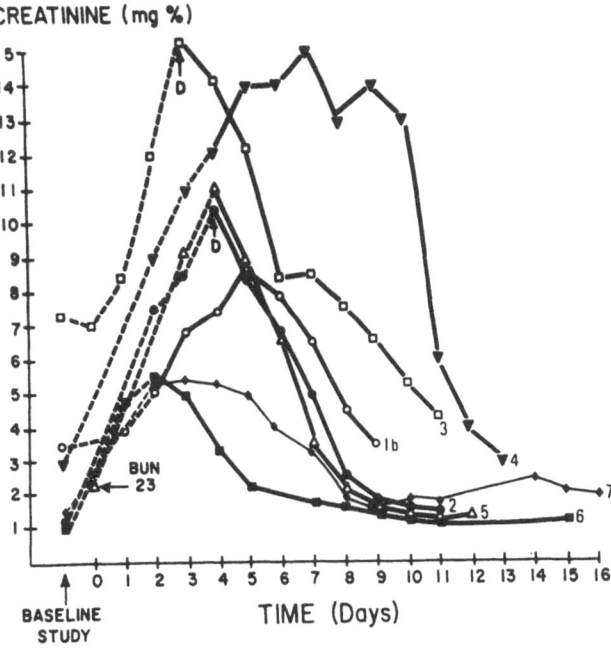

Fig. 10.5. Rise and fall in serum creatinine levels after use of contrast media in seven cases of contrast mediated renal failure (Alexander RD et al., Arch Intern Med 1978; 138:381-4). Oliguria phase of each patient's course is represented by dashed line. D indicates initiation of peritoneal dialysis. Only second episode of renal failure in patient 1 is represented.

SMALL VESSEL DISEASE

Causes

Table 10.3 lists the small arterial and arteriolar diseases that impair renal function. The most common of these, *benign arteriolar nephrosclerosis*, is a result of essential hypertension and produces chronic renal failure. The rarest of the conditions, *radiation nephritis*, produces acute or chronic renal failure. Fortunately, it has become uncommon thanks to modern radiotherapeutic methods.

Atheroembolic Renal Disease

Definition

This condition involves embolization of cholesterol crystals from eroded atherosclerotic plaques to small renal arteries (Figure 10.6).

Clinical picture

The typical patient is a white hypertensive male smoker over 60 years of age with underlying cerebral, coronary, aortic or peripheral vascular disease [73–75]. The emboli may be spontaneous, but usually follow one day to three weeks after arterial manipulation such as angiography or aortic surgery [74–78]. Anticoagulant or thrombolytic therapy probably increases the risk [79–80]. Systemic cholesterol crystal embolization may cause transient cerebral ischemic attacks, retinal ischemia, pancreatitis, ischemic colitis, polyneuritis, claudication, and muscle pain of the legs. However, the most common symptom is painful ischemic changes in the feet, e.g. livedo reticularis and purple, blue or gangrenous toes (Figure 10.7)

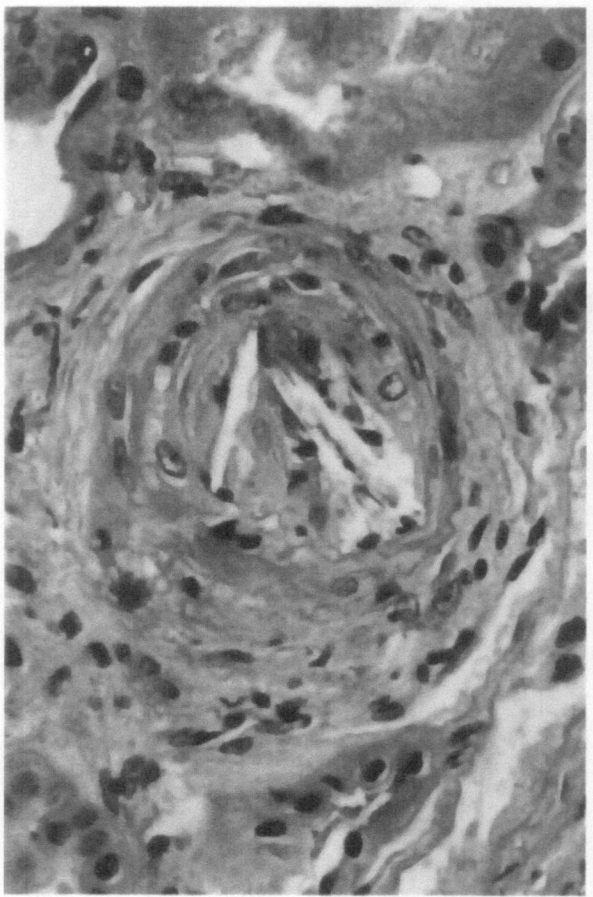

Fig. 10.6. Light micrograph of a renal biopsy from a patient with atheroembolic renal disease. A small artery is occluded by intimal thickening and fibrosis around cholesterol clefts. These are elongated spaces remaining after cholesterol crystals were dissolved during preparation of the specimen. (Courtesy of Dr. Alfredo Exparza.)

[74, 75, 77, 79, 81–84]. Despite these findings, the distal arterial pulses are often preserved [74]. The morbidity tends to be high, since the typical patient has diffuse atherosclerosis that may result in strokes, myocardial infarctions, amputations, and general debility [74, 75].

Flank or back pain may herald renal involvement [75]. Renal cholesterol emboli typically produce episodic or sustained hypertension [74, 75, 85, 86]. The Scr rises over weeks to months probably due to continuing embolization of crystals. Azotemia usually proceeds to end stage renal disease, but partial recovery can also be seen [77, 81, 85, 87]. The urine can be normal or can show microhematuria, gross hematuria [75], red cell casts

Table 10.3. Small vessel diseases that cause renal failure

Atheroembolic renal disease
Scleroderma
Malignant hypertension
Hemolytic uremic syndrome
    Childhood (classic) type
    Postpartum period
    Mitomycin C
    Other types
Thrombotic thrombocytopenic purpura
Acute cortical necrosis
Benign arteriolar nephrosclerosis
radiation nephritis

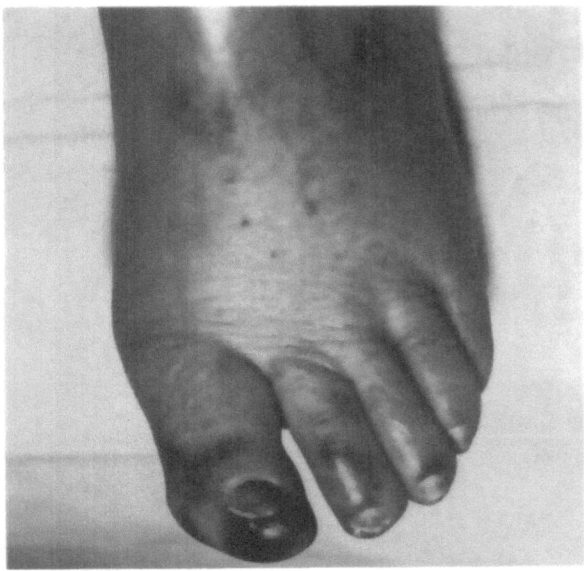

Fig. 10.7. Foot of patient with atheroembolic renal disease showing black tip of big toe and other ischemic skin changes.

[86], proteinuria below or within the nephrotic range [87–89], white cells with scant [90] to predominant eosinophils [91], or salt avidity [91]. Elevated erythrocyte sedimentation rate and eosinophilia with or without leukocytosis are common [75, 78, 85, 92].

Rare patients may have fever, malaise, weight loss and other constitutional symptoms [74]. Infarction of the bowel, spleen, adrenals or spinal cord are rare complications of atheroemboli [75]. Moderate reduction in platelet count, C3 and C4 occurs occasionally [86, 92]. Very high plasma renin levels have been observed [77]. High serum amylase levels due to pancreatitis, high creatine phosphokinase and aminotransferase values due to muscle and liver involvement, and frank or occult blood in the stool due to gastrointestinal embolization can be seen [74, 75, 93].

Diagnosis

A kidney biopsy showing intraarterial cholesterol crystal clefts confirms the diagnosis, but skin, muscle or bone marrow biopsies with intravascular clefts are also satisfactory for demonstrating cholesterol emboli and are less invasive [83]. In typical cases of atheroembolic renal disease with diffuse atherosclerotic vascular disease, eosinophilia and ischemic changes of the feet, a clinical diagnosis is acceptable without histologic confirmation.

Pitfalls. Atheroembolic renal disease in hypertensive patients without eosinophilia or ischemic changes of the feet may be misdiagnosed as benign arteriolar nephrosclerosis (if the rise in Scr is slow), as a primary glomerulopathy (if there is hematuria and proteinuria), or even as malignant hypertension (if the hypertension is severe). Physicians may also be misled by constitutional symptoms, multisystem involvement (kidney, skin, bowel and brain), high sedimentation rate, eosinophilia and low complement level and may erroneously diagnose vasculitis [91, 84]. In these situations, a renal biopsy will show the atheroemboli. Finally, collagen vascular and other diseases sometimes produce ischemic changes in the feet indistinguishable from those of atheroemboli [94].

Renal Scleroderma

Definition

Scleroderma or systemic sclerosis is an uncommon connective tissue disease characterized by Raynaud's phenomenon, and fibrosis and small vessel narrowing of the gastrointestinal tract, lungs, heart and especially the skin [95]. Most patients with scleroderma have characteristic lesions of small renal vessels (Figure 10.8) [96]. While this usually remains clinically inapparent, it can lead to acute renal failure in some patients.

Clinical picture

This complication, known as *scleroderma renal crisis*, is much more common in *diffuse* scleroderma than in limited scleroderma. It can affect either sex and be seen any time after early childhood; however, it typically occurs in women between the ages of 30 and 60 years one to seven years after the onset of scleroderma [97–99]. Renal involvement progresses rapidly to oliguric renal failure and is usually accompanied by abrupt onset or worsening of hypertension, grade 3 or 4 hypertensive retinopathy, high plasma renin activity, and microangiopathic anemia [97, 98, 100]. Hypertensive encephalopathy and heart failure are common [101]. The urine sediment is often benign [97, 101, 102], and proteinuria, if any, is moderate [97, 98]. Thrombocytopenia is common [103].

These patients also have typical laboratory findings of scleroderma. Antinuclear antibodies are almost always present and give a speckled or nucleolar pattern with immunofluorescent staining [104, 105]. Anticentromere, antinucleolar and anti-Scl-70 antibodies are each found in about 25% of

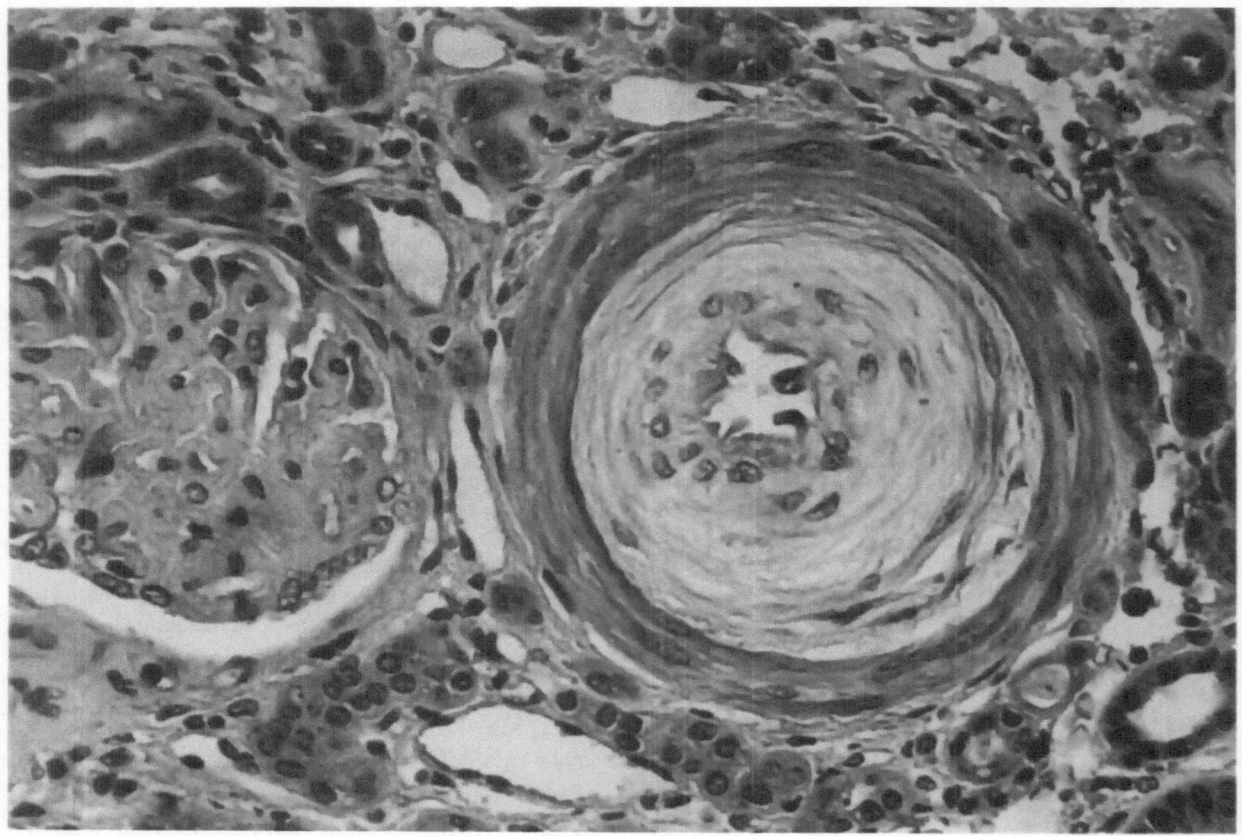

Fig. 10.8. Light micrograph of a renal biopsy from a patient with scleroderma renal crisis. An arteriole shows marked narrowing of the lumen due to subendothelial mucoid intimal proliferation. (Courtesy of Dr. Alfredo Esparza.)

patients with systemic sclerosis. These antibodies are relatively specific [105, 106] and are of diagnostic value if present. Nailfold capillaroscopy, using an ophthalmoscope at the bedside to look for capillary loss and enlargement, is both sensitive and specific in identifying patients with scleroderma [106].

Diagnosis

Scleroderma renal crisis is usually assumed to be the cause of renal failure in patients with scleroderma who develop sudden, severe hypertension and a rise in Scr. High renin activity and microangiopathic anemia support the diagnosis. The clinical picture is usually so typical that verification of the etiology with a renal biopsy is not indicated.

> *Pitfalls.* The diagnosis may be missed or in question in those unusual cases with mild or no hypertension [98, 107] or with scleroderma "sine scleroderma", in which patients have all

the features of scleroderma including the renal crisis without manifesting skin changes [108–110]. A renal biopsy is necessary for diagnosing such atypical cases. Consultation by a rheumatologist is often helpful in confirming the presence of scleroderma.

Thrombocytopenia and microangiopathic hemolytic anemia may suggest hemolytic uremic syndrome or thrombotic thrombocytopenic purpura (see below). However, the presence of Raynaud's phenomenon and typical skin changes of scleroderma should lead one to suspect the correct diagnosis.

Malignant Hypertension

Definition

Very high blood pressure produces fibrinoid necrosis and intimal thickening of small arteries and arterioles throughout the body, although the kidney, retina and brain are clinically the most important target organs. The renal lesion is known as malignant arteriolar nephrosclerosis. In about a third of cases, the marked rise in arterial pressure is an exacerbation of *essential* hypertension; in other patients it is a complication of one of the many forms of *secondary* hypertension, principally glomerulonephritis, other renal diseases, or renovascular hypertension (Table 10.4) [111–113].

Clinical picture
The typical patient with renal failure due to malignant hypertension has diastolic blood pressure higher than 130 mmHg and a history of hypertension [111, 113, 114], although some patients have had normal blood pressures documented days or weeks before [115, 116]. Throbbing headaches and blurred vision associated with retinal hemorrhages, exudates or papilledema are initial complaints in most patients [111, 113, 117]. Other common features are congestive heart failure, generalized weakness, nausea, vomiting, recent weight loss, oliguria and encephalopathy [111, 113, 114, 116, 117]. The latter includes dizziness, disturbances of consciousness, seizures, paresthesias, and focal deficits due to transient ischemic attacks and cerebrovascular accidents [111, 118]. Pancreatitis, gastrointestinal bleeding and an acute abdomen due to bowel ischemia have also been reported [119]. The urinalysis usually shows mild to moderate proteinuria, and about one-third of cases have microscopic or gross hematuria [111]. Red cell casts and nephrotic range proteinuria may be seen [111, 115, 119]. Microangiopathic anemia is common and mild thrombocytopenia can occur [115, 116, 119, 120]. A high renin state may produce a hypokalemic metabolic alkalosis [119, 121]. With effective blood pressure control renal function often worsens for a week or two and then may partly or completely recover even in patients who initially require dialysis (Figure 10.9) [116, 117, 122]. Proteinuria and hematuria may disappear [111].

Table 10.4. Etiologic classification in 66 patients with secondary malignant hypertension [112]

Diagnosis	Number
Renal diseases	54 (82%)
Primary glomerular lesions	25
Membranous GN	
Mesangial proliferative GN	
Membranoproliferative GN	
Focal segmental GN	
IgA GN	
Chronic GN	
Secondary glomerular lesions	16
Scleroderma	
Systemic lupus erythematosus	
Polyarteritis	
Goodpasture's syndrome	
Wegener's granulomatosis	
Hemolytic uremic syndrome	
Thrombotic thrombocytopenic purpura	
Diabetic nephropathy	
Interstitial disease	13
Analgesic nephropathy	
Reflux nephropathy	
Obstructive uropathy	
Polycystic kidney disease	
Familial interstitial nephropathy	
Renovascular disease	11 (17%)
Primary aldosteronism	1 (1%)

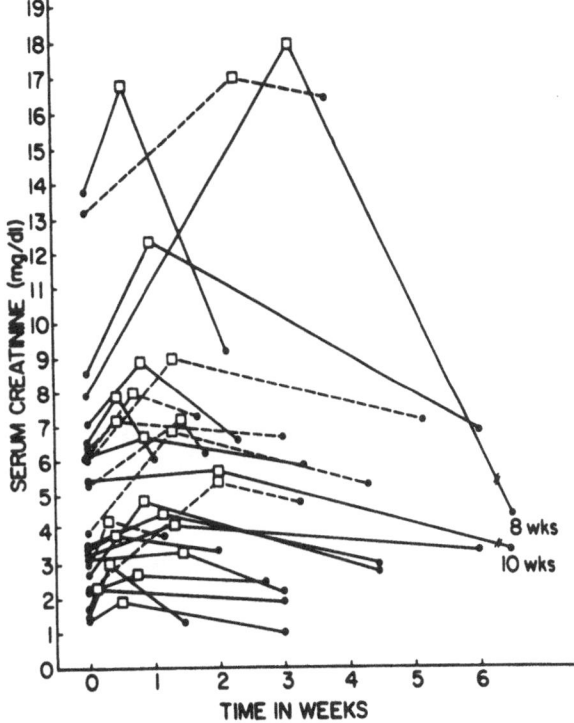

Fig. 10.9. Time course of serum creatinine in 24 patients with malignant hypertension in whom serum creatinine peaked and improved on antihypertensive therapy [117]. Patients with serum creatinine at discharge ---- equal to or less than admission serum creatinine, —— worse than admission serum creatinine, □ peak serum creatinine.

Diagnosis
The diagnosis of renal failure due to malignant hypertension is usually based on the presence of a typical clinical picture and a rise and subsequent fall in Scr with antihypertensive treatment. If renal function does not recover with lowering of the blood pressure or if certain features of the case do not fit with the diagnosis, a renal biopsy should be considered to identify a treatable renal lesion [112]. Renal arteriography or a screening test to detect renal artery stenosis (see below), and biochemical studies for primary aldosteronism and pheochromocytoma may also be indicated. Black patients generally have essential malignant hypertension, and evaluations for secondary hypertension may not be indicated as often [114, 123].

> *Pitfalls.* The diagnosis of malignant hypertension may be missed in patients without grade 3 or 4 hypertensive retinal changes [124–126] or without diastolic blood pressure above 130 mmHg. Renal failure may rarely be associated with diastolic blood pressure as low as 100 to 110 mmHg [112].

Hemolytic Uremic Syndrome

Definition
This syndrome consists clinically of microangiopathic hemolytic anemia, thrombocytopenia and acute renal failure, and histologically of glomerular and arterial thrombotic microangiopathy (Figure 10.10) [127–130].

Multiple causes
The variety of conditions that give rise to the hemolytic-uremic syndrome suggest that it is the common final pathway of several disease processes [128, 129]. The syndrome classically occurs in infants and preschool children usually after two days to two weeks of gastroenteritis often with abdominal pain and bloody stools [127, 128, 130–135]. Shiga-like toxin producing *E. coli*, especially serotype 0157 : H7, *Shigella dysenteriae* or other enteric pathogens may be found [131, 135–139]. Alternatively, the child may have a prodromal upper respiratory infection [127, 128].

The hemolytic uremic syndrome in adults is rare and is more heterogeneous than in children. It is seen most commonly one day [140] to six months [141–143] postpartum, and in malignancy treated with mitomycin C or other agents [144–147] or rarely untreated [148–150].

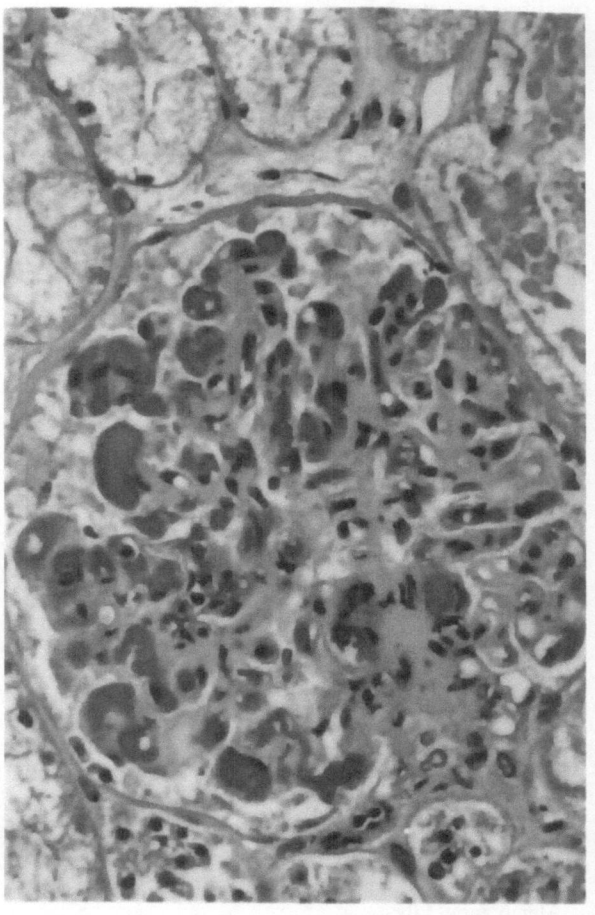

Fig. 10.10. Light micrograph of a renal biopsy from a patient with hemolytic uremic syndrome. The arteriole and the glomerular capillaries are narrowed by subendothelial deposition of fibrin. The arteriole and some glomerular capillaries also are occluded by fibrin thrombi. (Courtesy of Dr. Alfredo Esparza.)

> Adult hemolytic-uremic syndrome also occurs with oral contraceptives [151], conjugated estrogens [152], bacterial gastroenteritis [136, 139, 153–155], snakebite [156], glomerular disease [157], quinine [158, 159], cyclosporine A [160, 161], bone marrow, kidney, liver and lung transplantation [161–166], human immunodeficiency virus infection [167, 168] or in the absence of associated illness [169]. Familial, genetic and recurrent variants of hemolytic uremic syndrome have been described [128, 170–173].

Clinical picture
The typical patient has one of the predisposing factors or illnesses, and can present with a variety of manifestations. These include weakness, pallor, and jaundice due to hemolytic anemia, bleeding manifestations due to thrombocytopenia, gross

hematuria, oligoanuria and edema due to renal involvement, or fever [127, 128, 134, 169, 174]. Hypertension is common and can be malignant, especially in adults [134, 169, 175, 176]. Involvement of other organs can be part of the picture. Irritability, lethargy, confusion, convulsions or coma may occur unexplained by the severity of azotemia, and may be due to cerebral thrombotic microangiopathy [130, 134, 174, 177–179]. Noncardiogenic pulmonary edema is described in the cancer chemotherapy variant [180]. Pulmonary insufficiency, myocardial involvement, and perforation, gangrene, ulceration and strictures of the colon are rare complications in children [127, 179]. Stool culture may reveal *E. coli* 0157 : H7 in children or adults with prodromal diarrhea. Hematuria and proteinuria [134], and red cell casts [133, 181] may be seen on urinalysis, and the nephrotic syndrome [175, 182] is present in some cases. In children, serum uric acid concentration may be surprisingly high for the level of azotemia [183]. Leukocytosis is common [134, 181] and low serum C3 and CH5O can occur [143, 184].

Diagnosis
The possibility of hemolytic uremic syndrome in an azotemic patient should be suggested by certain settings, (e.g. postpartum period or mitomycin C treatment), by a prodrome with diarrhea, and especially by the hallmarks of the syndrome, thrombocytopenia and hemolytic anemia with schistocytes on smear. Usually this microangiopathic picture together with other typical features allow the physician to make a presumptive diagnosis without having to perform a renal biopsy.

Pitfalls. The diagnosis of hemolytic uremic syndrome may be missed if predisposing factors are absent or are not appreciated, if anemia, bleeding tendency or changes in consciousness are mistakenly ascribed to uremia, and, particularly, if thrombocytopenia or red cell fragments on the peripheral blood smear are overlooked. Rarely, thrombocytopenia and red cell fragments are absent and the diagnosis must be made by renal biopsy [185, 186].

Preeclamptic women sometimes develop the HELLP syndrome, which is characterized by nausea, upper abdominal pain, *H*emolysis, *E*levated *L*iver enzymes, and *L*ow *P*latelet count. Renal failure can also occur and, together with the hematologic abnormalities, mimics hemolytic uremic syndrome [187–191]. The renal failure in HELLP syndrome often develops as late as one to five days postpartum, which overlaps the usual onset of postpartum

hemolytic uremic syndrome, which may start as soon as one or two days after delivery. The diagnosis of HELLP syndrome will usually be clear when Scr falls within one to three weeks after delivery [187].

Thrombotic Thrombocytopenic Purpura

Definition
This disorder is a rare syndrome of unknown etiology characterized by a pentad of thrombocytopenia, microangiopathic anemia, neurologic dysfunction, renal abnormalities and fever. Hyaline microthrombi, containing fibrin and platelet aggregates, can be found in capillaries and arterioles of most visceral organs. The degree of involvement varies, but the brain and kidneys are among the organs most severely affected [192].

Clinical picture (Table 10.5)
The disease affects individuals of any age and either sex, but is most common in women between 20 and 50 years of age [192–195]. Drugs, pregnancy, collagen vascular diseases and infections (e.g. *E. coli* 0157 : H2 [139], HIV [195, 196]) are reported as precipitating causes in rare cases [192]. The typical patient with thrombotic thrombocytopenic purpura has severe thrombocytopenia with purpura and other bleeding symptoms, marked hemolytic anemia with pallor, weakness and fatigue, and variable neurologic manifestations [192, 193, 197–201]. These manifestations may be diffuse with headache, dizziness, confusion, and seizures or focal with dysarthria, aphasia, paresis, and paresthesias. Neurologic abnormalities are initially transient, but as the illness progresses, they often

Table 10.5. Clinical and laboratory features in thrombotic thrombocytopenia purpura [192]

Feature	Frequency (%)
Thrombocytopenia	100
Fragmented red cells	98
Anemia	98
CNS abnormalities	85
Hematuria	76
Fever	59
Azotemia	45
Triad (anemia + bleeding + CNS abnormalities)	*74*
Pentad (triad + renal abnormalities + fever)	*40*

proceed to coma and death [192, 198]. Most patients have fever [192, 193, 197–201].

> Some cases may have visual problems, nausea, vomiting, abdominal pain, jaundice, hepatic or splenic enlargement, cardiac conductive disturbances, myalgias, arthralgias and pancreatitis [192, 198, 202, 203]. Hypertension is unusual [197].

About 80% of patients have urinary abnormalities with gross or microscopic hematuria and with proteinuria varying from trace to the nephrotic range [192, 193, 197, 204]. Red cell casts can be seen in some individuals [197]. Scr is elevated in about half of cases [192, 197, 199–201], but severe renal failure is unusual. The BUN concentration may be disproportionately increased by volume depletion or protein breakdown giving a high BUN to creatinine ratio [197, 200]. Leukocytosis is common [192, 198]. Finally, one sees the expected laboratory findings of microangiopathic hemolytic anemia, including fragmented and nucleated red cells on peripheral blood smear, decreased haptoglobin concentration, elevated reticulocytes, and high lactic dehydrogenase and unconjugated bilirubin levels. Coagulation studies are usually normal or slightly altered; however, clearly raised fibrin-split products are found in 25% of patients [192].

Diagnosis

The recognition of thrombotic thrombocytopenia purpura in a patient with renal failure rests on the unexplained neurologic abnormalities and the hematologic findings of red cell fragments and low platelet count. Tissue confirmation is usually not necessary, but may be desired in atypical cases. Biopsy of a petechial skin lesion, the bone marrow, gingiva or the kidney, if not contraindicated by thrombocytopenia, may reveal the typical hyaline microthrombi [192, 193, 198, 200, 201].

> *Pitfalls.* In some patients, thrombotic thrombocytopenic purpura cannot be distinguished from hemolytic uremic syndrome, since the two conditions overlap clinically [192, 197]. In fact, recent case reports describe thrombotic thrombocytopenic purpura in patients with hemorrhagic colitis due to *E. coli* [139, 205]. Severe neurologic involvement and minimal to no hypertension or renal insufficiency are characteristic of thrombotic thrombocytopenic purpura, while mild to absent neurological findings and moderate to severe hypertension and renal failure favor the hemolytic uremic syndrome. Also onset in the postpartum period, after mitomycin C, or in early childhood after a diarrheal pro-

drome suggests hemolytic uremic syndrome, in contrast to thrombotic thrombocytopenic purpura, in which prodromal conditions are rare. Some authorities believe that both disorders are varied presentations of one disease referred to as "thrombotic microangiopathy" [206].

The diagnosis of thrombotic thrombocytopenic purpura may be missed at initial presentation, when cardinal manifestations are mild or have not yet appeared. Hematologic studies may need to be repeated, since schistocytes, anemia and marked thrombocytopenia may take several days to appear [206]. Early on, weakness, headache, myalgias, leukocytosis and fever can suggest an infectious illness. Even later the physician may not consider the real diagnosis. Uremia or cerebrovascular disease may be thought responsible for the neurological changes, the renal findings can easily be mistaken for glomerulonephritis, and the anemia may be ascribed to uremia or active bleeding. The failure to order a differential count with examination of the peripheral blood smear and a platelet count or the failure of an inexperienced technician to recognize red cell fragmentation on the blood smear may further delay the diagnosis.

If fibrin-split products are elevated, the low platelet count, anemia and schistocytes may be erroneously ascribed to disseminated intravascular coagulation. The finding of a normal fibrinogen level and other normal coagulation studies will rule out this diagnosis. Also, the thrombocytopenia and hemolytic anemia may be misdiagnosed as autoantibody mediated due to systemic lupus erythematosus or Evans syndrome. A negative Coomb's test will exclude these conditions.

Acute (Bilateral or Renal) Cortical Necrosis

Definition

This rare cause of renal failure results from thrombosis of the interlobular arteries, afferent arterioles and glomerular capillaries [207–209] and may involve total or patchy cortical necrosis. The arcuate and capsular arteries are unaffected, sparing the medullary, juxtamedullary and subcapsular regions of the kidney. The pathogenesis is obscure, but predisposing factors are blood loss, infection, shock, hemolysis and intravascular coagulation [207, 209].

Cause

In the past the most common setting was pregnancy complicated in different cases by induced septic abortion, puerperal sepsis, prolonged intrauterine fetal death, toxemia, and abruptio placenta or other peripartum hemorrhage [207, 208, 210, 211]. Presently, improved obstetric care prevents most of these cases. Other settings for acute cortical necrosis are severe gastroenteritis, sepsis, snake bites, nonsteroidal anti-inflammatory drugs, poisons and hemolytic uremic syndrome [207–209, 212–214].

Clinical picture
The classic patient is a multiparous woman with abruptio placenta or concealed hemorrhage, who develops prolonged oliguria or total anuria [207–209]. In some countries, induced septic abortion is still a common setting [208]. Many patients have abdominal or flank pain [215], and either *hypotension* from sepsis or hemorrhage or *hypertension* from fluid overload [208, 209, 216]. Gross hematuria may be noted [215, 217]. The urinalysis usually shows microscopic hematuria, granular casts and up to 4+ protein [209, 214], but may be normal [218] or show red blood cell casts [217, 219].

Diagnosis
The physician should consider acute cortical necrosis when oligoanuria occurs in a patient with a complication of pregnancy or with other predisposing factors. Previously, the diagnosis might have been confirmed by renal biopsy or by selective renal angiography that showed reduced blood flow to the cortical vessels, mottled or absent cortical nephrogram and prominent filling of the capsular arteries [207, 216]. However, contrast enhanced computed tomography is now the preferred study since it can diagnose acute cortical necrosis with less risk to the patient than biopsy or arteriography [217, 220–222]. Since scattered or linear radiopaque cortical calcification may occasionally occur after four weeks, the diagnosis may also be confirmed with an abdominal Xray and tomography of the kidneys in some patients with prolonged renal failure [208, 216, 219].

> *Pitfalls.* The diagnosis may be missed in patients with hypotension or sepsis who are mistakenly assumed to have acute tubular necrosis. The failure to recover after two to four weeks should raise the possibility of cortical necrosis. Also, the hematuria and proteinuria may suggest an acute glomerulonephritic picture, but a renal biopsy should provide the correct diagnosis.

LARGE VESSEL INVOLVEMENT

Definition

Total or near total occlusion of the main renal arteries causes renal failure, most often in older patients [223], and can be chronic or acute in nature. The chronic process, *renal artery stenosis*, is more common. It produces slowly progressive renal ischemia, which first manifests as hypertension and then months or years later as renal insufficiency. Atherosclerotic narrowing of the renal arteries or their ostia is the usual cause of the stenosis.

The acute process is abrupt renal artery occlusion. This produces sudden *renal infarction*, which often manifests as abdominal or flank pain and acute renal failure. Embolism of thrombi from the heart to the kidneys is the most common cause of acute occlusion.

Both renal artery stenosis and abrupt renal artery occlusion with infarction are usually unilateral processes, in which Scr remains below 2.0 to 2.5 mg/dl thanks to the remaining healthy kidney [224, 225]. In fact, with compensatory hypertrophy of the contralateral kidney Scr may rise only slightly and stay within the normal range. In the occasional patient, in whom the contralateral kidney is absent or functions poorly due to an unrelated condition, unilateral renal artery stenosis or infarction is able to produce severe renal failure [224, 226–228]. In other patients, *bilateral* renal artery stenosis or infarction seriously impair GFR [224, 229, 230].

Renal Artery Stenosis

Causes
Renal artery stenosis usually occurs as part of generalized atherosclerosis (Table 10.6). Renal blood flow may be compromised either by aortic plaques encroaching on the ostia of the renal arteries or by atherosclerosis of the renal artery itself. Stenosis due to a rare possibly hereditary disorder, fibromuscular hyperplasia [236], can also impair renal function [227, 231–233]. Both etiologies of renal artery stenosis usually begin unilaterally, but can progress to involve both sides [232, 237].

Table 10.6. Conditions that cause renal failure through renal artery stenosis

---

Atherosclerosis
Fibromuscular hyperplasia [227, 231–233]
Takayasu's arteritis* [234]
Cyclosporine-induced macroangiopathy* [235]

---

* Isolated case reports only.

Pathophysiology. Renal artery stenosis reduces perfusion pressure to the kidney, which initially maintains renal blood flow by dilating afferent glomerular arterioles and by raising systemic blood pressure through the release of renin. With progression of the stenosis renal blood flow slows, and glomerular filtration and urine output from that kidney fall and may eventually stop [238–240]. One usually sees worsening hypertension, but little or no azotemia, thanks to compensatory hypertrophy of the unaffected contralateral kidney.

With time tubules in the affected kidney atrophy, the interstitium fibroses, arterioles thicken and the kidney gets smaller. However, if blood flow is sufficient, glomeruli may survive even at this stage and restoration of perfusion may lead to recovery of function and increase in renal size [238, 241, 242]. Thus, the affected kidney initially receives enough blood to remain viable although nonfunctional. Collateral arterial supply may occasionally maintain this state even with total renal artery occlusion. Usually, however, as the stenosis gets progressively tighter, it causes an irreversibly atrophic kidney with obliterated glomeruli, focal infarcts [241] and sometimes with multiple cysts [243]. Atheromatous emboli to the renal parenchyma may further impair renal function [86].

Clinical picture

The typical patient with renal failure caused by renal artery stenosis is a hypertensive white male smoker over 50 years of age [223, 224, 229, 244]. One third of cases are women [224, 244–246]; few are black [229, 245, 247, 248]. Many patients have had cerebral, coronary, aortic or lower extremity vascular disease [223–225, 228, 240]. Presentation with severe hypertension or acceleration of hypertension after a period of good control is a hallmark of renal artery stenosis [225, 249]. In the past, this severe hypertension was often refractory to treatment, but now drugs, such as minoxidil, calcium channel blockers and ACE inhibitors, often permit control of blood pressure [224, 229]. Recurrent acute pulmonary edema can be another characteristic manifestation [250, 251].

Typically, slowly worsening azotemia evolves with progression of the vascular disease months or years after onset of renovascular hypertension.

However, if the hypertension has gone undetected, the Scr may be elevated at presentation. If a solitary kidney is involved, severe stenosis or thrombosis of a narrowed main renal artery may result in oliguria [228, 239]. The urinalysis typically shows negative to 1+ protein and no hematuria [86, 228, 238]. However, in rare cases proteinuria may be heavy [86, 238, 242, 252]. Urine sodium concentration is sometimes low in bilateral renal artery stenosis [238]. When renal artery stenosis causes renal failure, the peripheral vein renin activity is usually high and levels over 10 ng angiotensin-I/ml/h are seen in half of the reported cases [225, 227, 238, 253–256]. High renin activity raises aldosterone secretion, which may cause hypokalemia. Patients often have either a decreased size of one kidney relative to the other or (rarely) two small kidneys [224, 254]. The IVP [229, 238] or renogram [257] may show a differential in renal function even if renal size is equal. Occasionally a functional difference between kidneys is seen only after administration of an ACE inhibitor [258].

Diagnosis

Whom to evaluate. *Renal failure due to renal artery stenosis should be suspected in every hypertensive patient who has any manifestation of atherosclerosis, especially an abdominal bruit (Table 10.7). Similarly, one might also consider renal artery stenosis in hypertensive patients with risk factors for atherosclerosis such as age over 50 years, cigarette smoking, diabetes mellitus, hyperlipidemia, etc. In addition, the possibility of renal artery stenosis is increased by hypokalemia, atrophy of one kidney or discrepancy in renal size on ultrasound or IVP,[1] and certain unusual aspects of the hypertension [248, 259, 260]. These include onset of hypertension after the age of 50 years, recent acceleration of longstanding controlled hypertension, severe hypertension, grade 3 or 4 hypertensive retinopathy, and a rise in Scr during treatment with antihypertensive drugs (especially an ACE inhibitor) [254].*

Absence of hypertension excludes renal artery stenosis as a cause of renal failure.

Angiography. *When the physician feels that the evidence points to renal artery stenosis, confirmation requires angiography showing tight (more than 70–75%) stenosis [237, 249].[2] Definitive confirmation also requires evidence that the stenosis is causing the renal failure. If angiography is performed, vena*

Table 10.7. Clinical features suggestive of renal failure caused by renal artery stenosis

---

Hypertension – *a sine qua non*
Atherosclerosis of extrarenal vessels
    Especially, abdominal bruit
Atherosclerotic risk factors
"Unusual" hypertension
    Onset after age 50
    Escape from previous medical control
    Severe hypertension
    Refractory hypertension
    Grade 3 or 4 hypertensive retinopathy
    ↑ Scr after hypertension therapy
Hypokalemia
Solitary kidney or discrepancy in size of kidneys

---

cava and bilateral renal vein blood samples should be sent for renin levels. A ratio of renal vein renin to inferior vena cava renin greater than 2 : 1, and collateral circulation to the involved kidney seen on angiography suggest a reversible ischemic mechanism for the renal failure; however, the only real proof is recovery of renal function with correction of the lesion by angioplasty or surgery.

Angiography should only be done if the patient and the physician are willing to proceed to angioplasty or vascular surgery to correct any lesion that is found. While the possibility that angiography will reveal a treatable form of renal failure is attractive, one must take into consideration the fact that arteriography carries the risks of bleeding, contrast media nephrotoxicity and atheroembolic disease (rare), and that corrective treatment has additional risk. Percutaneous transluminal renal angioplasty has a complication rate of 5 to 10% and a mortality of 4% (Table 18.5) [237]. Surgery has a mortality rate of over 10% in some series (Table 18.5) [237]. Thus, one tends to consider arteriography in the youngest and healthiest of individuals and in patients whose blood pressure is poorly controlled by drugs or whose renal failure is severe or worsening. Conversely, one tends to avoid an aggressive approach in older, sicker individuals, and in patients whose hypertension is easily controlled and whose renal failure is mild and stable.

Whom to correct. *Once angiography reveals renal artery stenosis of greater than 70 to 75%, one needs to differentiate ischemic kidneys, whose function can improve after correction of the stenosis,*

from irreversibly atrophic kidneys. High renal vein renin level compared to the level in the vena cava, viable glomeruli on biopsy, function on radionuclide renal scan, and collateral circulation and a nephrogram on arteriography suggest reversibility of the renal impairment [238, 261, 262]. To have a good chance of success, vascular correction should be reserved for kidneys longer than 9 cm according to some [224], but good results are also reported with kidneys of 7 and 8 cm in length [250, 263].

If the renal failure seems curable by these guidelines, and if the benefits of correction outweigh the risks mentioned above, one should proceed with balloon angioplasty or vascular surgery (see Chapter 18, section on treatment of vascular causes of renal failure).

At times the physician will be only slightly suspicious of renal artery stenosis, and would like to have further evidence before undertaking arteriography.

Clinical Example. An asymptomatic 48-year-old white male smoker with a 15-year history of hypertension has a recent rise in Scr to 1.9 mg/dL. His father and a brother died of myocardial infarctions. Hypertension is well controlled with captopril and the kidneys are equal and normal in size. Although the patient has no evidence of vascular disease, the risk factors for atherosclerosis raise a concern about renal artery stenosis.

Two studies sometimes used in the evaluation of renovascular hypertension may be of some benefit in such situations, although they have not been evaluated in the diagnosis of renal failure from renal artery stenosis:

Renin. A peripheral vein renin determination should be ordered. A normal or low value tends to exclude the diagnosis. A high value is consistent with renal artery stenosis, but can also be seen in malignant hypertension, atheroembolic disease and scleroderma renal crisis.

Captopril (Renography) Radionuclide Scan. Captopril and other ACE inhibitors can acutely reduce GFR in kidneys with renal artery stenosis. Captopril renography uses radionuclide scanning to detect reduced GFR after a test dose. This test has been performed by different workers with various radionuclides, various criteria and various degrees of success [258, 264–267]. Its sensitivity in detecting *hypertension* caused by renal artery stenosis ranges from 71 to 96% and specificity ranges from 72 to 95%. However, its ability to detect *renal failure* caused by renal artery stenosis has not been studied. Nevertheless, if a physician is having difficulty deciding whether or not to perform an angiogram on a particular patient, a clearly positive or clearly negative captopril renogram might help in the decision.

New Tests Under Evaluation. Duplex sonography [267–270] *magnetic resonance angiography* [271–272] and *spiral CT angiography* [273–274] appear promising for detection of renal artery stenosis in some hands. Given the sparcity of reported experience with these new methods, they cannot be relied upon for a definitive diagnosis of renal artery stenosis, but might be used along with other information to decide on proceeding to angiography in certain patients.

Pitfalls. Severe renal failure may occur with tight renal stenosis on one side and a normal size kidney with a patent renal artery on the other side, i.e. with apparent unilateral disease [224, 261]. In these cases, the normal-looking kidney may have poor function due to malignant hypertension or cholesterol emboli.

In some cases the usual clues to renal artery stenosis are absent, and there is little or nothing to suggest the correct diagnosis. For example: The patient may not have difficult hypertension or extrarenal atherosclerotic manifestations [275]. Men with early atherosclerosis may be less than 50 years old and young women of any age can have fibromuscular hyperplasia. The kidneys may be of equal size [224, 239, 242] and function [228, 239]. Therefore, the physician needs a high index of suspicion for the clues listed in Table 10.7. Unfortunately, patients without any suggestive features may not be diagnosed unless clinical clues appear later.

Renal Infarction

Causes

Renal infarction is usually caused by large renal emboli from an intracardiac thrombus that is formed in the setting of atrial fibrillation or recent myocardial infarction.

Renal infarction due to the other etiologies is rare (Table 10.8). Extreme narrowing of atherosclerotic renal arteries, although not uncommon in the elderly, produces ischemic atrophy rather than infarction. Even when an acute thrombosis totally occludes a narrowed renal artery in this population, collaterals formed during the initial slow phase of stenosis can protect the kidney from frank infarction [300, 301]. In polyarteritis nodosa, occlusion of intrarenal arteries commonly produces multifocal ischemia and infarction [284, 302, 303], but the extent of infarction is sufficient to cause renal failure only in rare cases [283, 284]. Instead, renal failure in polyarteritis nodosa usually

Table 10.8. Conditions that cause renal failure through renal infarction

Renal artery embolism [230, 276, 277]
Atrial fibrillation
Post myocardial infarction
Myxoma [278]
Paradoxical embolism [279]
Dissecting aortic or renal aneurysm [280–282]
Renal artery vasculitis
Polyarteritis nodosa [283, 284]
Giant cell arteritis [285]
Renal artery thrombosis
Atherosclerosis [286]
Trauma [287]
Vascular neurofibromatosis [288]
Hypercoagulability [289, 290]
Vascular surgery [291, 292]
Catheterization or angioplasty [293–296]
Renal artery aneurysm [297]
Renal vein thrombosis [298, 299]

results from the associated glomerulitis. Even renal vein thrombosis is an uncommon cause of infarction, except in neonates [2, 3, 6, 7, 298, 299].

Renal Vein Thrombosis in the Nephrotic Syndrome. This complication is often seen in the nephrotic syndrome due to hypercoagulability, but almost never leads to infarction [304, 305]. Apparently the thrombus in the renal veins is not large enough to stop venous outflow from the kidney or stimulates adequate venous collateral circulation. Even in those cases where renal vein thrombosis reduces GFR, it produces mild or no renal failure thanks to the normal or hypertrophied contralateral kidney [304–307]. Thus, in nephrotic patients, severe renal failure due to renal vein thrombosis of a solitary or both kidneys is very unusual [308–310].

Pathophysiology. Emboli to the main renal arteries can seriously impair GFR by infarcting large portions of the renal parenchyma. In contrast, small emboli to segmental renal arteries as occur in bacterial endocarditis do not cause renal failure. Unilateral main renal artery embolism usually leads to mild renal insufficiency, when the other kidney is normal. However, some patients with unilateral embolism transiently have more severe azotemia than expected [277], perhaps due to reflex vasospasm or contrast media nephrotoxicity, which impairs contralateral renal function.

Clinical picture [276, 277, 311, 312]

The patient with renal infarction is usually of advanced age, reflecting the importance of cardiac disease as a source of the thrombus. While painless infarction can occur, most patients experience pain in the flank, abdomen, chest or low back. Nausea, vomiting and gross hematuria are other common presenting symptoms. Past history may show strokes or other embolic events [276]. In those rare cases of infarction not caused by renal artery embolism, the clinical setting may suggest another cause, e.g. recent renal angioplasty (which may trigger renal artery thrombosis). Similarly, pulmonary emboli or deep vein thrombosis in a patient with nephrotic syndrome should alert one to the possibility of renal vein thrombosis [305, 306].

On examination, one usually finds fever and abdominal or flank tenderness. The blood pressure may be higher than usual.

Most patients have leukocytosis and a urinalysis showing hematuria, mild pyuria and proteinuria as high as 4+. Serum lactic dehydrogenase levels are high in almost all cases, while serum aspartate aminotransferase, alanine aminotransferase and alkaline phosphatase rise less reliably. A radionuclide scan can show perfusion defects, poor perfusion or most often absent perfusion. Similarly, the IVP shows poor or absent function in the involved kidney. Arteriography shows occlusion of the main renal artery or of multiple segmental renal arteries.

Diagnosis

The diagnosis of renal infarction should be suggested in the setting of atrial fibrillation, recent myocardial infarction or renal artery manipulation. Presentation with flank or abdominal pain, unexplained nausea and vomiting, leukocytosis and gross hematuria also raise suspicion of this diagnosis. A serum lactic dehydrogenase should be ordered. If it is elevated, it supports the diagnosis; if it is normal in the acute phase of the illness, it virtually excludes the diagnosis. A renal sonogram should be obtained to rule out urinary obstruction. It will usually appear normal, but in the case of severe renal failure from unilateral embolism it could show an atrophic contralateral kidney destroyed by some previous process.

An IVP is not recommended because of the risk of contrast nephrotoxicity, but may have already been carried out to look for a renal stone. It will show poor function in the involved kidneys. An abdominal computed tomography with contrast enhancement is not recommended to diagnose renal infarction. However, if it has been obtained to investigate abdominal pain and fever or for some other reason, it will show the in-

farcted regions of the kidneys [313].

In most cases a renal arteriogram should be performed since it provides a definite diagnosis by showing the infarction and its cause. However, arteriography carries a certain risk and may be inappropriate in patients in whom the results will not affect management. This includes seriously ill patients in whom treatment with surgery, anticoagulation or thrombolytic therapy is contraindicated. It might also include a patient with atrial fibrillation and mild renal failure whose clinical picture leaves little doubt about the diagnosis and whose treatment already includes anticoagulation. A radionuclide scan can be ordered to show poor renal perfusion in such cases. Also, echocardiography is indicated to show the source of the embolus in the heart.

A vena cavagram and selective renal venogram should be carried out in patients suspected of having a renal vein thrombosis. If arterial or venous occlusions are suspected, a renal arteriogram with additional views of the venous phase will visualize both arteries and veins.

Pitfalls. The diagnosis of renal infarction may be missed in patients who present without the usual predisposing cardiac history or without abdominal or flank pain. The hematuria and proteinuria could be misinterpreted as a form of glomerulonephritis, and the diagnosis may be discovered on renal biopsy.

CONCLUSION

The conditions considered in this chapter can frequently be suspected by their characteristic clinical and laboratory manifestations, e.g. they might occur in certain settings such as the postpartum period for hemolytic uremic syndrome. Often the overall picture is typical enough to make a presumptive diagnosis; in other cases, additional tests will be needed. Table 10.9 summarizes the clinical features that should suggest a vascular cause of renal failure.

NOTES

1. One should not order an IVP to determine renal size, but an old IVP may be available.
2. *Intravenous* digital subtraction angiography does not reliably provide adequate visualization. Instead, standard

Table 10.9. Clinical clues to vascular causes of renal failure

Condition	Clues
Vasomotor disturbance	Severe liver disease, ↑ Ca, sepsis, contrast media Drugs: NSAID's, nifedipine, ACE inhibitors, cyclosporine A
Small vessel disease Atheroembolic disease	Atherosclerosis, recent angiography, ischemic toes, livedo reticularis, eosinophilia
Renal scleroderma	Raynaud's phenomenon, scleroderma, ↑ hypertension
Malignant hypertension	Diastolic BP > 130 mmHg, ↓ vision, grade 3 or 4 retinopathy, headaches or CNS changes, ↓ K
Hemolytic uremic syndrome	Postpartum period, mitomycin C, diarrhea, hemolytic anemia, RBC fragments, ↑ LDH, ↓ platelets
Thrombotic thrombocytopenic purpura	Fever, CNS changes, hemolytic anemia, RBC fragments, ↑ LDH, ↓ platelets
Acute cortical necrosis	Complications of pregnancy, shock, DIC, failure to recover from ATN
Large vessel disease Renal artery stenosis	Atherosclerosis, abdominal bruits, "unusual" hypertension, hypertensive Rx → ↑ Scr, small kidney, ↓ K$^+$
Renal infarction	Recent MI, atrial fibrillation, abdominal or flank pain, gross hematuria, ↑ LDH

ACE – angiotensin-converting enzyme, ATN – acute tubular necrosis, CNS – central nervous sytem, DIC – disseminated intravascular coagulation, LDH – lactic dehydrogenase.

angiography or, preferably, *intra-arterial* digital subtraction angiography should be used to reveal the stenosis.

REFERENCES

1. Davidman M, Olson P, Kohen J, Leither T and Kjellstrand C. Iatrogenic renal disease. Arch Intern Med 1991; 151:1809–12.
2. Niaudet P, Haj-Ibrahim M, Gagnadoux M-F and Broyer M. Outcome of children with acute renal failure. Kidney Int 1985; 28:S148–51.
3. Hodson EM, Kjellstrand CM and Mauer SM. Acute renal failure in infants and children: outcome of 53 patients requiring hemodialysis. J Pediatr 1976; 93:756–61.
4. Counahan R, Cameron JS, Ogg CS, Spurgeon P, Williams DG, Winder E and Chantler C. Presentation, management, complications and outcome of acute renal failure in childhood: five years' experience. Br Med J 1977; 1:599–602.
5. Rengel M, Caro P, Fdez-Llebrez J, Vargas-Z F, Gomes F and Garcia L. Acute renal failure in children. Kidney Int 1985; 28:299.
6. Stapleton FB, Jones DP and Green RS. Acute renal failure in neonates: incidence, etiology and outcome. Pediatr Nephrol 1987; 1:314–20.
7. Jones AS, James E, Bland H and Groshong T. Renal failure in the newborn. Clin Pediat 1979; 18:286–91.
8. Davidson EW and Dunn MJ. Pathogenesis of the hepatorenal syndrome. Ann Rev Med 1987; 38:361–72.
9. Mahnensmith RL. Hypercalcemia, hypernatremia, and reversible renal insufficiency. Am J Kidney Dis 1992; 19:604–8.
10. Bennett WM. Management of acute renal failure in sepsis – clinical considerations. Circ Shock 1983; 11:261–7.
11. Vaz AJ. Low fractional excretion of urine sodium in acute renal failure due to sepsis. Arch Intern Med 1983; 143:738–9.
12. Badr KF, Kelley VE, Rennke HG and Brenner BM. Roles for thromboxane A_2 and leukotrienes in endotoxin-induced acute renal failure. Kidney Int 1986; 30:474–80.
13. Packer M, Lee WH, Medina N, Yushak M and Kessler PD. Functional renal insufficiency during long-term therapy with captopril and enalapril in severe chronic heart failure. Ann Intern Med 1987; 106:346–54.
14. Hricik DE and Dunn MJ. Angiotensin-converting enzyme inhibitor-induced renal failure: causes, consequences, and diagnostic uses. J Am Soc Nephrol 1990; 1:845–58.
15. Diamond JR, Cheung JY and Fang LST. Nifedipine-induced renal dysfunction. Am J Med 1984; 77:905–9.
16. Eicher JC, Morelon P, Chalopin JM, Tanter Y, Louis P and Rifle G. Acute renal failure during nifedipine therapy in a patient with congestive heart failure. Crit Care Med 1988; 16:1163–4.

17. Cacoub P, Deray JY, Deray G, Grosgogeat Y and Jacobs C. Nifedipine-induced acute renal failure. Clin Nephrol 1988; 29:272-3.
18. Conte G, Dal Canton A, Sabbatini M, Napodano P, De Nicola L, Gigliotti G et al. Acute cyclosporine renal dysfunction reversed by dopamine infusion in healthy subjects. Kidney Int 1989; 36:1086-92.
19. Skorecki KL, Rutledge WP and Schrier RW. Acute cyclosporine nephrotoxicity – prototype for a renal membrane signalling disorder. Kidney Int 1992; 42:1-10.
20. Morales JM, Andres A, Prieto C, Arenas J, Ortuno B, Praga M et al. Severe reversible cyclosporine-induced acute renal failure. Transplantation 1988; 46:163-4.
21. Kone BC, Watson AJ, Gimenez LF and Kadir S. Acute renal failure following percutaneous transhepatic cholangiography. Arch Intern Med 1986; 146:1405-7.
22. Anzari Z and Baldwin DS. Acute renal failure due to radiocontrast agents. Nephron 1975; 17:28-40.
23. Nora N and Berns AS. Renal failure following cardiac angiography: a prospective study of diatrizoate and iopamidol. Kidney Int 1989; 35:414.
24. Taliercio CP, McCallister SH, Holmes DR, Ilstrup DM and Vlietstra RE. Nephrotoxicity of nonionic contrast media after cardiac angiography. Am J Cardiol 1989; 64:815-6.
25. Gomes RE, Lois JF, Baker JD, McGlade CT, Bunnell DH and Hartzman S. Acute renal dysfunction in high-risk patients after angiography: comparison of ionic and nonionic contrast media. Radiology 1989; 170:65-8.
26. Aron NB, Feinfeld DA, Peters AT and Lynn RI. Acute renal failure associated with ioxaglate, a low-osmolality radiocontrast agent. Am J Kidney Dis 1989; 13:189-93.
27. Barrett BJ and Carlisle EJ. Metaanalysis of the relative nephrotoxicity of high- and low-osmolality iodinated contrast media. Radiology 1993; 188:171-8.
28. Clive DM and Stoff JS. Renal syndromes associated with non-steroidal anti-inflammatory drugs. N Engl J Med 1984; 310:563-72.
29. Gurwitz JH, Avorn J, Ross-Degnan D and Lipsitz LA. Nonsteroidal anti-inflammatory drug-associated azotemia in the very old. JAMA 1990; 264:471-5.
30. Carmichael J and Shankel SW. Effects of nonsteroidal anti-inflammatory drugs on prostaglandins and renal function. Am J Med 1985; 78:992-1000.
31. Blackshear JL, Davidman M and Stillman T. Identification of risk for renal insufficiency from nonsteroid anti-inflammatory drugs. Arch Intern Med 1983; 143:1130-4.
32. Hricik DE. Captopril-induced renal insufficiency and the role of sodium balance. Ann Intern Med 1985; 103:222-3.
33. Schwartz D, Averbuch M, Pines A, Kornowski R and Levo Y. Renal toxicity of enalapril in very elderly patients with progressive, severe congestive heart failure. Chest 1991; 100:1558-61.
34. Taliercio CP, Vlietstra RE, Fisher LD and Burnett JC. Risks for renal dysfunction with cardiac angiography. Ann Intern Med 1986; 104:501-4.
35. Levenson DJ, Skorecki KL, Newell GC and Narins RG. Acute renal failure associated with hepatobiliary disease. In: Brenner BM and Lazarus JM, editors. Acute renal failure. New York, Churchill Livingstone, 1988; 535-80.
36. Gentilini P and Laffi G. Renal functional impairment and sodium retention in liver cirrhosis. Digestion 1989; 43:1-32.
37. Gines A, Escorsell A, Gines P, Salo J, Jimenez W, Inglada L et al. Incidence, predictive factors, and prognosis of the hepatorenal syndrome in cirrhosis with ascites. Gastroenterol 1993; 105:229-36.
38. Lenz K, Hortnagl H, Druml W, Grimm G, Laggner A, Schneewesisz B et al. Beneficial effect of 8-ornithin vasopressin on renal dysfunction in decompensated cirrhosis. Gut 1989; 30:90-6.
39. Parrillo JE. Pathogenetic mechanisms of septic shock. N Engl J Med 1993; 328:1471-7.
40. Whelton A, Stout RL, Spilman PS and Klassen DK. Renal effects of ibuprofen, piroxican, and sulindac in patients with asymptomatic renal failure. Ann Intern Med 1990; 112:568-76.
41. Toto RD, Mitchell HC, Lee H-C, Milam C and Pettinger WA. Reversible renal insufficiency due to angiotensin converting enzyme inhibitors in hypertensive nephrosclerosis. Ann Intern Med 1991; 115:513-9.
42. Chapman AB, Gabow PA and Schrier RW. Reversible renal failure associated with angiotensin-converting enzyme inhibitors in polycystic kidney disease. Ann Intern Med 1991; 115:769-73.
43. Murray BM, Venuto RC, Kohli R and Cunningham EE. Enalapril-associated acute renal failure in renal transplants: possible role of cyclosporine. Am J Kidney Dis 1990; 16:66-9.
44. Deray G, Le Hoang P, Aupetit B, Achour A, Rottembourg J, and Baumelou A. Enhancement of cyclosporine A nephrotoxicity by diclofenac. Clin Nephrol 1987; 27:213.
45. Harris KP, Jenkins D and Walls J. Nonsteroidal anti-inflammatory drugs and cyclosporine. Transplantation 1988; 46:598-9.
46. Berg KJ, Forre O, Djoseland O, Mikkelsen M, Narverud J and Rugstad HE. Renal side effects of high and low cyclosporin A doses in patients with rheumatoid arthritis. Clin Nephrol 1989; 31:232-8.
47. Epstein M. Renal prostaglandins and the control of renal function in liver disease. Am J Med 1986; 80:46-54.
48. Reams GP, Bauer JH and Gaddy P. Use of the converting enzyme inhibitor enalapril in renovascular hypertension. Hypertension 1986; 8:290-7.
49. Textor SC, Biscardi A, Bravo EL, Tarazi RC and Fouad FM. Acute renal failure during converting enzyme inhibition in patients with renal artery stenosis. American Soc Nephrol (abstract) 1982:45.
50. Zarich S, Fang LST and Diamond JR. Fractional excretion of sodium. Exceptions to its diagnostic value. Arch Intern Med 1985; 145:108-12.
51. Fang LST, Sirota RA, Ebert TH and Lichtenstein NS. Low fractional excretion of sodium with contrast media-induced acute renal failure. Arch Intern Med 1980; 140:531-3.
52. Greenberg A, Egel J, Thompson M, Bahnson H, Griffith B, Hardesty R et al. Renal failure in heart transplant patients receiving cyclosporin A. Clin Res 1983; 31:429A.
53. Agus ZS and Goldfarb S. Calcium metabolism: normal and abnormal. In Arieff AI and DeFronzo RA, editors. Fluid, electrolyte, and acid-base disorders. New York, Churchill

Livingstone, 1985; 511–74.

54. Wilkinson SP, Hirst D, Day DW and Williams R. Spectrum of renal tubular damage in renal failure secondary to cirrhosis and fulminant hepatic failure. J Clin Pathol 1978; 31:101–7.

55. Dudley FJ, Kanel GC, Wood LJ and Reynolds TB. Hepatorenal syndrome without avid sodium retention. Hepatology 1986; 6:248–51.

56. Baldus WP, Feichter RN and Summerskill WHJ. The Kidney in cirrhosis. I. Clinical and biochemical features of azotemia in hepatic failure. Ann Intern Med 1964; 60:353–65.

57. Papper S. Hepatorenal syndrome. In: Epstein M, editor. The kidney in liver disease. Elsevier Biomedical, New York, 1983:2nd ed., 87–106.

58. Ring-Larsen H and Palazzo U. Renal failure in fulminant hepatic failure and terminal cirrhosis: a comparison between incidence, types, and prognosis. Gut 1981; 22:585–91.

59. Wilkinson SP, Blendis LM and Williams R. Frequency and type of renal and electrolyte disorders in fulminant hepatic failure. BMJ 1974;1:186–9.

60. Cade R, Wagemaker H, Vogel S, Mars D, Hood-Lewis D, Privette M et al. Hepatorenal syndrome. Am J Med 1987; 82:427–38.

61. Davenport A and Finn R. Paracetamol (Acetaminophen) poisoning resulting in acute renal failure without hepatic coma. Nephron 1988; 50:55–6.

62. Newell GC. Cirrhotic glomerulonephritis: incidence, morphology, clinical features, and pathogenesis. Am J Kidney Dis 1987; 9:183–90.

63. Byrd L and Sherman RL. Radiocontrast-induced acute renal failure: a clinical and pathophysiological review. Medicine 1979; 58:270–9.

64. Teruel JL, Marcen R, Onaindia JM, Serrano A, Quereda C and Ortuno J. Renal function impairment caused by intravenous urography. A prospective study. Arch Intern Med 1981; 141:1271–4.

65. Shafi T, Chou S-Y, Porush JG and Shapiro WB. Infusion intravenous pyelography and renal function. Effect in patients with chronic renal insufficiency. Arch Intern Med 1978; 138:1218–21.

66. Van Zee BE, Hoy WE, Talley TE and Jaenike JR. Renal injury associated with intravenous pyelography in nondiabetic and diabetic patients. Ann Intern Med 1978; 89:51–4.

67. Carvalho A, Rakowski TA, Argy WP and Schreiner GE. Acute renal failure following drip infusion pyelography. Am J Med 1978; 65:38–45.

68. Martin-Paredero V, Dixon SM, Baker JD, Takiff H, Gomes AS, Busuttil RW et al. Risk of renal failure after major angiography. Arch Surg 1983; 118:1417–20.

69. Lautin EM, Freeman NJ, Schoenfeld AH, Bakal CW, Haramati N, Friedman AC et al. Radiocontrast-associated renal dysfunction: incidence and risk factors. AJR 1991; 157:49–58.

70. Rich MW and Crecelius CA. Incidence, risk factors, and clinical course of acute renal insufficiency after cardiac catheterization in patients 70 years of age or older. Arch Intern Med 1990; 150:1237–42.

71. Moore RD, Steinberg EP, Powe NR, Brinker JA, Fishman EK, Graziano S et al. Nephrotoxicity of high-osmolality versus low-osmolality contrast media: randomized clinical trial. Radiology 1992; 182:649–55.

72. Lautin EM, Freeman NJ, Schoenfeld AH, Bakal CW, Haramati N, Friedman AC et al. Radiocontrast-associated renal dysfunction: a comparison of lower-osmolality and conventional high-osmolality contrast media. AJR 1991; 157:59–65.

73. Saklayen MG. Atheroembolic renal disease: preferential occurrence in whites only. Am J Nephrol 1989; 9:87–8.

74. Fine MJ, Kapoor W and Falanga V. Cholesterol crystal embolization: a review of 221 cases in the English literature. J Vasc Dis 1987; 38:769–84

75. Dahlberg PJ, Frecentese DF, Cogbill TH. Cholesterol embolism: experience with 22 histologically proven cases. Surgery 1989; 105:737–46.

76. Baxter BT, McGee GS, Flinn WR, McCarthy WJ, Pearce WH and Yao JST. Distal embolization as a presenting symptom of aortic aneurysms. Am J Surg 1990; 160:197–201.

77. Colt HG, Begg RJ, Saporito JJ, Cooper WM and Shapiro AP. Cholesterol emboli after cardiac catheterization. Medicine 1988; 67:389–400.

78. Fraser I, Ihle B and Kincaid-Smith P. Renal failure due to cholesterol emboli. Aust NZ J Med 1991; 21:418–21.

79. Hyman BT, Landas SK, Ashman RF, Schelper RL and Robinson RA. Warfarin-related purple toes syndrome and cholesterol microembolization. Am J Med 1987; 82:1233–7.

80. Case Records of the Massachusetts General Hospital, Case 38-1993. N Engl J Med 1993; 329:948–55.

81. Mannesse CK, Blankestijn PJ, Man In't Veld AJ and Schalekamp MADH. Renal failure and cholesterol crystal embolization: a report of 4 surviving cases and a review of the literature. Clin Nephrol 1991; 36:240–5.

82. Kaufman JL, Stark K and Brolin RE. Disseminated atheroembolism from extensive degenerative atherosclerosis of the aorta. Surgery 1987; 102:63–9.

83. McGowan JA and Greenberg A. Cholesterol atheroembolic renal disease. Am J Nephrol 1986; 6:135–9.

84. Cosserat J, Bletry O, Frances C, Wechsler B, Piette JC, Kieffer E et al. Embolies multiples de cholesterol simulant une periarterite noueuse. Presse Med 1992; 21:557–64.

85. Smith MC, Ghose MK and Henry AR. The clinical spectrum of renal cholesterol embolization. Am J Med 1981; 71:171–80.

86. Meyrier A, Buchet P, Simon P, Fernet M, Rainfray M and Callard P. Atheromatous renal disease. Am J Med 1988; 85:139–46.

87. Ludmerer KM and Kissane JM. Progressive renal failure with hematuria in a 62 year old man. Am J Med 1981; 71:468–74.

88. Endreny RG, Zipin S, Chazan J and King B. Atheroembolic renal disease – presentation and clinical course in ten patients. Am J Kidney Dis 1988; 11:A6

89. Williams HH, Wall BM and Cooke CR. Case report: reversible nephrotic range proteinuria and renal failure in atheroembolic renal disease. Am J Med Sci 1990; 299:58–61.

90. Wilson DM, Salazer TL, Farkouh ME. Eosinophiluria in atheroembolic renal disease. Am J Med 1991; 91:186–90.

91. Case Records of the Massachusetts General Hospital, Case

30-1986. N Engl J Med 1986; 315:308–15.

92. Cosio FG, Zager RA and Sharma HM. Atheroembolic renal disease causes hypocomplementaemia. Lancet 1985; 1:118–22.

93. Hendel RC, Cuenoud HF, Giansiracusa DF and Alpert JS. Multiple cholesterol emboli syndrome. Arch Intern Med 1989; 149:2371–4.

94. O'Keeffe ST, Woods BO'B, Breslin DJ and Tsapatsaris NP. Blue toe syndrome. Arch Intern Med 1992; 152:2197–202.

95. Donohoe JF. Scleroderma and the kidney. Kidney Int 1992; 41:462–77.

96. Kovalchik MT, Guggenheim SJ, Silverman MH, Robertson JS and Steigerwald JC. The kidney in progressive systemic sclerosis. Ann Intern Med 1978; 89:881–7.

97. LeRoy EC and Fleischmann RM. The management of renal scleroderma. Am J Med 1978; 64:974–8.

98. Traub YM, Shapiro AP, Rodnan GP, Medsger TA, McDonald RH Jr., Steen VD et al. Hypertension and renal failure (scleroderma renal crisis) in progressive systemic sclerosis. Medicine 1983; 62:335–52.

99. Steen VD, Medsger TA Jr., Osial TA Jr., Ziegler GL, Shapiro AP and Rodnan GP. Factors predicting development of renal involvement in progressive systemic sclerosis. Am J Med 1984; 76:779–86.

100. Gavras H, Gavras I, Cannon PJ, Brunner HR and Laragh JH. Is elevated plasma renin activity of prognostic importance in progressive systemic sclerosis. Arch Intern Med 1977; 137:1554–8.

101. Oliver JA and Cannon PJ. The kidney in scleroderma. Nephron 1977; 18:141–50.

102. Cannon PJ, Hassar M, Case DB, Casarella WJ, Sommers SC and LeRoy EC. The relationship of hypertension and renal failure in scleroderma (progressive systemic sclerosis) to structural and functional abnormalities of the renal cortical circulation. Medicine 1974; 53:1–46.

103. Salyer WR, Salyer DC and Heptinstall RH. Scleroderma and microangiopathic hemolytic anemia. Ann Intern Med 1973; 78:895–7.

104. Hultman P, Enestron S, Pollard KM and Tan EM. Antifibrillarin autoantibodies in mercury-treated mice. Clin Exp Immunol 1989; 78:470–2.

105. Tan EM. Systemic autoimmunity and antinuclear antibodies. Clin Aspects Autoimmunity 1986; 1:2–8.

106. Ferri C, Bernini L, Cecchetti R, Latorraca A, Marotta G, Pasero G et al. Cutaneous and serologic subsets of systemic sclerosis. J Rheumatol 1991; 18:1826–32.

107. Kagan A, Nissim F, Green L and Bar-Khayim Y. Scleroderma renal crisis without hypertension. J Rheumatol 1989; 16:707–8.

108. Gouge SF, Wilder K, Welch P, Sabnis SG and Antonovich TT. Scleroderma renal crisis prior to scleroderma. Am J Kidney Dis 1989; 14:236–8.

109. Sanders PW, Herrera GA and Ball GV. Acute renal failure without fibrotic skin changes in progressive systemic sclerosis. Nephron 1988; 48:121–5.

110. Zwettler U, Andrassy K, Waldherr R and Ritz E. Scleroderma renal crisis as a presenting feature in the absence of skin involvement. Am J Kidney Dis 1993; 22:53–6.

111. Guelpa G, Lucsko M, Chaignon M and Guedon J. Hypertension arterielle maligne, aspect semiologique et prognostique. Schweiz med Wschr 1984; 114:1870–7.

112. Yu S-H, Whitworth JA and Kincaid-Smith PS. Malignant hypertension: aetiology and outcome in 83 patients. Clin and Exper Theory and Pract 1986; A8:1211–30.

113. Gudbrandsson T, Hansson L, Herlitz H and Andren L. Malignant hypertension – improving prognosis in a rare disease. Acta Med Scand 1979; 206:495–9.

114. Pitcock JA, Johnson JG, Hatch FE, Acchiardo S, Muirhead EE and Brown PS. Malignant hypertension in blacks. Human Pathol 1976; 7:333–46.

115. Mattern WD, Sommers SC and Kassirer JP. Oliguric acute renal failure in malignant hypertension. Am J Med 1972; 52:187–97.

116. Isles CG, McLay A and Jones JMB. Recovery in malignant hypertension presenting as acute renal failure. Quart J Med 1984; 23:439–52.

117. Lawton WJ. The short-term course of renal function in malignant hypertensives with renal insufficiency. Clin Nephrol 1982; 17:277–83.

118. Krogsgaard AR, McNair A, Hilden T and Nielsen PE. Reversibility of cerebral symptoms in severe hypertension in relation to acute antihypertensive therapy. Acta Med Scand 1986; 220:25–31.

119. Nolan CR III and Linas SL. Accelerated and malignant hypertension. In: Shrier RW and Gottschalk CW, editors. Diseases of the kidney. Little Brown and Company, Boston. 1988:1703–1826.

120. Gavras H, Oliver N, Aitchison J, Begg C, Briggs JD, Brown JJ et al. Abnormalities of coagulation and the development of malignant phase hypertension. Kidney Int 1975; 8:S252–61.

121. Laragh JH, Ulick S, Januszewicz V, Deming QB, Kelly WG and Lieberman S. Aldosterone secretion and primary and malignant hypertension. J Clin Invest 1960; 39:1091–106.

122. Mroczek WJ, Davidov M, Gavrilovich L, Finnerty FA Jr. et al. The value of aggressive therapy in the hypertensive patient with azotemia. Circulation 1969; 40:893–904.

123. Patel R, Ansari A and Grim CE. Prognosis and predisposing factors for essential malignant hypertension in predominantly black patients. Am J Cardiol 1990; 66:868–9.

124. Sevitt LH, Evans DJ and Wrong OM. Acute oliguric renal failure due to accelerated (malignant) hypertension. Quart J Med 1971; 40:127–44.

125. Brown JJ, Davies DL, Lever AF and Robertson JIS. Plasma renin concentration in human hypertension. 1: Relationship between renin, sodium, and potassium. BMJ 1965; 2:144–8.

126. McNair A, Krogsgaard AR, Hilden T and Nielsen PE. Severe hypertension with cerebral symptoms treated with furosemide, fractionated diazoxide or dihydralazine. Acta Med Scand 1986; 220:15–23.

127. Fong JSC, de Chadarevian J-P and Kaplan BS. Hemolytic uremic syndrome. Current concepts and management. Pediatr Clin N Amer 1982; 29:835–56.

128. Goldstein MH, Churg J, Strauss L and Gribetz D. Hemolytic-uremic syndrome. Nephron 1979; 23:263–72.

129. Neild G. The haemolytic uraemic syndrome: a review. Quart J Med 1987; 63:367–76.

130. Van Damme-Lombaerts, Proesmans W, Van Damme B, Eeckels R, Binda ki Muaka P, Mercieca V et al. Heparin plus dipyridamole in childhood hemolytic-uremic syndrome: a prospective, randomized study. J Pediatr 1988; 113:913–8.

131. Martin DL, MacDonald KL, White KE, Soler JT and Osterholm MT. The epidemiology and clinical aspects of the hemolytic uremic syndrome in Minnesota. N Engl J Med 1990; 323:1161–7.

132. van Wieringen PMV, Monnens LAH and Schretlen EDAM. Haemolytic-uraemic syndrome. Arch Dis Child 1974; 49:432–7.

133. Dolislager D and Tune B. The hemolytic-uremic syndrome. Am J Dis Child 1978; 132:55–8.

134. Sorrenti Y and Lewy PR. The hemolytic-uremic syndrome. Am J Dis Child 1978; 132:59–62.

135. Besser RE, Lett SM, Weber JT, Doyle MP, Barrett TJ, Wells JG et al. An outbreak of diarrhea and hemolytic uremic syndrome from *Escherichia coli* 0157 : H7 in fresh-pressed apple cider. JAMA 1993; 269:2217–20.

136. Pavia AT, Nichols CR, Green DP, Tzuxe RV. Mottice S, Greene KD et al. Hemolytic-uremic syndrome during an outbreak of *Escherichia coli* 0157 : H7 infections in institutions for mentally retarded persons: clinical and epidemiologic observations. J Pediatr 1990; 116:544–51.

137. Rowe PC, Orrbine E, Wells GA and McLaine PN, and members of the Canadian Pediatric Kidney Disease Reference Centre: epidemiology of hemolytic-uremic syndrome in Canadian children from 1986 to 1988. J Pediatr 1991; 119:218–24.

138. Ostroff SM, Kobayashi JM and Lewis JH. Infections with *Escherichia coli* 0157 : H7 in Washington State. JAMA 1989; 262:355–9.

139. Griffin PM and Tauxe RV. The epidemiology of infections caused by *Escherichia coli* 0157 : H7, other enterohemorrhagic *E. coli*, and the associated hemolytic uremic syndrome. Epidemiologic Reviews 1991; 13:60–98.

140. Brandt P, Jespersen J and Gregersen G. Post partum haemolytic-uraemic syndrome treated with antithrombin-III. Nephron 1981; 27:15–8.

141. Hayslett JP. Postpartum renal failure. N Engl J Med 1985; 312:1556–9.

142. Souquiyyeh MZ and Kabir MZ. Postpartum hemolytic-uremic syndrome. Saudi Kidney Dis and Transplant Bull 1991; 2:90–2.

143. Segonds A, Louradour N, Suc JM and Orfila C. Postpartum hemolytic uremic syndrome: a study of three cases with a review of the literature. Clin Nephrol 1979; 12:229–42.

144. Lesesne JB, Rothschild N, Erickson B, Korec S, Sisk R, Keller J et al. Cancer-associated hemolytic-uremic syndrome: Analysis of 85 cases from a national registry. J Clin Oncol 1989; 7:781–9.

145. Murgo AJ. Thrombotic microangiopathy in the cancer patient including those induced by chemotherapeutic agents. Semin Hematol 1987; 24:161–77.

146. Giroux L, Bettez P and Giroux L. Mitomycin-C nephrotoxicity: a clinico-pathologic study of 17 cases. Am J Kidney Dis 1985; 6:28–39.

147. Khansur T and Kennedy A. Case Report: cisplatin-induced hemolytic uremic syndrome. Am J Med Sci 1991; 301:390–2.

148. Eugene M, Deray G, Cacoub P, Achour A and Baumelou A. Hemolytic uremic syndrome and prostatic adenocarcinoma. Clin Nephrol 1987; 27:46.

149. Avvento L, Gordon S, Silberberg JM, Zarrabi MH and Zucker S. Hemolytic uremic syndrome in a patient with small cell lung cancer. Am J Hematol 1988; 27:221–3.

150. Ortega Marcos O, Escuin F, Miguel JL, Gomez Fernandez P, Perez Fontan M, Selgas R et al. Hemolytic uremic syndrome in a patient with gastric adenocarcinoma: partial recovery of renal function after gastrectomy. Clin Nephrol 1985; 24:265–8.

151. Hauglustaine D, Van Damme B, Vanrenterghem Y and Michielsen P. Recurrent hemolytic uremic syndrome during oral contraception. Clin Nephrol 1981; 15:148–53.

152. Ashouri OS, Marbury TC, Fuller TJ, Gaffney E, Grubb WG and Cade JR. Hemolytic uremic syndrome in two postmenopausal women taking a conjugated estrogen preparation. Clin Nephrol 1982; 17:212–15.

153. Neill MA, Agosti J and Rosen H. Hemorrhagic colitis with *Escherichia coli* 0157 : H7 preceding adult hemolytic uremic syndrome. Arch Intern Med 1985; 145:2215–7.

154. Allan A, Keighley MRB and Thompson H. Beware of hemolytic uremic syndrome presenting as colorectal disease in adults. Dis Colon Rectum 1989; 32:426–8.

155. White DJ. Haemolytic uraemic syndrome in adults. BMJ 1988; 296:899.

156. Date A, Pulimood R, Jacob CK, Kirubakaran MG and Shastry JCM. Haemolytic-uraemic syndrome complicating snake bite. Nephron 1986; 42:89–90.

157. Siegler RL, Brewer ED and Pysher TJ. Hemolytic uremic syndrome associated with glomerular disease. Am J Kidney Dis 1989; 13:144–7.

158. Hagley MT, Hosney IA, Hulisz DT and Davis HH. Hemolytic-uremic syndrome associated with ingestion of quinine. Am J Nephrol 1992; 12:192–5.

159. Maguire RB, Stroncek DF and Campbell AC. Recurrent pancytopenia, coagulopathy, and renal failure associated with multiple quinine-dependent antibodies. Ann Intern Med 1993; 119:215–7.

160. Beaufils H, DeGroc F, Gubler MC, Wechsler B, LeHoang P, Baumelou A et al. Hemolytic uremic syndrome in patients with Behcet's disease treated with cyclosporin A: report of 2 cases. Clin Nephrol 1990; 34:157–62.

161. Remuzzi G and Bertani T. Renal vascular and thrombotic effects of cyclosporine. Am J Kidney Dis 1989; 13:261–72.

162. Bonsib SM, Ercolani L, Ngheim D and Hamilton HE. Recurrent thrombotic microangiopathy in a renal allograft. Am J Med 1985; 79:520–7.

163. Butkus DE, Herrera GA and Raju SS. Successful renal transplantation after cyclosporine-associated hemolytic-uremic syndrome following bilateral lung transplantation. Transplantation 1992; 54:159–89.

164. Loomis LJ, Aronson AJ, Rudinsky R and Spargo BH. Hemolytic uremic syndrome following bone marrow

transplantation: a case report and review of the literature. Am J Kidney Dis 1989; 14:324–8.

165. Cohen EP, Lawton CA, Moulder JE, Becker CG and Ash RC. Clinical course of late-onset bone marrow transplant nephropathy. Nephron 1993; 64:626–36.

166. Oursler DP, Holley KE and Wagoner RD. Hemolytic uremic syndrome after bone marrow transplantation without total body irradiation. Am J Nephrol 1993; 13:167–70.

167. Esforzado N, Poch E, Almirall J, Lopez-Pedret J and Revert L. Hemolytic uremic syndrome associated with HIV infection. AIDS 1991; 5:1041–2.

168. Frem GJ, Rennke HG and Sayegh MH. Late renal allograft failure secondary to thrombotic microangiopathy-human immunodeficiency virus nephropathy. J Am Soc Nephrol 1994; 4:1643–8.

169. Ponticelli C, Rivolta E, Imbasciati E, Rossi E and Mannucci PM. Hemolytic uremic syndrome in adults. Arch Intern Med 1980; 140:353–7.

170. Kaplan S. Hemolytic uremic syndrome with recurrent episodes: an important subset. Clin Nephrol 1977; 8:495–8.

171. Kaplan BS, Chesney RW and Drummond KN. Hemolytic uremic syndrome in families. N Engl J Med 1975; 292:1090–3.

172. Mattoo TK, Mahmood MA, Al-Harbi MS and Mikail I. Familial, recurrent hemolytic-uremic syndrome. J Pediat 1989; 114:814–6.

173. Pirson Y, Lefebvre C, Arnout C and van Ypersele de Strihou C. Hemolytic uremic syndrome in three adult siblings: a familial study and evolution. Clin Nephrol 1987; 28:250–5.

174. Hakim RM, Schulman G, Churchill WH Jr. and Lazarus JM. Successful management of thrombocytopenia, microangiopathic anemia, and acute renal failure by plasmapheresis. Am J Kidney Dis 1985; 5:170–6.

175. Kaplan BS, Thomson PD and de Chadarevian J-P. The hemolytic uremic syndrome. Pediatr Clin N Amer 1976; 23:761–77.

176. Morel-Maroger L, Kanfer A, Solez K, Sraer J-D and Richet G. Prognostic importance of vascular lesions in acute renal failure with microangiopathic hemolytic anemia (hemolytic-uremic syndrome): Clinicopathologic study in 20 adults. Kidney Int 1979; 15:548–58.

177. Bale JF Jr., Brasher C and Siegler RL. CNS manifestations of the hemolytic-uremic syndrome. Am J Dis Child 1980; 134:869–72.

178. Trevathan E and Dooling EC. Large thrombotic strokes in hemolytic-uremic syndrome. J Pediatr 1987; 111:863–6.

179. Upadhyaya K, Barwick K, Fishaut M, Kashgarian M and Siegel NJ. The importance of nonrenal involvement in hemolytic-uremic syndrome. Pediatr 1980; 65:115–20.

180. Jolivet J, Giroux L, Laurin S, Gruber J, Bettez P and Band PR. Microangiopathic hemolytic anemia, renal failure, and noncardiogenic pulmonary edema: A chemotherapy-induced syndrome. Cancer Treatment Reports 1983; 67:429–34.

181. Clarkson AR, Lawrence JR, Meadows R and Seymour AE. The haemolytic uraemic syndrome in adults. Quart J Med 1970; 39:227–44.

182. Habib R. Hemolytic uremic syndrome. In: Royer P, Habib R, Mathieu H and Broyer M, editors. Pediatric nephrology. W.B. Saunders Company, Philadelphia, 1974;291–301.

183. O'Regan S and Rousseau E. Hemolytic uremic syndrome: urate nephropathy superimposed on an acute glomerulopathy? A hypothesis. Clin Nephrol 1988; 30:207–10.

184. Gonzalo A, Mampaso F, Gallego N, Bellas C, Segut J and Ortuno J. Hemolytic uremic syndrome with hypocomplementemia and deposits of IgM and C3 in the involved renal tissue. Clin Nephrol 1981; 16:193–9.

185. Poch E, Gonzalez-Clemente JM, Torras A, Darnell A, Botey A and Revert L. Silent renal microangiopathy after mitomycin C therapy. Am J Nephrol 1990; 10:514–7.

186. Case Records of the Massachusetts General Hospital, Case 41-1990. N Engl J Med 1990; 323:1050–61.

187. Sibai BM, Villar MA and Mabie BC. Acute renal failure in hypertensive disorders of pregnancy. Pregnancy outcome and remote prognosis in thirty-one. Am J Obstet Gynecol 1990; 162:777–83.

188. Sibai BM, Taslimi MM, El-Nazer A, Amon E, Mabie BC and Ryan GM. Maternal-perinatal outcome associated with the syndrome of hemolysis, elevated liver enzymes, and low platelets in severe preeclampsia-eclampsia. Am J Obstet Gynecol 1986; 155:501–9.

189. Thiagarajah S, Bourgeois FJ, Harbert GM Jr. and Caudle MR. Thrombocytopenia in preeclampsia: associated abnormalities and management principles. Am J Obstet Gynecol 1984; 150:1–7.

190. Krane NK. Acute renal failure in pregnancy. Arch Intern Med 1988; 148:2347–57.

191. McCrae KR, Samuels P and Schreiber AD. Pregnancy-associated thrombocytopenia: pathogenesis and management. Blood 1992; 80:2697–714.

192. Ridolfi RL and Bell WR. Thrombotic thrombocytopenic purpura. Medicine 1981; 60:413–28.

193. Kennedy SS, Zacharski LR and Beck JR. Thrombotic thrombocytopenic purpura: analysis of 48 unselected cases. Semin Thrombosis and Hemostasis 1980; 6:341–9.

194. Rock GA, Shumak KH, Buskard NA, Blanchette VS, Kelton JG, Nair RC, Spasoff RA and The Canadian Apheresis Study Group. Comparison of plasma exchange with plasma infusion in the treatment of thrombotic thrombocytopenic purpura. N Engl J Med 1991; 325:393–7.

195. Bell WR, Braine HG, Ness PM and Kickler TS. Improved survival in thrombotic thrombocytopenic purpura-hemolytic uremic syndrome. N Engl J Med 1991; 325:398–403.

196. Rarick MU, Espina B, Mocharnuk R, Trilling Y and Levine AM. Thrombotic thrombocytopenic purpura in patients with human immunodeficiency virus infection: a report of three cases and review of the literature. Am J Hematol 1992; 40:103–9.

197. Eknoyan G and Riggs SA. Renal involvement in patients with thrombotic thrombocytopenic purpura. Am J Nephrol 1986; 6:117–31.

198. Amorosi EL and Ultmann JE. Thrombotic thrombocytopenic purpura: Report of 16 cases and review of the literature. Medicine 1966; 45:139–59.

199. Petitt RM. Thrombotic thrombocytopenic purpura: a thirty year review. Semin Thrombosis and Hemostasis 1980; 6:350–5.

200. Pisciotta AV and Gottschall JL. Clinical features of thrombotic thrombocytopenic purpura. Semin Thrombosis and Hemostasis 1980; 6:330–40.

201. Evans TL, Winkelstein A, Zeigler ZR, Shadduck RK and Mangan KF. Thrombotic thrombocytopenic purpura: clinical course and response to therapy in eight patients. Am J Hematol 1984; 17:401–7.

202. Kwaan HC. Clinicopathologic features of thrombotic thrombocytopenic purpura. Semin Hematol 1987; 24:71–81.

203. Webb JG, Butany J, Langer G, Scott G and Liu PP. Myocarditis and myocardial hemorrhage associated with thrombotic thrombocytopenic purpura. Arch Intern Med 1990; 150:1535–7.

204. Bukowski RM. Thrombotic thrombocytopenic purpura: a review. Prog Hemost Thromb 1982; 6:287–337.

205. Kovacs MJ, Roddy J, Gregoire S, Cameron W, Eidus L and Drouin J. Thrombotic thrombocytopenic purpura following hemorrhagic colitis due to *Escherichia coli* 0157 : H7. Am J Med 1990; 88:177–9.

206. Case Records of the Massachusetts General Hospital, Case 30-1991. N Engl J Med 1991; 325:265–73.

207. Kleinknecht D, Grunfeld J-P, Cia Gomez P, Moreau J-F and Garcia-Torres R. Diagnostic procedures and long-term prognosis in bilateral renal cortical necrosis. Kidney Int 1973; 4:390–400.

208. Chugh KS, Singhal PC, Kher VK, Gupta VK, Malik GH, Narayan G et al. Spectrum of acute cortical necrosis in Indian patients. Am J Med Sci 1983; 286:10–20.

209. Matlin RA and Gary NE. Acute cortical necrosis. Am J Med 1974; 56:110–8.

210. Stratta P, Canavese C, Colla L, Dogliani M, Bussolino F, Bianco O, Gagliardi L, Todros T, Iberti M, Veronesi GV and Bianchi GM. Acute renal failure in preeclampsia. Gynecol Obstet Invest. 1987; 24:225–32.

211. Grunfeld J-P, Ganeval D and Bournerias F. Acute renal failure in pregnancy. Kidney Int 1980; 18:179–91.

212. Darwish R, Vaziri ND, Gupta S, Novey H, Spear GS, Licorish K et al. Focal renal cortical necrosis associated with zomepirac. Am J Med 1984; 76:1113–7.

213. Amaral CFS, Da Silva OA, Godoy P and Miranda D. Renal cortical necrosis following Bothrops Jararaca and B. Jararacussu snake bite. Toxicon 1985; 23:877–85.

214. Schneider PD. Nonsteroidal anti-inflammatory drugs and acute cortical necrosis. Ann Intern Med 1986; 105:303–4.

215. Wells JD, Gordon Margolin E and Gall EA. Renal cortical necrosis. Am J Med 1960; 29:257–67.

216. Deutsch V, Frankl O, Drory Y, Eliahou H and Braf ZF. Bilateral renal cortical necrosis with survival through the acute phase with a note on the value of selective nephroangiography. Am J Med 1971; 50:828–33.

217. Goergen TG, Lindstrom RR, Tan H and Lilley JJ. CT appearance of acute renal cortical necrosis. AJR 1981; 137:176–7.

218. Cohen AH. Renal pathology forum. Am J Nephrol 1985; 5:305–11.

219. Whelan JG Jr., Ling JT and Davis LA. Antemortem roentgen manifestations of bilateral renal cortical necrosis. Radiology 1967; 89:682–9.

220. Papo J, Peer G, Aviram A and Paizer R. Acute renal cortical necrosis as revealed by computerized tomography. Isr J Med Sci 1985; 21:862–3.

221. Jordan J, Low R and Jeffrey RB Jr. CT findings in acute renal cortical necrosis. J Computer Assisted Tomography 1990; 14:155–6.

222. Agarwal A, Sakhuja V, Malik N, Joshi K and Chugh KS. The diagnostic value of CT scan in acute renal cortical necrosis. Renal Failure 1992; 14:193–6.

223. Scoble JE, Maher ER, Hamilton G, Dick R, Sweny P and Moorhead JF. Atherosclerotic renovascular disease causing renal impairment – a case for treatment. Clin Nephrol 1989; 31:119–22.

224. Novick AC, Pohl MA, Schreiber M, Gifford RW Jr. and Vidt DG. Revascularization for preservation of renal function in patients with atherosclerotic renovascular disease. J Urol 1983; 129:907–12.

225. Madias NE, Ball JT and Millan VG. Percutaneous transluminal renal angioplasty in the treatment of unilateral atherosclerotic renovascular hypertension. Am J Med 1981; 70:1078–84.

226. De La Rocha AG, Zorn M and Downs AR. Acute renal failure as a consequence of sudden renal artery occlusion. Canad J Surg 1981; 24:218–22.

227. de Jong PE, van Bockel JH and de Zeeuw D. Unilateral renal parenchymal disease with contralateral renal artery stenosis of the fibrodysplasia type. Ann Intern Med 1989; 110:438–46.

228. Wasser WG, Krakoff LR, Haimov M, Glabman S and Mitty HA. Restoration of renal function after bilateral renal artery occlusion. Arch Intern Med 1981; 141:1647–51.

229. Madias NE, Kwon OJ and Millan VG. Percutaneous transluminal renal angioplasty. A potential effective treatment for preservation of renal function. Arch Intern Med 1983; 142:693–7.

230. Jones RE, Tribble CG, Tegtmeyer CJ, Craddock GB Jr. and Mentzer RM Jr. Bilateral renal artery embolism: a diagnostic and therapeutic problem. J Vasc Surg 1987; 5:479–82.

231. Tegtmeyer CJ, Elson J, Glass TA, Ayers CR, Chevalier RL, Wellons HA Jr. et al. Percutaneous transluminal angioplasty: the treatment of choice for renovascular hypertension due to fibromuscular dysplasia. Radiology 1982; 143:631–7.

232. Sheps SG, Kincaid OW and Hunt JC. Serial renal function and angiographic observations in idiopathic fibrous and fibromuscular stenoses of the renal arteries. Am J Cardiol. 1972; 30:55–60.

233. Mestres CA, Campistol JM, Ninot S, Botey A, Abad C, Guerola M et al. Improvement of renal function in azotaemic hypertensive patients after surgical revascularization. Br J Surg 1988; 75:578–80.

234. Weiss RA, Jodorkovsky R, Weiner S, Bennett B, Kogan S, Greifer I and Bernstein R. Chronic renal failure due to Takayasu's arteritis: recovery of renal function after nine

months of dialysis. Clin Nephrol 1982; 17:104–7.

235. Sawaya B, Provenzano R, Kupin WL and Venkat KK. Cyclosporine-induced renal macroangiopathy. Am J Kidney Dis 1988; 12:534–7.

236. Rushton AR The genetics of fibromuscular dysplasia. Arch Intern Med 1980; 140:233–6.

237. Jacobson HR. Ischemic renal disease: an overlooked clinical entity? Kidney Int 1988; 34:729–43.

238. Besarab A, Brown RS, Rubin NT, Salzman E, Wirthlin L, Steinman T et al. Reversible renal failure following bilateral renal artery occlusive disease: clinical features, pathology, and the role of surgical revascularization. JAMA 1976; 235:2838–41.

239. Heaney D, Kupor LR, Noon GP and Suki WN. Bilateral renal artery stenosis causing acute oliguric renal failure. Arch Surg 1977; 112:641–3.

240. Kaylor WM, Novick AC, Ziegelbaum M and Vidt DG. Reversal of end stage renal failure with surgical revascularization in patients with atherosclerotic renal artery occlusion. J Urol 1989; 141:486–8.

241. May J, Ross Sheil AG, Horvath J, Tiller DJ and Johnson JR. Reversal of renal failure and control of hypertension in patients with occlusion of the renal artery. Surgery 1976; 143:411–13.

242. Libertino JA, Zinman L, Breslin DJ, Swinton NW Jr. and Legg MA. Renal artery revascularization. JAMA 1980; 244:1340–2.

243. Cohen EP and Elliott WC Jr. The role of ischemia in acquired cystic kidney disease. Am J Kidney Dis 1990; 15:55–60.

244. Bardram L, Helgstrand U, Bentzen MH, Hansen HJB and Engell HC. Late results after surgical treatment of renovascular hypertension. Ann Surg 1985; 201:219–24.

245. Grim CE, Luft FC, Yune HY, Klatte EC and Weinberger MH. Percutaneous transluminal dilatation in the treatment of renal vascular hypertension. Ann Intern Med 1981; 95:439–42.

246. Sos TA, Pickering TG, Phil D, Sniderman K, Saddekni S, Case DB et al. Percutaneous transluminal renal angioplasty in renovascular hypertension due to atheroma or fibromuscular dysplasia. N Engl J Med 1983; 309: 274–9.

247. Dean RH, Oates JA, Wilson JP, Rhamy RK, Hollifield JW, Burko H et al. Bilateral renal artery stenosis and renovascular hypertension. Surgery 1977; 81:53–62.

248. Simon N, Franklin SS, Bleifer KH and Maxwell MH. Clinical characteristics of renovascular hypertension. JAMA 1972; 220:1209–18.

249. Ying CY, Tifft CP, Gavras H and Chobanian AV. Renal revascularization in the azotemic hypertensive patient resistant to therapy. N Engl J Med 1984; 311:1070–5.

250. Messina LM, Zelenock GB, Yao KA and Stanley JC. Renal revascularization for recurrent pulmonary edema in patients with poorly controlled hypertension and renal insufficiency: a distinct subgroup of patients with arteriosclerotic renal artery occlusive disease. J Vasc Surg 1992; 15:73–82.

251. Diamond JR. Flash pulmonary edema and the diagnostic suspicion of occult renal artery stenosis. Am J Kidney Dis 1993; 21:328–30.

252. Remuzzi A, Schieppati A, Battaglia C and Remuzzi G. Angiotensin-converting enzyme inhibition ameliorates the defect in glomerular size selectivity in hyponatremic hypertensive syndrome. Am J Kidney Dis 1989; 14:170–7.

253. Steensma-Vegter AJ, Krediet RT, Westra D and Tegzess AM. Reversible stenosis of the renal artery in cadaver kidney grafts: a report of three cases. Clin Nephrol 1981; 15:102–6.

254. Textor SC, Novick AC, Tarazi RC, Klimas V, Vidt DG and Pohl M. Critical perfusion pressure for renal function in patients with bilateral atherosclerotic renal vascular disease. Ann Intern Med 1985;102:308–14.

255. Gerlock AJ Jr., MacDonell RC Jr., Smith CW, Muhletaler CA, Parris WCV, Johnson HK et al. Renal transplant arterial stenosis: Percutaneous transluminal angioplasty. AJR 1983; 140:325–31.

256. Muller FB, Sealey JE, Case DB, Atlas SA, Pickering TG, Pecker MS et al. The captopril test for identifying renovascular disease in hypertensive patients. Am J Med 1986; 80:633–44.

257. Morris GC, Jr., DeBakey ME and Cooley DA. Surgical treatment of renal failure of renovascular origin. JAMA 1962; 182:609–12.

258. Mann SJ, Pickering TG, Sos TA, RG Uzzo, S Sarkar, K Friend et al. Captopril renography in the diagnosis of renal artery stenosis: accuracy and limitations. Am J Med 1991; 90:30–40.

259. Carmichael DJS, Mathias CJ, Snell ME and Peart S. Detection and investigation of renal artery stenosis. Lancet 1986; 1:667–70.

260. Kaufman JJ. Renovascular hypertension: the UCLA experience. J Urol. 1979; 121:139–44.

261. Zinman L and Libertino JA. Revascularization of the chronic totally occluded renal artery with restoration of renal function. J Urol 1977; 118:517–21.

262. Schefft P, Novick AC, Stewart BH and Straffon RA. Renal revascularization in patients with total occlusion of the renal artery. J Urol 1980; 124:184–6.

263. Mercier C, Piquet P, Alimi Y, Tournigand P and Albrand J-J. Occlusive disease of the renal arteries and chronic renal failure: the limits of reconstructive surgery. Ann Vasc Surg 1990; 4:166–70.

264. Setaro JF, Saddler MC, Chen CC, Hoffer PB, Roer DA, Markowitz DM et al. Simplified captopril renography in diagnosis and treatment of renal artery stenosis. Hypertension 1991; 18:289–98.

265. Postma CT, van Oijen AHAM, Barentsz JO, de Boo T, Hoefnagels WHL, Corstens FHM et al. The value of tests predicting renovascular hypertension in patients with renal artery stenosis treated by angioplasty. Arch Intern Med 1991; 151:1531–5.

266. Erbsloh-Moller B, Dumas A, Roth D, Sfakianakis GN and Bourgoignie JJ. Furosemide-^{131}I-hippuran renography after angiotensin-converting enzyme inhibition for the diagnosis of renovascular hypertension. Am J Med 1991; 90:23–40.

267. Distler A and Spies K-P. Diagnostic procedure in renovascular hypertension. Clin Nephrol 1991; 36:174–80.

268. Hoffmann U, Edwards JM, Carter S, Goldman ML, Harley JD, Zaccardi MJ et al. Role of duplex scanning for the detection of atherosclerotic renal artery disease. Kidney Int 1991; 39:1232–9.

269. Middleton WD. Doppler US evaluation of renal artery stenosis: past, present, and future. Radiology 1992; 184:307–8.

270. Kliewer MA, Tupler RH, Carroll BA, Paine SS, Kriegshauser JS, Hertzberg BS et al. Renal artery stenosis: analysis of Doppler waveform parameters and tardus-parvus pattern. Radiology 1993; 189:779–87.

271. Farrugia E, King BF and Larson TS. Magnetic resonance angiography and detection of renal artery stenosis in a patient with impaired renal function. Mayo Clin Proc 1993; 68:157–60.

272. Postma CT, Hartog O, Rosenbusch G and Thien T. Magnetic resonance angiography in the diagnosis of renal artery stenosis. J Hypertension 1993; 11:S204–S205.

273. Galanski M, Prokop M, Chavan A, Schaefer CM, Jandeleit K and Nischelsky JE. Renal arterial stenoses: spiral CT angiography. Radiology 1993; 189:185–92.

274. Rubin GD, Dake MD, Napel S, Jeffrey RB Jr., McDonnell CH, Sommer FG et al. Spiral CT of renal artery stenosis: comparison of three-dimensional rendering techniques. Radiology 1994; 190:181–9.

275. Roche Z, Rutecki G, Cox J and Whittier FC. Reversible acute renal failure as an atypical presentation of ischemic nephropathy. Am J Kidney Dis 1993; 22:662–7.

276. Zucchelli P, Fabbri L, Cagnoli L, Grimaldi C, Pavlica P and Losinno F. Acute renal failure due to renal artery occlusion. In: Eliahou HE, editor. Acute renal failure. John Libbey & Company Limited, London, 1982:152–5.

277. Lessman RK, Johnson SF, Coburn JW and Kaufman JJ. Renal artery embolism: clinical features and long term follow-up of 17 cases. Ann Intern Med 1978; 89:477–82.

278. Mignon F, Meyrier A, Cuvelier R, Morel-Maroger L and Dewilde J. Reno-vascular complications of left atrial myxoma: report of two patients. Kidney Int 1982; 22:327.

279. Gill TJ and Dammin GJ. Paradoxical embolism with renal failure caused by occlusion of the renal arteries. Am J Med 1958; 25:780–7.

280. Gewertz BL, Stanley JC and Fry WJ. Renal artery dissections. Arch Surg 1977; 112:409–14.

281. Hasday JD, Sterns RH and Karch FE. Renal infarction due to renal artery dysplasia with dissection. Am J Med 1984; 76:943–6.

282. Hirst AE Jr., Johns VJ Jr. and Kime SW Jr. Dissecting aneurysm of the aorta: a review of 505 cases. Medicine 1958; 37:217–79.

283. Hoover LA, Hall-Craggs M and Dagher FJ. Polyarteritis nodosa involving only the main renal arteries. Am J Kidney Dis 1988; 11:66–9.

284. Templeton PA and Pais SO. Renal artery occlusion in PAN. Radiology 1985; 156:308.

285. Elling H and Kristensen IB. Fatal renal failure in polymyalgia rheumatica caused by disseminated giant cell arteritis. Scand J Rheumatol 1980; 9:206–8.

286. Fogel RI, Endreny RG, Cronan JJ and Chazan JA. Acute renal failure with anuria caused by aortic thrombosis and bilateral renal artery occlusion. A report of two cases. RI Med J 1987; 70:501–4.

287. Cosby RL, Miller PD and Schrier RW. Traumatic renal artery thrombosis. Am J Med 1986; 81:890–4.

288. DiPrete DA, Abuelo JG, Abuelo DN and Cronan JJ. Acute renal failure due to renal infarctions in a patient with neurofibromatosis. Am J Kidney Dis 1990; 15:357–60.

289. Bello Nicolau I, Conde Zurita JM, Barrientos Guzman A, Gutierrez Millet V, Ruilope Urioste LM, Prieto Carles C et al. Essential thrombocytosis with acute renal failure due to bilateral thrombosis of the renal arteries and veins. Nephron 1982; 32:73–4.

290. Ames PRJ, Cianciaruso B, Bellizzi V, Balletta M, Lubrano E, Scarpa R et al. Bilateral renal artery occlusion in a patient with primary antiphospholipid antibody syndrome: thrombosis, vasculitis or both? J Rheumatol 1992; 19:1802–6.

291. Franklin SS, Young JD Jr., Maxwell MH, Foster JH, Palmer JM, Cerny J et al. Operative morbidity and mortality in renovascular disease. JAMA 1975; 231:1148–53.

292. Johansen K, Voci V, Cohen D and Fleet P. Acute bilateral renal artery occlusion. Arch Surg 1981; 116:1232–5.

293. Lacombe M and Couffinhal J-C. Thromboses aigues de l'artere renale apres angiographie abdominale. La Nouv Presse med 1978; 7:3333–6.

294. Kuhlmann U, Greminger P, Gruntzig A, Schneider E, Pouliadis G, Luscher T et al. Long-term experience in percutaneous transluminal dilatation of renal artery stenosis. Am J Med 1985; 79:692–8.

295. Mahler F, Triller J, Weidmann P and Nachbur B. Complications in percutaneous transluminal dilatation of renal arteries. Nephron 1986; 44:60–3.

296. Baciewicz B. Bilateral renal artery thrombotic occlusion – a unique complication following removal of a transthoracic intraaortic balloon. Ann Thoracic Surg 1982; 33:631–4.

297. Scully RE, Mark EJ, McNeely WF and McNeely BU. Case records of the Massachusetts General Hospital, Case 39-1987. N Engl J Med 1987; 317:819–28.

298. Asherson RA, Buchanan N, Baguley E and Hughes GRV. Postpartum bilateral renal vein thrombosis in the primary antiphospholipid syndrome. J Rheumatol 1993; 20:874–6.

299. Ricci MA and Lloyd DA. Renal venous thrombosis in infants and children. Arch Surg 1990; 125:1195–9.

300. Pontremoli R, Rampoldi V, Morbidelli A, Fiorini F, Ranise A and Garibotto G. Acute renal failure due to acute bilateral renal artery thrombosis: successful surgical revascularization after prolonged anuria. Nephron 1990; 56:322–4.

301. O'Donohoe MK, Donohoe J and Corrigan TP. Acute renal failure of renovascular origin: cure by aortorenal reconstruction after 25 days of anuria. Nephron 1990; 56:92–3.

302. Ewald EA, Griffin D and McCune J. Correlation of angiographic abnormalities with disease manifestations and disease severity in polyarteritis nodosa. J Rheumatol 1987; 14:952–6.

303. Travers RL, Allison DJ, Brettle RP and Hughes GRV.

Polyarteritis nodosa: a clinical and angiographic analysis of 17 cases. Sem in Arth Rheum 1979; 8:184–99.

304. Llach F and Papper S. The clinical spectrum of renal vein thrombosis: Acute and chronic. Am J Med 1980; 69:819–27.

305. Wagoner RD, Stanson AW, Holley KE and Winter CS. Renal vein thrombosis in idiopathic membranous glomerulopathy and nephrotic syndrome: incidence and significance. Kidney Int 1983; 23:368–74.

306. Trew PA, Biava CG, Jacobs RP and Hopper J Jr. Renal vein thrombosis in membranous glomerulonephropathy: Incidence and association. Medicine 1978; 57:69–82.

307. Schwartz MM and Lewis EJ. Immunopathology of the nephrotic syndrome associated with renal vein thrombosis. Am J Med 1973; 54:528–34.

308. Burrow CR, Walker WG, Bell WR and Gatewood OB. Streptokinase salvage of renal function after renal vein thrombosis. Ann Intern Med 1984; 100:237–8.

309. Rowe JM, Rasmussen RL, Mader SL, Dimarco PL, Cockett ATK and Marder VJ. Successful thrombolytic therapy in two patients with renal vein thrombosis. Am J Med 1984; 77:1111–4.

310. Vogelzang RL, Moel DI, Cohn RA, Donaldson JS, Langman CB and Nemcek AA. Acute renal vein thrombosis: successful treatment with intraarterial urokinase. Radiology 1988; 169:681–2.

311. Gasparini M, Hofmann R and Stoller M. Renal artery embolism: clinical features and therapeutic options. J Urol 1992; 147:567–72.

312. Ouriel K, Andrus CH, Ricotta JJ, DeWeese JA and Green RM. Acute renal artery occlusion: when is revascularization justified? J Vasc Surg 1987; 5:348–55.

313. Choyke PL and Pollack HM. The role of MRI in diseases of the kidney. Radiol Clin N Amer 1988; 26:617–31.

11. Glomerular causes of renal failure

J. GARY ABUELO

INTRODUCTION

Glomerulopathies cause about 10% of cases of acute renal failure due to intrinsic renal diseases (Table 2.2), and are the most common etiology of chronic renal failure [1, 2].

Classification

Glomerular causes of renal failure fall into two categories:

(1) *Acute nephritic diseases*, like poststreptococcal glomerulonephritis (GN), are characterized by hematuria, proteinuria and acute or subacute renal failure.

(2) *Nephrotic diseases* are characterized by heavy proteinuria, and usually present with normal or near normal Scr. Worsening renal function may be observed when the underlying disease pursues a rapidly destructive course, as with HIV nephropathy, or when a sequela of the nephrotic pathophysiology itself, such as renal vein thrombosis, impairs GFR.

The glomerular diseases are subclassified as to whether they are *primary* renal diseases, i.e. only the kidneys are involved, or are *secondary* diseases, i.e. a component of a multisystem disorder like polyarteritis nodosa. Most primary glomerular diseases are idiopathic, and probably immune-mediated. The diseases may be further characterized by etiology and histology. Examples of glomerular causes of renal failure are shown on Table 11.1.

Table 11.1. Examples of glomerular causes of renal failure

Disease	Etiology	Histology	1°/2°
Acute nephritic disease			
Idiopathic crescentic GN	Idiopathic	NCGN	1°
GN of endocarditis	Bacterial infection	FPGN	2°
Nephrotic diseases			
Rapid progression of FSGS	Idiopathic	Advanced FSGS	1°
Renal vein thrombosis complicating diabetic nephropathy	Diabetes mellitus	Diabetic nephropathy	2°

FPGN – focal proliferative GN, FSGS – focal segmental glomerulosclerosis, NCGN – necrotizing and crescentic GN, 1°/2° – primary or secondary glomerulopathy.

ACUTE NEPHRITIC DISEASES

Definition

The *acute nephritic syndrome* refers to the clinical picture of hematuria, proteinuria and variable hypervolemia and renal impairment typically seen in acute glomerulonephritis.

The acute nephritic syndrome should not be confused with the *nephrotic syndrome*, which is *heavy proteinuria* (greater than 3g/day) that leads to *hypoalbuminemia* (less than 3 g/dl) and *edema*. Hematuria may or may not be present in the nephrotic syndrome, and acute renal failure is rare, but it does occur as discussed later in this chapter.

The pathophysiologic processes in the acute nephritic and the nephrotic syndromes are different. In the acute nephritic syndrome arteriolar vasoconstriction reduces blood flow, while glomerular damage reduces glomerular capillary permeability and filtering surface area, thereby decreasing GFR. The damaged glomerular capillaries probably also develop holes that are the source of the hematuria. In contrast, in the nephrotic syndrome glomerular capillary

J.G. Abuelo (ed.), Renal Failure, 93–116.
© 1995 *Kluwer Academic Publishers.*

damage may cause little or no hematuria, but diffusely increases permeability to macromolecules, and allows massive loss of albumin and other plasma proteins into the urine. GFR is usually preserved initially, although it may progressively decline in chronic nephrotic diseases.

The specific conditions that produce the acute nephritic and nephrotic syndromes are also different as can be seen by comparing Tables 11.2 and 11.12. However, when severe, all the nephritic diseases may cause the nephrotic syndrome; membranoproliferative GN and lupus nephritis are particularly likely to produce both syndromes simultaneously.

Causes

The various types of acute nephritic diseases are shown in detail on Table 11.2. The most common primary acute nephritic disease is idiopathic crescentic glomerulonephritis, while the leading secondary nephritic diseases are lupus nephritis, polyarteritis nodosa and Wegener's granulomatosis [41a–41c].

Primary Glomerular Diseases

Pathology

The primary acute nephritic diseases have some differences in clinical presentation, but are mainly distinguished by their histologic appearance.

Idiopathic Crescentic GN. This is characterized by the presence of crescent shaped masses of cells in Bowman's space in more than 30–50% of the glomeruli. These "crescents" initially contain monocytes and glomerular epithelial cells, but with time become less cellular and more fibrous (Figure 11.1). The glomerular tufts themselves may appear normal or may have cellular proliferation or necrosis, for which the term *necrotizing and crescentic GN* may be used. By immunofluorescent staining for IgG and C3, cases of crescentic GN are subcategorized as having a linear capillary pattern associated with anti-glomerular basement membrane (GBM) antibodies (type I), a granular pattern associated with circulating immune complexes (type II) or minimal or negative staining, so-called *pauci-immune GN*, associated with anti-neutrophil cytoplasmic antibodies (ANCA) (type III).

IgA Nephropathy or *Berger's Disease.* This is characterized by mesangial immune complex deposits with IgA as the predominant immunoglobulin. Mesangial cellularity and matrix are variably increased. Crescents may occur in more damaged glomeruli.

Membranoproliferative GN. This is also known as mesangiocapillary GN. It is characterized by mesangial hypercellularity, thickening of the capillary wall by subendothelial infiltration of mesangial matrix and cells, and by deposition of C3 and sometimes immunoglobulins along the capillary wall and in the mesangium. The circumferential deposition of mesangial matrix produces an apparent duplication of the capillary wall, known as a double contour, tram track or splitting. The type I variant has subendothelial electron dense (immune complex) deposits, while the type II variant, *dense deposit disease*, has sausage-shaped or fusiform deposits within the basement membrane of the glomerular capillaries, tubules and Bowman's capsule.

Clinical Picture

Renal Manifestations. The clinical picture of primary GN is mainly that of the acute nephritic syndrome. In contrast, patients with secondary GN also have signs and symptoms of their underlying disorder, such as fever and murmur in bacterial endocarditis.

The acute nephritic syndrome classically presents with gross hematuria, oliguria, anuria, flank pain [42–45], or hypervolemia, which may be severe enough to produce acute pulmonary edema or malignant hypertension. Less often patients come to the physician when uremic symptoms develop (e.g. fatigability and anorexia) or when an unrelated medical problem leads to the discovery of microscopic hematuria or an increased Scr. The physical examination is normal in some patients, and in others shows hypertension and peripheral edema. Hypervolemia is more common in poststreptococcal GN (85% of cases) [42] and less common in idiopathic crescentic GN (0–33% of cases) [46–48]. Patients who also have nephrotic syndrome may have marked edema. Scr can rise rapidly from one day to the next or gradually from one week or month to the next. Urine output may be normal initially, but can decrease or stop over several days. Hematuria, either microscopic or gross, is present in all cases, although rarely it is intermittent [49]. Gross hematuria does not necessarily signify severe damage; IgA nephropathy is noted for episodes of gross hematuria despite normal GFR. Red cell casts are a common, but not a universal finding. Proteinuria is usually moderate (1 to 2+; 30 to 100 mg/dL; 1 to 3 g/day), but may be in the nephrotic range (3 to 4+; 300 to 1000 mg/dL; greater than 3 g/day) or in rare cases *may be absent.* Slight pyuria is not unusual.

Extrarenal Manifestations. These often occur in primary GN, but tend to be non-specific. The underlying immunologic mechanism is triggered by

Table 11.2. Glomerular causes of an acute nephritic picture

Disease	Etiology	Histology*
Primary glomerular disease		
Idiopathic crescentic GN	Idiopathic	NCGN
IgA Nephropathy (Berger's Disease)	Idiopathic	DPGN + lgA mesangial deposits
Membranoproliferative GN	Idiopathic	MPGN
Secondary glomerular disease		
GN Associated with infection		
Streptococcal pharyngitis or pyoderma [3]	Group A streptococcus	DPGN
Bacterial endocarditis [4]	*S. aureus, S.viridans, and others*	FPGN or DPGN
Visceral abscesses [5]	*S.aureus, P. aeruginosa, and others*	FPGN or MPGN + crescents
Ventriculo-atrial shunts [6]	*S. albus and others*	DPGN or MPGN
Other infections (rare)	Variety of bacteria, viruses, fungi and parasites [6]	various lesions
GN associated with collagen or autoimmune disease		
Systemic lupus erythematosus	Idiopathic	FPGN, DPGN
Polyarteritis nodosa	Usually idiopathic, rare: allergic hyposensitization [7], hepatitis B [8], otitis media [9], streptococcus [10], silicosis [11], sulfa [12, 13], penicillin [14], neoplasm [15]	NCGN
Wegener's granulomatosis	Idiopathic	NCGN
Henoch-Schonlein purpura [16]	Idiopathic	NCGN + lgA mesangial deposits
Essential mixed cryoglobulinemia [17]	Hepatitis C virus	DPGN or MPGN
Goodpasture's syndrome	Usually idiopathic; rare: influenza A [18], hydrocarbons [19, 20]	NCGN, linear IgG by IF
Mixed connective tissue disease [21, 22]	Idiopathic	Various lesions
Churg-Strauss syndrome [23]	Idiopathic	Various lesions
Hypocomplementemic vasculitis [24, 25]	Idiopathic	Various lesions
Temporal arteritis [26–28]	Idiopathic	Various lesions
Takayasu's arteritis [29]	Idiopathic	Various lesions
Behcet's disease [30]	Idiopathic	Various lesions
Sarcoidosis [31, 32]	Idiopathic	Various lesions
GN associated with malignancy		
Lymphoma [33, 34]	Idopathic	NCGN
Angioimmunoblastic lymphadenopathy [35, 36]	idiopathic	MPGN
Monoclonal gammopathy [37, 38]	Idiopathic	DPGN or NCGN
Cancer [37, 39]	Idiopathic	NCGN
Cirrhosis [40, 41]	Alcohol	MPGN + lgA mesangial deposits

* DPGN – diffuse proliferative GN, FPGN – focal proliferative GN, MPGN – membranoproliferative GN, NCGN – necrotizing and crescentic GN.

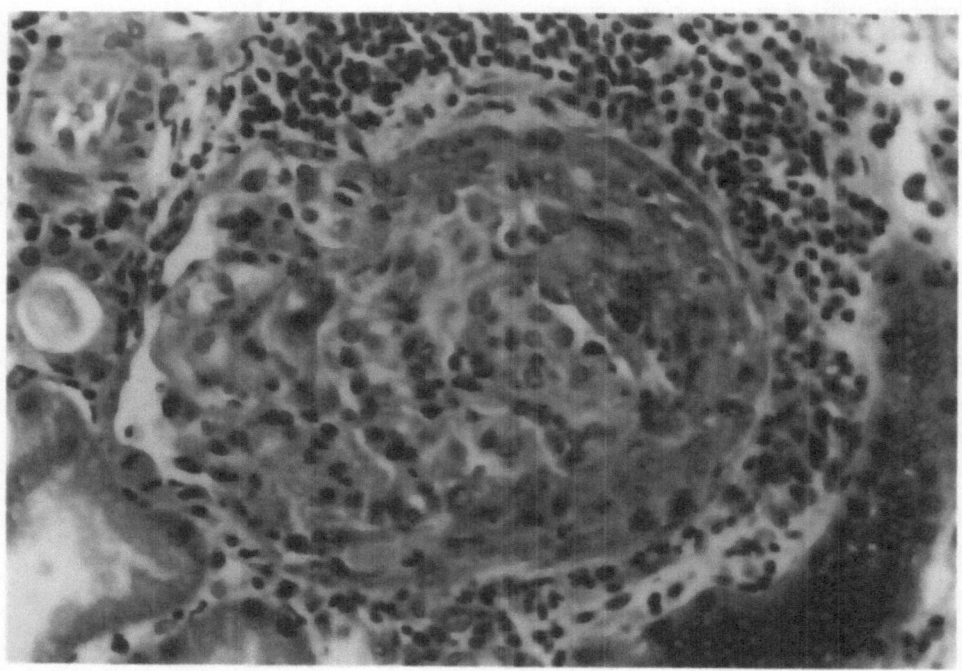

Fig. 11.1. Renal biopsy from a patient with idiopathic crescentic GN. Note the large cellular crescent and collapsed glomerular tuft. There is a red blood cell cast in the tubule at the lower right hand corner. (Courtesy of Dr. Alfredo Esparza.)

a viral infection in some patients, who report prodromal sore throats and other viral symptoms. Also, this immunologic mechanism may produce vasculitis-like symptoms such as malaise, fever, rash and arthralgias. Investigation of extrarenal symptoms is of little help in diagnosis.

Idiopathic Crescentic GN. This can occur at any age, but is most common between ages 30 and 60 [50], and exhibits a slight male predominance [51–55]. Exposure to hydrocarbons or penicillamine administration plays a causative role in some patients [51–57]. A rash or constitutional or joint symptoms may suggest an underlying collagen vascular disease, but subsequent development of a specific disorder is rare [52, 53, 55, 58, 59].

Patients often have viral-like or "flu-like" prodrome consisting of fever, myalgias, malaise, sore throat and upper respiratory symptoms [51–55, 58, 60, 61]. Anemia [52, 60, 62] and an elevated erythrocyte sedimentation rate [60] are common; C3 or CH50 serum complement levels are occasionally depressed [52, 55, 60, 63]. Most patients have *anti-neutrophil cytoplasmic antibodies (ANCA)* present [64, 65].

IgA Nephropathy (Berger's Disease). This is the most common type of GN; it usually presents as either asymptomatic microscopic hematuria with proteinuria or episodes of gross hematuria that are often triggered by upper respiratory infections and last several hours to days [66]. Renal failure is

not observed in most patients with IgA nephropathy, but can occur: *chronic* renal failure in 20% or more of cases [66], *subacute* renal failure in about 5% of cases and *transient* acute renal failure in about 10% of cases [67–74].

Patients with a *subacute* nephritic picture range in age from 7 to 60 years and are predominantly male. A long history of asymptomatic urinary abnormalities may precede the renal failure, and fever and upper respiratory infections may trigger the nephritic episode. Hypertension and the nephrotic syndrome are common. There is usually no response to therapy and progression to end-stage renal disease occurs over a few months to years [74, 75].

Patients with *transient* acute renal failure, are predominantly male [70, 73, 75a] and range in age from 6 to 71 years [70, 72]. Typically Scr rises during an episode of gross hematuria, peaks after 3 to 10 days [75a] and decreases over a few weeks to several months [70, 72, 75a]. A prodrome of pharyngitis is usually observed [68, 75a] and flank pain may be a prominent complaint [43]. Dialysis is occasionally **necessary [43, 70]. Recurrent episodes of gross hematuria** and acute renal failure have been reported in some patients [70, 75a]. Recent studies suggest that the renal failure results from tubular damage and obstruction by red cell casts [75a, 75b].

Membranoproliferative (or Mesangiocapillary) GN. This disease occurs equally in both sexes and affects individuals of all ages with a peak prevalence in adolescence [44, 76–83]. Patients most commonly come to medical attention with nephrotic syndrome, but the disease may also present with recurrent gross hematuria or asymptomatic proteinuria and hematuria. About one third of patients have an upper respiratory infection or sore throat either before or at the time of presentation [76, 82–84]; some of these cases have evidence of a streptococcal infection [82, 84]. Other infections, non-specific febrile illness, rash and flank pain are occasionally present [44, 45, 76, 82, 84]. Some cases have hepatitis C virus infection with or without mildly elevated aminotransferase levels [85, 86]. The type II or dense deposit disease form may be associated with partial lipodystrophy, a rare condition characterized by loss of fat from the face, arms and trunk [76, 81, 83, 87].

Profound anemia has been reported in some cases [84, 88]. The serum C3 concentration is commonly decreased, while C4 concentrations are low in rare cases [77, 78, 81, 84, 88, 89].

About a third of patients have an increased Scr at initial presentation [77–81]. This usually reflects a chronic process that goes on to severe renal failure, but sometimes an *acute nephritic picture* is responsible for the azotemia [76–79, 81]. This acute renal failure may be transient or progressive [44, 45, 84].

Diagnosis
The investigation for an acute nephritic cause of renal failure starts when the urinalysis shows proteinuria and hematuria. Acute nephritis should also be considered in the patient who presents with anuria and has no urine for analysis. A primary GN is suggested by non-specific or no extrarenal manifestations, and can only be diagnosed by renal biopsy. The physician should quantitate the protein excretion with a 24-hour urine for protein or a random urine protein to creatinine ratio, and should obtain serum complement levels (CH50, C3 and C4), and antineutrophil cytoplasmic antibodies (ANCA). Antinuclear antibodies (ANA), antiglomerular basement membrane (GBM) antibodies, and antistreptococcal antibodies are not economical in the absence of specific clinical clues. They may be obtained later if indicated by renal biopsy findings. A renal sonogram should be ordered to exclude urinary obstruction and confirm normal renal anatomy. If two normal size kidneys are present, and if screening for a bleeding diathesis is negative, a percutaneous renal biopsy should be performed to determine the type of GN and the severity of acute and chronic changes.

Pitfalls. Renal failure associated with hematuria and proteinuria can result from renal diseases other than GN. Most cases of *small vessel diseases*, *renal infarction*, *acute tubular necrosis* and *acute interstitial nephritis* should be suspected

from the clinical picture, and may be confirmed as outlined in Chapters 11, 12 and 13. Red cell casts, proteinuria over 2.5 g/d and gross hematuria or greater than 100 red cells per high power field typify glomerulopathies. These "nephritic" urinary findings are evidence against tubular or interstitial disease, but can also be seen in renal infarction and most of the small vessel diseases.

The rare absence of proteinuria or intermittence of hematuria in cases of acute nephritic diseases must be kept in mind. In patients without proteinuria other clues, such as hematuria with red cell casts, usually point to the diagnosis.

Secondary Glomerular Diseases

The extrarenal manifestations of these secondary conditions are often specific enough to permit the physician to make a diagnosis on clinical grounds alone. Thus, a renal biopsy may not be necessary to identify the type of GN, although it may help by indicating its severity or reversibility.

Poststreptococcal GN
This disease is the result of glomerular deposition of streptococcal antigens, antibodies and complement.

Pathology. Poststreptococcal GN is characterized histologically by diffuse proliferation of mesangial and endothelial cells. An exudative stage with variable infiltration by polymorphonuclear and mononuclear leukocytes occurs in the first two to three weeks of disease. Immune complexes containing IgG and complement deposit along the capillary wall and in the mesangium. They take on the characteristic appearance of a *hump* when located subepithelially.

Clinical Picture. Although poststreptococcal GN is mainly seen in children between 2 and 10 years of age, cases occur up to the ninth decade of life [90, 91]. Poststreptococcal GN typically follows a pharyngitis caused by certain *nephritogenic* strains of group A streptococcus [90, 92]. It may also complicate streptococcal pyoderma (*impetigo*), which occurs more often in the summer and early fall, and in the tropics [90, 93–97].'

Occasional patients with poststreptococcal GN have an asymptomatic infection only evidenced by a serological response [96, 98]. Rarely, GN may complicate streptococcal infections that involve other organs (e.g. otitis, pneumonia) or that involve other streptococcal groups (C or G) [93, 98, 99, 100]. Most cases of GN are sporadic, but epidemics of poststreptococcal GN may occur in communities with poor hygiene [93, 101]. The risk of GN after a streptococcal infection with a nephritogenic strain is 5 to 25% [90, 94], and is probably not reduced by antibiotic treatment of the infection [102, 103]. The occurrence of azotemia in poststreptococcal GN is about 60% [96, 104, 105].

A latent period of one to three weeks usually passes between the streptococcal infection and the onset of GN; by this time most patients no longer have an active infection and cultures are often negative [95–97]. However, 95% of patients have antibodies to at least one of five streptococcal enzymes [90, 95] (Table 11.3). Antistreptolysin O titers increase in two-thirds of throat infections, but less often after skin infections [90, 93, 94, 96, 105].

Serum total hemolytic complement (CH50) and C3 levels are low for two weeks after the onset of GN in over 90% of cases, but they return to normal over several weeks [90, 93, 95, 96, 98]. Concentrations of C4 and other early components are usually normal [93]. The erythrocyte sedimentation rate (ESR) is typically increased and may be greater than 100 mm/h [90]. Cryoglobulins may be present [42, 106, 107].

Diagnosis
For poststreptococcal GN the key clinical clues are the recent pharyngitis or impetigo, and the 1 to 3 week latent period. One should obtain serum complement levels, cultures of the throat or skin lesions, and order a combined antibody assay, the streptozyme test, or antibody titers against as many steptococcal enzymes as possible. The diagnosis is made by a compatible clinical picture, serologic or culture evidence of a streptococcal infection, low complement levels, and renal function that begins to improve in a few days and returns to normal by 2 weeks. If any of these elements is atypical, a renal biopsy is indicated.

Table 11.3. Serologic response in poststreptococcal GN [90]

Antibody to:	Pharyngitis	Pyoderma
Streptolysin O	+	+/−
DNAase B	+	+
NADase	+	+/−
Hyaluronidase	+	+
Streptokinase	+/−	+/−

GN due to bacterial endocarditis

Clinical Picture. This condition is a result of glomerular deposition of bacterial antigen, antibody and complement. Urinary abnormalities occur in half of endocarditis cases and some develop renal failure [108, 109].

Initially, the manifestations of the infected heart valves predominate over the renal manifestations. The hallmarks of bacterial endocarditis are fever and cardiac murmurs, although in rare cases the fever is absent or the murmur develops late. Patients typically have a history of valve disease, valve replacement or intravenous drug abuse. Ruptured cordae tendineae or perforated valves may produce congestive heart failure, and pericarditis is sometimes observed.

Acute bacterial endocarditis is caused by *S. aureus* or other invasive organisms. It frequently occurs in intravenous drug addicts, typically involves normal heart valves, and is characterized by new or changing murmurs. It presents with chills, high fever, myalgias and often back pain, and runs a fulminant course. Focal abscesses may occur in the lungs, brain and other sites.

Subacute bacterial endocarditis is caused by *S. viridans* and other less virulent organisms. It affects abnormal valves, begins with insidious symptoms and runs a long course. Extracardiac manifestations predominate initially with malaise, fatigue, anorexia, night sweats and intermittent fever going on for weeks or months. Myalgias, arthralgias and arthritis are often present and may mimic a rheumatologic disorder. Emboli may produce a stroke, myocardial or pulmonary infarction or sudden pain from embolization to an abdominal organ. Mycotic aneurysms sometimes rupture and cause hemorrhage in the brain or elsewhere. Rare cases present with gross hematuria or uremic symptoms [110].

Physical examination will reveal fever and one or more murmurs. Congestive heart failure, splenomegaly, splinter hemorrhages under the distal third of the nails and mucocutaneous petechiae of the mouth, conjunctivae or upper chest are frequent physical findings. Less often the patient has a purpuric rash, Roth's spots (retinae), Osler's nodes (painful nodules on pulp of fingers), Janeway's lesions (palms and soles) or clubbing [111].

Typical laboratory findings include anemia, leukocytosis, raised ESR and the *sine qua non*, positive blood cultures.

Blood cultures usually reveal *S. aureus* or a relatively avirulent streptococcus. In occasional cases other bacteria may be responsible [109]. Antibiotic therapy or fastidious organisms may cause negative or delayed growth in blood cultures.

Most patients with GN associated with bacterial endocarditis have cryoglobulinemia and low CH50 or C3. Rheumatoid factor is present in half of patients, as is depression of C1q and C4 [108, 111]. Thrombocytopenia has been described [111].

Diagnosis
The main clues to GN due to bacterial endocarditis are fever and a heart murmur. The diagnosis of bacterial endocarditis depends on a positive blood culture. Three cultures of 10 to 20 ml of blood should be drawn on the first day. If there is no growth after 24 hours, three further cultures should be ordered. If the patient is taking an antibiotic, it should be stopped and additional blood cultures sent during the next several days. The cultures need to be incubated for at least three weeks. The detection of vegetations on echocardiography supports the diagnosis.

Blood specimens should be sent for ESR, rheumatoid factor and complement levels. The physician may attribute azotemia to a secondary GN in patients with bacterial endocarditis, if the urinalysis reflects an acute nephritic picture and if the complement levels are depressed. A fall in Scr with response of the infection to antibiotic treatment supports the diagnosis. A worsening of Scr despite resolution of the infection or any atypical features should make the physician consider other diagnoses and a renal biopsy.

Pitfalls. Causes of renal failure other than GN may be seen in the setting of bacterial endocarditis. Nephrotoxic acute tubular necrosis, especially from aminoglycosides, allergic interstitial nephritis from other antibiotics, ischemic acute tubular necrosis from sepsis, and pre-renal azotemia from cardiogenic shock are examples.

GN due to visceral abscesses [6, 112]

This rare immune complex GN is a complication of pyogenic infections in the thorax, abdomen or other locations caused by *S. aureus* or one of the gram-negative bacteria. The duration of the infection at the onset of GN ranges from one week to over a year. Patients typically are febrile and appear critically ill. Blood cultures may or may not be positive. Most patients have cryoglobulins; some have depressed CH50 and C3.

GN due to infected ventriculoatrial shunts

On rare occasion an immune complex GN with renal failure can complicate infections of these shunts, which were used in the past to treat hydrocephalus [113, 114]. Infections of the ventriculo*peritoneal* shunts now employed may cause a mild GN, but not azotemia [113, 115]. Since some patients still have ventriculoatrial shunts and since infections complicated by secondary GN may occur years after shunt placement, this cause of renal failure is still observed [116]. A variety of bacteria may be responsible, but *S. epidermitis* is found in over 70% of cases on blood or spinal fluid culture. The typical patient is a child or young adult with fever, anemia and hepatosplenomegaly. Malaise, lethargy, anorexia, nausea and vomiting are common and purpura, skin rash and arthralgia may occur. In addition to manifestations of the nephritic syndrome and a positive culture of the organism, laboratory studies usually show cryoglobulins, depressed C3 and C4, and an elevated ESR [114].

Lupus nephritis
Renal disease is one of the common complications of systemic lupus erythematosis (SLE) and is a major cause of morbidity and mortality [117].

Pathology. Lupus nephritis is an immune complex disease, which always manifests electron dense deposits on electron microscopy, and IgG, C3 and usually other immunoglobulin and complement components on immunofluorescent microscopy. It may have several pathologic appearances. In *mesangial* GN there are mesangial immune complex deposits and sometimes mesangial hypercellularity, but azotemia is rare (Table 11.4).

Membranous GN has uniform thickening of the capillary walls due to subepithelial immune deposits. Slight mesangial hypercellularity may be seen. In *focal proliferative* GN, 50 percent or less of the glomeruli have subendothelial immune complex deposits, hypercellularity and often segmental necrosis. These two forms occasionally produce azotemia.

The most common form of lupus nephritis in patients with azotemia is *diffuse proliferative* GN. Over 50 percent of glomeruli have hypercellularity, segmental necrosis, and capillary wall thickening by large subendothelial immune complex deposits. Crescentic formation may occur.

Some degree of *interstitial nephritis* with peritubular immune complex deposits often accompanies the glomerular lesions of lupus nephritis, but in rare cases it may occur in the absence of glomerular lesions and produce azotemia (see Interstitial Causes of Renal Failure, Chapter 13).

There are several typical pathologic features of lupus nephritis. *Hematoxylin bodies* are ill-defined, lilac-stained nuclear remnants derived from leukocytes. They are pathognomonic of lupus nephritis, but are seen only in a minority of cases. Suggestive, but not diagnostic of lupus nephritis, are a *fingerprint-like pattern* in the grain of electron dense deposits, tubuloreticular inclusions in endothelial cells (so-called *virus-like particles*), and massive suben-

Table 11.4. Renal manifestations of lupus nephritis: percent incidence by histologic class [118, 119]

	MSGN[†]	FPGN[†]	DPGN[†]	MGN[†]
Total patients	34	27	53	34
No abnormality (%)	41	7	0	3
Proteinuria (%)	50	81	98	97
Hematuria (%)	24	56	89	41
Nephrotic syndrome (%)	3	19	87	74
Azotemia (%)	9	19	72	21

†. MSGN – mesangial GN, FPGN – focal proliferative GN, DPGN – diffuse proliferative GN, MGN – membranous GN.

Table 11.5. Clinical features of SLE in 49 patients with membranous or diffuse proliferative lupus nephritis[†][126]

Finding	Percentage of patients
Arthritis	69
Facial erythema	57
Alopecia	22
Pericarditis	18
Pleuritis	18
Vasculitis	18
Lymph nodes	16
Raynaud's phenomenon	12
Myocarditis	8
Photosensitivity	8
Oral or nasal ulceration	6

† No significant difference between the two groups.

dothelial immune deposits in the form of either *"wire loop"* capillary wall thickening or intracapillary *"hyaline thrombi"*.

Clinical Picture.

Lupus nephritis affects about 35% of individuals with SLE and, if not a presenting feature of lupus in these patients, usually appears during the first three years of disease [117–122]. Ninety percent of patients with lupus nephritis are female. The average age of disease onset is about 28 years with many cases in adolescents and only rare cases before 10 years of age or after 60 [119–125]. Patients develop lupus nephritis during periods of lupus activity, and typically exhibit various extrarenal manifestations of SLE, such as fever, malar rash, arthralgias and arthritis (Table 11.5) [119, 124, 126, 127]. Laboratory studies also reflect active disease with leukopenia, anemia, thrombocytopenia and an elevated ESR [119, 120, 128]. A positive antinuclear antibody test (ANA) is a *sine qua non* for active SLE, and most patients also have anti-double-stranded DNA antibodies and depressed complement levels (CH50, C3 and C4) [119–121, 127, 129–131]. Serum cryoglobulins are often positive [129].

The clinical manifestations of lupus nephritis differ with the histologic class (Table 11.4), and, therefore, the course of the disease depends on the evolution of the pathologic lesions. With progression to a more severe class, azotemia may appear *de novo* in patients who initially have asymptomatic urinary abnormalities or nephrotic syndrome (118, 119). While azotemia early in the course of lupus nephritis is associated with active disease and extrarenal manifestations of SLE, its onset after years of quiescent lupus nephritis may occur despite the absence of lupus activity [132–134].

Diagnosis

Lupus nephritis should be suspected when an individual with an acute nephritic picture has extrarenal manifestations compatible with SLE, especially fever, rash and arthralgias. Blood samples should be obtained for an ESR, rheumatoid factor, ANA, ANCA, cryoglobulins and complement studies (CH50, C3, C4). If the ANA is positive, an anti-double-stranded DNA antibody test should be ordered. Blood cultures are indicated in febrile patients. Patients with typical multisystem findings, low complement levels, an acute nephritic picture, and a positive ANA and anti-double-stranded DNA antibody can be assumed to have lupus nephritis. Despite the near certainty of this diagnosis, many patients need a renal biopsy to guide therapy by determining the histologic form of lupus nephritis and by estimating its reversibility.

Pitfalls. In some patients with lupus nephritis, the extrarenal manifestations of SLE are absent [135] or so atypical that the physician either does not perform an ANA initially or is not sure how to interpret a positive test. Such confusing cases require a renal biopsy for diagnosis.

Patients with lupus nephritis may occasionally have a positive ANCA [136, 137]. The renal biopsy will dispel any doubt created about the diagnosis.

A positive ANA, usually in low titer (less than 1 : 320), are found in 10 percent of the normal population after age 50 and in 20 percent after age 70. A positive ANA also may be induced by procainamide, hydralazine or other drugs. Some cases with drug-induced seropositivity develop a reversible lupus syndrome, but renal involvement is rare [138]. If a patient appears to have drug-induced lupus nephritis with azotemia, one should consider other possibilities, if Scr does not fall after stopping the drug.

RENAL VASCULITIS – A CAPSULE DESCRIPTION.

The next four conditions, polyarteritis nodosa, Wegener's granulomatosis, Henoch-Schonlein purpura and essential mixed cryoglobulinemia, are rare systemic vasculitides. They are similar in that, in addition to an acute nephritic picture, they produce fever and other constitutional symptoms, and tend to involve multiple organs. *Upper or lower respiratory tract lesions* are the hallmark of Wegener's granulomatosis, and a *purpuric rash* the hallmark of Henoch-Schonlein purpura. The diagnosis of these diseases is suspected from the clinical picture, and is mainly confirmed through biopsy of the kidney or other involved organs.

Polyarteritis nodosa

This rare cause of renal failure usually impairs GFR through its accompanying GN. Renal infarcts from vasculitis of medium-sized arteries [139, 140], and urinary obstruction from retroperitoneal vasculitis [141] produce renal failure in very rare cases.

Pathologists split this disease into *microscopic* polyarteritis nodosa, which affects small vessels (small arteries and arterioles) and the less common, *classic* polyarteritis nodosa, which affects medium-sized arteries (and often small vessels as well). The classic variety can produce tissue infarcts and often manifests typical arterial aneurysms on arteriography. The distinction between the two variants has little clinical relevance. First, both produce renal failure as a result of GN, usually a pauci-immune necrotizing and crescentic GN. Furthermore, the clinical pictures are similar, and treatment is the same. Some authors maintain that idiopathic crescentic GN of the pauci-immune type (see above) is a renal-limited form of microscopic polyarteritis nodosa [47, 142], but other workers believe that this conclusion is as yet unproven or incorrect [48, 143].

Clinical Picture.
Polyarteritis nodosa may occur at any age, but is mainly a disease of the middle years. It is somewhat more common in males and less common in blacks [47, 142–146]. The disease typically presents with constitutional symptoms, such as fever, malaise, fatigue, anorexia and weight loss, or a flu-like illness with sore throat, myalgias or arthralgias. Usually one also sees involvement of the skin, musculoskeletal, gastrointestinal, respiratory or other organ systems (Table 10.6) [47, 143–147]. Renal manifestations may be part of the initial clinical picture, but more often begin weeks to months later [47, 143, 145, 146]. Occasionally the disease presents with an acute nephritic picture in the absence of systemic symptoms [47, 143].

Anemia, high white blood cell count (with granulocytosis), hypoalbuminemia, a markedly elevated ESR, and a *positive ANCA* occur in many patients. Some cases have a positive rheumatoid factor, hepatitis B surface antigen, or eosinophilia, while low complement levels are rare, and cryoglobulins, antistreptolysin O titers and ANA are usually negative [142–144, 146–150].

Diagnosis
Polyarteritis nodosa is suggested by constitutional symptoms and multisystem findings in an individual with an acute nephritic picture. The physician should order an ESR, rheumatoid factor, ANA, ANCA, cryoglobulin, and complement studies. Blood cultures may be needed to evaluate fever. One should biopsy the kidney or other involved tissue, such as a tender muscle, a necrotic skin nodule or an affected sural nerve, since this is the usual means of diagnosis (Table 11.7) [47, 143–145]. Any recent surgical specimen, e.g. gallbladder, ought to be reexamined for affected vessels. Unfortunately, the kidney biopsy is often not diagnostic, and usually shows a pauci-immune GN without vasculitis [142, 143].

If no tissue specimens reveal vasculitis, renal and celiac arteriography should be considered, although the risk of contrast-mediated renal failure needs to be considered in azotemic patients. Arteriographic diagnoses have been reported in patients with renal failure [48, 145], and in classic polyarteritis nodosa more than half of cases have multiple aneurysms on celiac or renal arteriography [150–152]. However, in patients with renal polyarteritis nodosa, the yield of arteriography is probably lower [143], since few have the classic type. Alternatively, one may biopsy asymptomatic muscle, which has a yield as high as 29% [152].

Pitfalls. Frequently, patients with suspected vasculitis have no involved extrarenal organ available for biopsy or none of the biopsies have been diagnostic. Consequently, suspected vasculitis cannot be confirmed or is only demonstrated at autopsy (Table 11.8) [143].

Table 11.6. Extrarenal manifestations of polyarteritis nodosa affecting the kidney [143]

System	Percent of cases	System	Percent of cases
Constitutional symptoms	78	Neurologic	36
Fever	75	Mononeuritis multiplex	
Musculoskeletal	72	CVA	
Myalgias		Convulsions	
Arthralgia		Headache	
Arthritis		Change in sensorium	
Gastrointestinal	58	Ataxia	
Abnormal liver function tests		Vertigo	
G.I. bleeding		Ear, nose and throat	36
Abdominal pain		Epistaxis	
Pancreatitis		Sore throat	
Skin	58	Sinusitis	
Purpura		Otitis media	
Erythematous rash		Ear chondritis	
Ulcers		Cardiovascular	30
Hemorrhagic vesicles		Hypertension	
Splinter hemorrhage		Pericarditis	
Erythema nodosum		ECG changes	
Pulmonary	56	Eye	28
Infiltrates		Conjunctivitis	
Hemoptysis		Retinopathy	
Pleurisy		Uveitis	
Effusions		Episcleritis	
Asthma		Proptosis	

Table 11.7. Vasculitis on biopsy in 71 cases with polyarteritis nodosa affecting the kidney [47, 143–145][*]

Tissue	Number of cases
Kidney	43
Skin	13
Muscle	7
Lung	2
Nose	2
Liver	1

* Several diagnoses made at autopsy.

Table 11.8. Vasculitis at autopsy in 15 cases with polyarteritis nodosa affecting the kidney [143]

Tissue	Number of cases
Kidney	14
Spleen	5
Lung	4
Muscle	3
Adrenal	3
Pancreas	2
Heart	2
Gastrointestinal	1
Pericardium	1
Central nervous system	1
Bone marrow	1
Testis	1
Uterus	1

Wegener's granulomatosis

This rare idiopathic disease is characterized pathologically by a triad of vasculitis, parenchymal necrosis and granulomatous inflammation, and clinically by a triad of GN, upper and lower respiratory tract lesions.

Clinical Picture. The mean age of onset is 40 to 50 years (range: 9 to 83 years) [153, 154]. Patients typically present with constitutional symptoms (fever, malaise, anorexia, weight loss and fatigue), upper or lower respiratory complaints, and musculoskeletal manifestations (Table 11.9). Symptoms from disease in other organs occur with no consistent pattern. Some patients give a long history of chronic upper or lower respiratory infection, including sinusitis, otitis, bronchiectasis or tuberculosis [155]. In one study 77% of cases developed GN, some initially, but most during the first two years of disease [153]. Common laboratory abnormalities include leukocytosis, thrombocytosis, raised alkaline phosphatase, markedly elevated ESR and, in more than 90% of cases with active disease, *a positive ANCA* [153–155].

Some individuals with renal involvement have eosinophilia or a positive rheumatoid factor, while hypocomplementemia, HBs Ag, positive ANA and raised antistreptolysin O titer are normally not seen [147, 155–157].

Diagnosis

Wegener's granulomatosis is suggested by the onset of a nephritic picture in a patient with upper or lower respiratory symptoms. The physician should order chest and sinus X-rays, appropriate cultures, ESR, ANA, ANCA, complement studies and, in cases with pulmonary symptoms, anti-glomerular basement membrane (GBM) antibodies. In patients with upper respiratory disease, an otolaryngologist should be consulted and biopsies obtained from the affected area. Patients with suggestive lung findings should be seen by a pulmonary specialist, and a lung biopsy obtained. Although transbronchial biopsy specimens can be diagnostic, the yield is so low that open lung biopsies are recommended [153, 158]. A diagnosis is made from the clinical picture, the exclusion of infection through cultures and special stains, and from characteristic histology on biopsy of the lung, nose or paranasal sinuses. In rare cases, tissue from other affected organs (e.g. parotid gland, breast) may be diagnostic [153, 154, 156].

Pitfalls. Unfortunately, biopsies with inconclusive results are common (Table 11.10). Kidney biopsies are usually not specific for Wegener's granulomatosis, since they typically show a pauci-immune necrotizing and crescentic glomerulonephritis, and only rarely have characteristic granulomas and vasculitis [47, 147, 153–156, 159]. A positive ANCA test with a "cytoplasmic pattern" (or antiproteinase 3 positivity) has a sensitivity for active Wegener's granulomatosis of greater than 80% and a specificity of 90% [148, 160]. However, it is not considered reliable for diagnosis in the absence of tissue confirmation, because of occasional positive results in certain infections and other diseases.

Henoch-Schonlein purpura

This is an IgA-immune complex-mediated vasculitis that by definition affects the skin, and usually involves the joints, gastrointestinal tract and kidney.

Pathology. In the kidney one sees an IgA mesangial deposit disease indistinguishable on biopsy from IgA nephropathy (see above).

Clinical Picture. While Henoch-Schonlein purpura can develop at any age, well over 90% of cases occur in children [161–164]. A pharyngitis, other infection, or variety of drugs may precede the disease, which usually begins with a purpuric rash over the buttocks, and extensor surfaces of the arms and legs (Figure 11.2) [161, 162, 164]. The rash can involve other areas, and initially may be urticarial or erythematous [161]. Most patients have arthralgias or arthritis, mainly of the ankles and knees, and abdominal pain, occasionally with gastrointestinal bleeding [161–165]. Disease in other organs, although rare, is reported [161]. Some renal involvement occurs in about half of patients, but among adults only one third of these cases have renal impairment [161–165].

Diagnosis

Henoch-Schonlein purpura is usually suggested by the constellation of organs affected. The physician should obtain an ESR, rheumatoid factor, cryoglobulins, ANA, ANCA, complement levels, and a dermatologic consultation. If a fresh skin lesion is available, a biopsy for histology and immunofluorescence is recommended. A renal biopsy should be performed in azotemic patients, unless renal failure is mild and transient. The diagnosis is confirmed on immunofluorescence by demonstrating

Table 11.9. Extrarenal disease in 158 patients with Wegener's granulomatosis [153]

Organ system	Total % of cases	Organ system	Total % of cases
Upper airway	92	Ocular	52
Sinusitis		Conjunctivitis	
Epistaxis		Dacrocystitis	
Rhinorrhea		Scleritis	
Mucosal ulcerations		Proptosis/diplopia	
Nasal deformity		Eye pain	
Perforated septum		Visual loss	
Otitis media		Retinopathy	
Hearing loss		Cutaneous	46
Earache		Palpable purpura	
Subglottic stenosis		Erythematous rash	
Oral lesions		Ulcers/vesicles	
Pharyngitis		Papules	
Lower airway	85	Subcutaneous nodules	
Infiltrate		Neurological	15
Nodules		Mononeuritis multiplex	
Cavitation		Stroke	
Cough		Cranial neuropathy	
Sputum production		Cardiac	6
Hemoptysis		Pericarditis/myocarditis	
Dyspnea		Coronary vasculitis	
Pleuritis		Parotid Gland	<1
Musculoskeletal	67	Breast	<1
Arthralgias		Urethra	<1
Myalgias		Cervix	<1
Polyarteritis		Vagina	<1

Table 11.10. Histologic confirmation of Wegener's granulomatosis in 109 patients [154]

Tissue	Number of biopsies	
	Total	Diagnostic
Upper airway		
Nasal	68	38
Oral	7	1
Glottis	6	1
Ear	3	0
Lung	37	29
Renal	40	6
Skin	16	2
Liver	5	1
Other	8	2

IgA deposition in skin lesions or in mesangial deposits [161, 164, 166].

Essential mixed cryoglobulinemia

Cryoglobulins are abnormal circulating immunoglobulins that precipitate in the cold. Clinically, they can produce GN and diffuse vasculitis. When associated with lymphoproliferative disorders, such as macroglobulinemia, cryoglobulins are monoclonal immunoglobulins that either cryoprecipitate alone (*type I*) or only with another immunoglobulin (*type II*). These latter, *mixed* cryoglobulins commonly have a monoclonal IgM *x*, acting as an antibody with anti-IgG (rheumatoid factor) activity, and polyclonal IgG, acting as the antigen. Type II cryoglobulins can also be associated with autoimmune or infectious disease or with no specific disorder, which is known as *essential mixed cryoglobulinemia* (Table 11.11) [167, 168, 170]. *Type III* cryoglobulins are also mixed cryoglobulins with an IgM anti-IgG, but the IgM is polyclonal. Type III cryoglobulins also are usually associated with autoimmune or infectious disease or are idiopathic (essential). Up to 58% of cases of type II essential mixed cryoglobulinemia have GN, and a third or more of these develop azotemia [167–169, 171, 172]. Type III cryoglobulins cause GN less often [167–169, 173, 174].

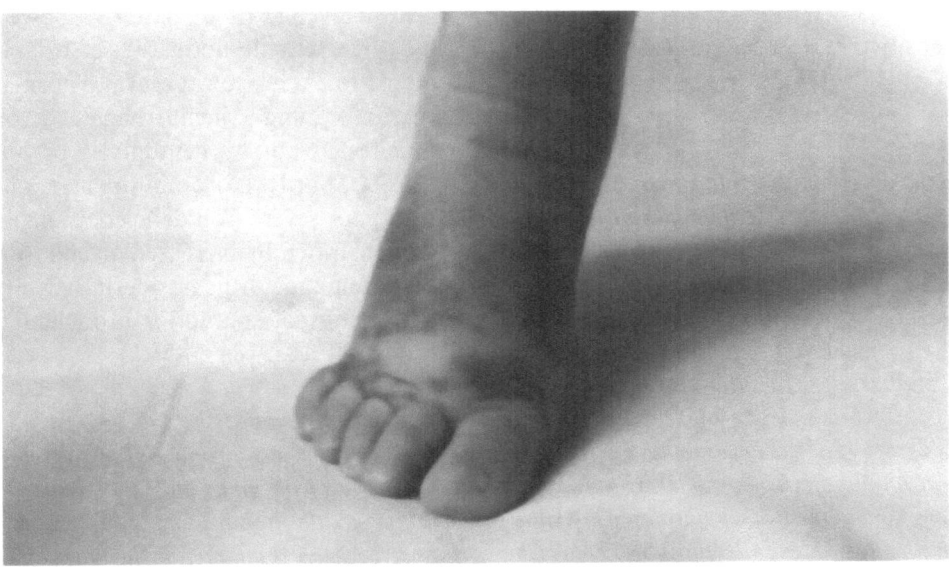

Fig. 11.2. Purpuric papules coalescing into plaques on the dorsum of the foot of a child with Henoch-Schonlein purpura. (Courtesy of Dr. Andrew Brem.)

Table 11.11. Differences between types I, II and III cryoglobulinemia

	Type I monoclonal CG	Type II mixed CG with monoclonal component	Type III mixed polyclonal CG
Usual composition	M IgM or M IgG	M IgM ϰ (RF) + P IgG	P IgM (RF) + P IgG
Associated diseases:			
Lymphoproliferative	+	+	−
Autoimmune	−	+	+
Infectious	−	+	+
None (essential)	−	+	+
Incidence of GN*	<25%	>50%	<25%

CG – cryoglobulin, M – monoclonal, P – polyclonal, RF – rheumatoid factor.

* Estimate from [167–169].

Pathology. The GN may appear either as a diffuse proliferative or membranoproliferative type. A characteristic feature superimposed in one-third of cases is eosinophilic masses in the glomerular capillaries. These masses may be large enough to occlude the capillary lumen, and appear to be mainly cryoglobulin. Like purified cryoprecipitate, they stain on immunofluorescence for IgM, IgG, ϰ chain, and sometimes complement components, and by electron microscopy they often have a crystalloid structure in the form of cylinders. The same immune components and crystalloid structure seen in these masses occur in subendothelial deposits in most cases [171, 173, 174].

Clinical Picture. Essential mixed cryoglobulinemia usually presents with systemic manifestations, and any nephritic picture appears months or years later [168, 171, 174]. The typical extrarenal features are palpable purpura over the lower extremities, arthralgias, and hepatomegaly or elevated liver enzymes [168, 171, 172]. Less common are weakness, fever, splenomegaly, leg ulcers, Raynaud's phenomenon, abdominal pain, peripheral neuropathy, lymphadenopathy and pulmonary involvement [168, 169, 171]. Laboratory findings usually include a positive rheumatoid factor, depressed complement levels (C4 and CH50, often, and C3, sometimes), raised ESR, anemia and, the *sine qua non*, cryoglobulins [168, 169, 174, 175]. Hepatitis C studies are positive in over 80% of cases, implying a viral etiology [172, 176].

Diagnosis

Essential mixed cryoglobulinemia is suggested by the constellation of lower extremity purpura, multisystem complaints, acute nephritic syndrome and signs of liver disease. The physician should order cryoglobulins (collected with equipment warmed to 37 °C), ESR, rheumatoid factor, ANA, ANCA, complement studies, liver function tests and hepatitis C studies (viral RNA may be more sensitive than serology [172, 176]). If a cryoglobulin is present, serum protein immunofixation at 37 °C will detect any monoclonal component. Dermatologic consultation is recommended. The constellation of purpura, arthralgias, a nephritic urine, positive rheumatoid factor and cryoglobulins is considered diagnostic of this condition. A renal biopsy should be carried out, if therapy for the GN is planned or if doubt exists about the diagnosis. A skin biopsy with immunofluorescent studies [167, 168, 171], and immunochemical analysis of the cryoprecipitate may also prove confirmatory [170].

Goodpasture's syndrome

This condition is the association of GN and diffuse pulmonary hemorrhage, both mediated by anti-GBM antibodies.

> *Pathology.* Goodpasture's syndrome manifests necrotizing and crescentic GN or occasionally other non-specific lesions by light microscopy, but on immunofluorescent microscopy displays its hallmark: linear staining for IgG.

Clinical Picture. Patients' ages range from early adolescence to over 80 years, but the prevalence peaks between 17 and 25 years; men predominate by 2.5 : 1 [177–181]. An antecedent upper respiratory infection is sometimes reported [180, 181]. Most cases present with hemoptysis, cough or dyspnea, which may be recurrent for weeks or rarely for years before diagnosis [180–183]. The nephritic picture is seen initially or first appears months after the pulmonary symptoms. In rare cases, the nephritic manifestations precede the lung hemorrhage. Examination typically reveals inspiratory crackles and pallor, reflecting severe

anemia [180, 181]. Chest X-ray shows a bilateral central alveolar filling pattern followed after 2 or 3 days by a reticulo-nodular interstitial infiltrate and after 1 to 2 weeks by a return to normal, if bleeding ceases. Lung hemorrhage occasionally is manifested not by hemoptysis or pulmonary infiltrates, but by a drop in the hemoglobin concentration or severe iron deficiency anemia. It may be demonstrated by increased alveolar uptake of carbon monoxide or hemosiderin-laden macrophages in cytology of sputum or bronchoalveolar lavage fluid [180, 182, 184, 185].

Diagnosis

Goodpasture' syndrome is suggested by an acute nephritic syndrome and pulmonary hemorrhage, known as the pulmonary renal syndrome. *To demonstrate covert pulmonary hemorrhage in cases with unexplained pulmonary manifestations or iron deficiency anemia, sputum cytology and lung uptake of carbon monoxide should be ordered. The investigation of pulmonary hemorrhage requires a consideration of pulmonary emboli, malignancies, infections, heart failure, and collagen vascular diseases. A pulmonary consultation is recommended to assist in this investigation. Blood should be drawn for ANCA, ANA, cryoglobulins, complement levels and anti-GBM antibody. A renal biopsy should be carried out. The* sine qua non *for the diagnosis is anti-GBM antibodies. Since the results of anti-GBM antibody assays are usually delayed up to a week, these antibodies are most quickly demonstrated by a renal biopsy showing IgG in a linear pattern along the glomerular capillaries. The antibodies may also be seen on transbronchial lung biopsies, showing a linear IgG pattern along the alveolar capillary wall, but only a minority of biopsies are positive [182, 184].*

> *Pitfalls.* Goodpasture's syndrome is responsible for less than half of cases of pulmonary renal syndrome; other causes include bacterial endocarditis, SLE, Wegener's and other vasculitides [185–187]. A renal biopsy helps distinguish these conditions.

> Some patients with Goodpasture's syndrome have fever and a skin rash or other multisystem complaints [179–181]. Many of these cases have features of a complicating vasculitis as evidenced by positive ANCA (in addition to the anti-GBM antibodies), and by granulomas and vasculitis on renal biopsy [177, 178, 188].

DIAGNOSING SECONDARY GLOMERULONEPHRITIDES – A RECAPITULATION.

While these conditions often have typical presentations which usually lead the physician to carry out the right confirmatory studies, the clinical picture may be incomplete or unusual. In many of these disorders the patient can have a non-specific "vasculitis-like" picture, comprising fever, other constitutional symptoms, rash, arthralgias, multiorgan symptoms and an acute nephritic syndrome. A general diagnostic approach is to obtain an ESR, rheumatoid factor, ANA, ANCA, cryoglobulins and complement studies (CH50, C3, C4). In addition, blood cultures are usually indicated for fever, anti-GBM antibodies for pulmonary symptoms, and dermatologic consultation and skin biopsy with immunofluorescent studies for rash. Often patients need a renal biopsy either for diagnosis or as a prerequisite for therapy, but there are many exceptions. For example, the diagnosis may be made from the clinical picture as in postinfectious or lupus GN or from a biopsy of other tissue, like lung, as in Wegener's granulomatosis. Even in situations where a renal biopsy is usually desirable to guide therapy such as lupus nephritis, this may not be necessary if the patient will get immunosuppressive therapy for extrarenal disease. Thus, in all of these examples, a renal biopsy might be needed only if the Scr does not fall with the treatment.

NEPHROTIC DISEASES

The nephrotic syndrome is characterized by massive loss of plasma albumin into the urine and edema. Nephrotic patients typically manifest little or no azotemia at presentation, although they may later progress to chronic renal failure. For some patients, however, renal failure is an early feature, and a rise in Scr may occur from one month to the next or faster.

Causes (Table 11.12)

Rapid Progression of Underlying Disease. For unknown reasons some nephrotic patients may have an unusually aggressive disease process, whereby

Table 11.12. Complications of nephrotic diseases that cause renal failure

---

Rapid progression of underlying disease
Primary diseases
    Membranous GN [189–191]
    Membranoproliferative GN [84, 192]
    Focal segmental glomerulosclerosis [193, 194]
    Fibrillary/ Immunotactoid GN [195–197]
Secondary diseases
    Diabetic nephropathy [198, 199, 200]
    Amyloidosis [201, 202]
    Light chain deposition disease [203–206]
    Heroin nephropathy [207–208]
    HIV nephropathy [209–213]

Sequela of the nephrotic pathophysiology
Tubulointerstitial nephritis in lipoid nephrosis [214]
Hypovolemia from severe hypoalbuminemia [215]
Renal vein thrombosis [216, 217]

---

they develop renal failure early and progress to end stage over several months to a few years.

Sequela of the Nephrotic Pathophysiology. Three conditions are included here. First, a transient *tubulointerstitial nephritis* with renal failure can occur in severe cases of lipoid nephrosis[1] [214]. The mechanism is unknown. Second, severe hypoalbuminemia has been postulated to reduce blood volume in some patients, and cause renal failure through *hypotension* and decreased renal perfusion [215]. However, a fall in blood pressure low enough to raise Scr occurs rarely, if ever, in nephrotic patients, unless it is due to sepsis or diuretics. Finally, the nephrotic syndrome produces hypercoagulability, which may lead to *renal vein thrombosis*. This can impair renal function in rare cases [216, 217].

Clinical picture

Rapid Progression of Underlying Disease. These patients generally present with edema, and the Scr, if not elevated initially, begins to climb within a few months. Laboratory studies show proteinuria greater than 3 g per day, a serum albumin level less than 3 g/dL, and in many cases microscopic hematuria. Alternatively, patients may come to medical attention because of proteinuria or azotemia accidentally detected during evaluation of another complaint. Such patients may have proteinuria less than 3 g per day, a serum albumin level over 3 g/dL, and no edema. One half of patients with membranoproliferative GN have a reduced C3 or CH50 [77, 78, 81, 84, 88, 89].

With regard to secondary glomerulopathies, diabetes mellitus and heroin addiction have usually been recognized by the time that secondary renal disease develops. In contrast, amyloidosis, light chain deposition disease, and HIV infection [212] may or may not have been diagnosed from extrarenal findings at the time that renal manifestations appear.

> Light chain *amyloidosis* and *light chain deposition disease* result from deposition of monoclonal light chains produced by multiple myeloma or by an otherwise asymptomatic monoclonal gammopathy. In amyloidosis, the light chains deposit in the form of fine fibrils that stain with Congo red; in light chain deposition disease, the deposits are granular and do not stain with Congo red. Light chain amyloidosis is usually caused by lambda chains, while light chain deposition disease mostly involves kappa chains.
>
> Secondary amyloid results from deposition of an AA protein probably derived from serum amyloid A protein; this *AA form* of amyloidosis is seen in chronic inflammatory diseases.

Affected patients are usually greater than 50 years of age in light chain amyloidosis and greater than 40 years of age in light chain deposition disease, and they may already have a diagnosis or symptoms of multiple myeloma. Patients with secondary or the *AA form* of amyloidosis have an underlying chronic infection, such as tuberculosis, or a chronic inflammatory condition, such as ankylosing spondylitis [202]; such patients may be younger than those with light chain amyloidosis. Light chain deposition disease and both forms of amyloidosis may involve the heart, liver and other organs as well as the kidneys [206].

Sequela of the Nephrotic Pathophysiology. When azotemia due to tubulointerstitial nephritis complicates lipoid nephrosis, it occurs one to four weeks or more after the onset of nephrotic syndrome. While the age range is adolescence to old age and either sex is affected, the typical patient is a mildly hypertensive man in his fifties or sixties, with severe nephrotic syndrome (average urine protein 12 g/24 hours; average serum albumin 1.9 g/dL) [214].

Prerenal azotemia or acute tubular necrosis due to severe hypoalbuminemia with hypovolemia is rare, if it occurs at all. One should see severe nephrotic syndrome with a serum albumin level below 1.0 to 1.5 g/dL and hypotension.

Renal vein thrombosis is a common sequela of the *hypercoagulable state* seen in the nephrotic syndrome. Although it affects a significant minority of nephrotic patients, it usually produces partial venous obstruction and is clinically silent [217]. Rare cases, however, can develop pulmonary emboli or sufficient venous obstruction to impair GFR. The latter patients often manifest back, flank or abdominal pain at the time the Scr rises [216, 217].

Diagnosis

Renal failure due to a nephrotic disease is suggested by azotemia in the setting of heavy proteinuria (>3+ or 300 mg/dL by dipstick, >3.0 mg/mg (0.34 g/mmol) protein to creatinine ratio or >3 g per 24 hour) and with or without hematuria. Serum albumin, cholesterol and complement levels, and renal sonography should be ordered. An ANCA is indicated in patients with hematuria. Funduscopy is important in diabetics, since retinopathy is almost a sine qua non for diabetic nephropathy. If retinopathy is present in a diabetic patient and the Scr is rising slowly, no more quickly than from month to month, the physician may limit his investigation to excluding non-diabetic causes of renal failure, if any are suggested by the initial evaluation. If the Scr is rising more rapidly, diabetic nephropathy is not as likely and a renal biopsy might be indicated. Patients over 50 years of age should have a needle biopsy of the abdominal fat pad with staining for amyloid. If the diagnosis of amyloidosis is made, a renal biopsy is not needed [202]. Chronic inflammatory diseases also raise the question of amyloidosis, and are indications for fat pad biopsies with amyloid staining. Bone marrow biopsies may also be used to diagnose secondary amyloidosis [219]. HIV risk factors should be sought and testing performed, if appropriate. Renal venography should be considered in nephrotic patients with back, flank or abdominal pain, keeping in mind the rarity of renal vein thrombosis as a cause of renal failure. With the exception of cases diagnosed as diabetic nephropathy with the aid of funduscopy, amyloidosis by fat pad biopsy, and renal vein thrombosis by venography, other nephrotic patients with rapidly progressive renal failure require a renal biopsy.

Pitfalls. Nonsteroidal anti-inflammatory drugs can produce nephrotic syndrome with acute renal failure, which mimics the renal failure caused by complications of nephrotic diseases. Renal biopsy shows lipoid nephrosis together with acute interstitial nephritis (see Chapter 13).

CHRONIC GLOMERULAR DISEASES

Definition
Most glomerular diseases can produce chronic renal failure, even in cases where the initial GFR was normal. Patients may present with asymptomatic hematuria and proteinuria as in IgA nephropathy, a full-blown nephritic picture as in diffuse proliferative lupus nephritis or with nephrotic syndrome as in membranous GN. With continued activity the disease enters a chronic progressive phase characterized by *proteinuria*, and *azotemia* that is stable or worsening so slowly that a change in Scr is observed only over several months. Many patients also have hematuria. The progression of renal failure can be a result of "smoldering" activity of the primary disease or of a poorly understood sclerosing process that is independent of the primary disease. This sclerosing process is usually triggered by renal damage with loss of renal function, and is thought to be mediated by glomerular capillary hypertension [220, 221].

Causes
Glomerular etiologies of chronic renal failure are listed on Table 7.2, and encompass all the acute nephritic diseases covered at the beginning of this chapter and all the diseases that commonly produce the nephrotic syndrome, with the exception of lipoid nephrosis. In some cases nephrotic conditions, such as membranous GN and diabetic nephropathy, produce chronic renal failure, despite *less-than-nephrotic range* proteinuria.

Diagnosis
Chronic renal failure accompanied by proteinuria and, occasionally, hematuria suggests chronic glomerulonephritis. The evaluation of such cases is the same as that described for other types of chronic renal failure in Chapter 7.

CONCLUSION

The large number of conditions described in this chapter constitute a confusing array for the nonspecialist. A simplified overview is, therefore, offered to help the physician approach the evaluation of these patients.

One first should sort cases into *nephritic* patients with hematuria, proteinuria and a rise in Scr from one month to the next or faster, *nephrotic* patients with proteinuria near or in the nephrotic range and a rise in Scr from one month to the next or faster, and *chronic GN* patients with proteinuria and a rise in Scr only over several months or slower. Any extrarenal manifestations should be investigated with an eye to identifying multisystem disease. Common clues to these conditions are listed on Table 11.13. Consultations with rheumatologists and other subspecialists may be appropriate in different cases. Nephritic and nephrotic patients who cannot be diagnosed from their extrarenal manifestations require a renal biopsy. Patients with chronic GN generally do not need a tissue diagnosis, given the lack of effective treatment for the conditions involved.

NOTES

1. This also occurs in focal segmental glomerulosclerosis and IgM nephropathy, two conditions that are related to lipoid nephrosis.

REFERENCES

1. Malangone JM, Abuelo JG, Pezzullo JC, Lund K and McGloin CA. Clinical and laboratory features of patients with chronic renal disease at the start of dialysis. Clin Nephrol 1989; 31:77–87.
2. US Renal Data System, USRDS 1993 Annual Data Report, The National Institutes of Health, National Institute of Diabetes and Digestive and Kidney Diseases, Bethesda, MD, March 1993, p 24.
3. Rodriguez-Iturbe B. Epidemic poststreptococcal glomerulonephritis. Kidney Int 1984; 25:129–36.
4. Feinstein EI and Eknoyan G. Renal complications of bacterial endocarditis. Am J Nephrol 1985; 5:457–69.
5. Beaufils M, Morel-Maroger L, Sraer JD, Kanfer A, Kourilsky O and Richet G. Acute renal failure of glomerular origin during visceral abscesses. N Engl J Med 1976; 295:185–9.
6. Levy M. Infections and glomerular diseases. Clin Immunol and Allergy 1986; 6:255–85.

Table 11.13. Clinical clues to glomerular causes of renal failure

Condition	Clues
Acute Nephritic Diseases	*Hematuria, proteinuria, RBC casts, ↑ Scr (over 1 month or less)*
Primary Glomerular Disease	
Idiopathic crescentic GN	CS, "flu-like" prodrome
IgA nephropathy (Berger's disease)	Recurrent gross hematuria triggered by a common cold
Membranoproliferative GN	Partial lipodystrophy, ↑ aminotransferase
Secondary Glomerular Disease	
Poststreptococcal GN	Sore throat, impetigo, 1-3 week latent period
GN due to bacterial endocarditis	CS, heart murmur, splenomegaly, rash, joint sx, petechiae
GN due to visceral abscesses	Fever, critically ill patient
GN due to infected VA shunt	History of a VA shunt, fever, rash, arthralgias
Lupus nephritis	CS, malar rash, joint sx, serositis, ↓ platelets, ↓ wbc
Polyarteritis nodosa	CS, multisystem sx
Wegener's granulomatosis	CS, upper or lower respiratory sx, multisystem sx
Henoch-Schonlein purpura	Purpuric rash, arthralgias, GI pain or bleeding
Essential mixed cryoglobulinemia	CS, purpuric rash, joint sx, ↑ LFT's, ↑ liver size, multisystem sx
Goodpasture's syndrome	Cough, hemoptysis, dyspnea, infiltrates, ↓ Fe-anemia
Nephrotic Diseases	*Nephrotic syndrome + ↑ Scr (over 1 month or less)*
Rapid Progression of Disease	
Diabetic Nephropathy	↑ blood glucose, retinopathy
Amyloidosis	Chronic inflammation, old age, myeloma sx, multisystem sx
HIV nephropathy	HIV risk factors, sx of ARC/AIDS
Sequela of Nephrotic Pathophysiology	
Renal vein thrombosis	Back, flank or abdominal pain, pulmonary emboli
Chronic Glomerular Disease	*Proteinuria (+/– hematuria), ↑ Scr (over several months)*
Various primary and secondary diseases	

CS – constitutional symptoms: fever, malaise, fatigue, anorexia, weight loss, sx – symptoms, VA – ventriculoatrial.

7. Phanuphak P and Kohler PF. Onset of polyarteritis nodosa during allergic hyposensitization treatment. Am J Med 1980; 68:479–85.

8. Johnson RJ and Couser WG. Hepatitis B infection and renal disease: clinical, immunopathogenetic and therapeutic considerations. Kidney Int 1990; 37:663–76.

9. Sergent JS and Christian CL. Necrotizing vasculitis after acute serous otitis media. Ann Intern Med 1974; 81:195–9.

10. Case Records of the Massachusetts General Hospital, Case 22-1983. N Engl J Med 1983; 308:1343–53.

11. Arnalich F, Lahoz C, Picazo ML, Monereo A, Arribas JR, Martinez Ara J et al. Polyarteritis nodosa and necrotizing glomerulonephritis associated with long-standing silicosis. Nephron 1989; 51:544–7.

12. Mullick, FG, McAlliste, HA Jr., Wagner BM and Fenoglio JJ Jr. Drug related vasculitis. Human Pathol 1979; 10:313–25.

13. Minetti L, diBelgioioso GB and Busnach G. Immuno-histological diagnosis of drug-induced hypersensitivity nephritis. Contr Nephrol 1978; 10:15–29.

14. Schrier RW, Bulger RJ and VanArsdel PP Jr. Nephropathy associated with penicillin and homologues. Ann Intern Med 1966; 64:116–27.

15. Godeau P, Guillevin L, Herreman G, Wecschler B and Bletry O. Periarterite noueuse et syndromes paraneoplasiques ischemiques. Nouv Presse Med 1979; 8:2419.

16. Fogazzi GB, Pasquali S, Moriggi M, Casanova S, Damilano I, Mihatsch MJ et al. Long-term outcome of Schonlein-Henoch nephritis in the adult. Clin Nephrol 1989; 31:60–6.

17. D'Amico G and Fornasieri A. Cryoglobulinemic glomerulonephritis: a membranoproliferative glomerulonephritis induced by hepatitis C virus. Am J Kidney Dis 1995; 25:361–9.

18. Wilson CB and Smith RC. Goodpasture's syndrome associated with influenza A2 virus infection. Ann Intern Med 1972; 76:91–4.

19. Churchill DN, Fine A and Gault MH. Association between hydrocarbon exposure and glomerulonephritis. An appraisal of the evidence. Nephron 1983; 33:169–72.

20. Kleinknecht D, Morel-Maroger L, Callard P, Adhemar J-P

and Mahieu P. Antiglomerular basement membrane nephritis after solvent exposure. Arch Intern Med 1980; 140:230-2.

21. Lazaro MA, Maldonado Cocco JA, Catoggio LJ, Babini SM, Messina OD and Garcia Morteo O. Clinical and serologic characteristics of patients with overlap syndrome: is mixed connective tissue disease a distinct clinical entity? Medicine 1989; 68:58-65.

22. Savouret J-F, Chudwin DS, Wara DW, Ammann AJ, Cowan MJ and Miller WL. Clinical and laboratory findings in childhood mixed connective tissue disease: Presence of antibody to ribonucleoprotein containing the small nuclear ribonucleic acid U1. J Pediatr 1983; 102:841-6.

23. Lanham JG, Elkon KB, Pusey CD and Hughes GR. Systemic vasculitis with asthma and eosinophilia: a clinical approach to the Churg-Strauss syndrome. Medicine 1984; 63:65-81.

24. Moorthy AV and Pringle D. Urticaria, vasculitis, hypocomplementemia, and immune-complex glomerulonephritis. Arch Pathol Lab Med 1982; 106:68-70.

25. Waldo F, Leist PA, Strife F, Forristal J and West CD. Atypical hypocomplementemic vasculitis syndrome in a child. J Pediat 1985; 106:745-50.

26. Droz D, Noel LH, Leibowitch M and Barbanel C. Glomerulonephritis and necrotizing angiitis. Adv Nephrol 1979; 8:343-63.

27. O'Neill WM Jr., Hammar SP and Bloomer A. Giant cell arteritis with visceral angiitis. Arch Intern Med 1976; 136:1157-60.

28. Canton CG, Bernis C, Paraiso V, Barril G, Garcia A, Osorio C et al. Renal failure in temporal arteritis. Am J Nephrol 1992; 12:380-3.

29. Koumi S, Endo T, Okumura H, Yoneyama K, Fukuda Y and Masugi Y. A case of Takayasu's arteritis associated with membranoproliferative glomerulonephritis and nephrotic syndrome. Nephron 1990; 54:344-6.

30. Donnelly S, Jothy S and Barre P. Crescentic glomerulonephritis in Behcet's syndrome – results of therapy and review of the literature. Clin Nephrol 1989; 31:213-8.

31. Ducret F, Pointet P, Lambert C and Chevalier JP. Insuffisance rénale sévère révélatrice d'une sarcoidose. La Presse Med 1989; 18:1979.

32. Singer DRJ and Evans DJ. Renal impairment in sarcoidosis: granulomatous nephritis as an isolated cause (two case reports and review of the literature). Clin Nephrol 1986; 26:250-6.

33. Moulin B, Ronco PM, Mougenot B, Francois A, Fillastre J-P and Mignon F. Glomerulonephritis in chronic lymphocytic leukemia and related B-cell lymphomas. Kidney Int 1992; 42:127-35.

34. Weinstein T, Chagnac A, Gafter U, Zevin D, Gal R, Djaldetti M et al. Unusual case of crescentic glomerulonephritis associated with malignant lymphoma. Am J Nephrol 1990; 10:329-32.

35. Wood WG and Harkins MM. Nephropathy in angioimmunoblastic lymphadenopathy. Am J Clin Pathol 1979; 71:58-63.

36. Jenkins P, Schrager M, Lodish J and Hall R. Acute glomerulonephritis (AGN) causing acute renal failure (ARF) in angioimmunoblastic lymphadenopathy with disproteinuria (AILD). Kidney Int 1983; 23:127 (abstract).

37. Alpers CE and Cotran RS. Neoplasia and glomerular injury. Kidney Int 1986; 30:465-73.

38. Rollino C, Coppo R, Mazzucco G, Roccatello D, Amore A, Basolo B et al. Monoclonal gammopathy and glomerulonephritis with organized microtubular deposits. Am J Kidney Dis 1990; 15:276-80.

39. Haskell LP, Fusco, S Wadler, LB Sablay and Mennemeyer RP. Crescentic glomerulonephritis associated with prostatic carcinoma: evidence of immune-mediated glomerular injury. Am J Med 1990; 88:189-92.

40. Newell GC. Cirrhotic glomerulonephritis: incidence, morphology, clinical features, and pathogenesis. Am J Kidney Dis 1987; 9:183-90.

41. Montoliu J, Darnell A, Torras A and Revert L. Glomerular disease in cirrhosis of the liver: low frequency of IgA deposits. Am J Nephrol 1986; 6:199-205.

41a. Mustonen J, Pasternack A, Helin H, Pystynen S, Tuominen T. Renal biopsy in acute renal failure. Am J Nephrol 1984; 4:27-31.

41b. Duhoux P, Kourilsky O, Kanfer A, Sraer JD, Morel-Maroger L, Richet G. Les insuffisances renales aigues necessitant un traitement etiopathologenique. In: Seminaires D'Uro-Nephrologie, Masson: Paris 1981: 226-40.

41c. Turney JH, Marshall DH, Brownjohn AM, Ellis CM and Parsons FM. The evolution of acute renal failure, 1956-1988. Quart J Med 1990; 74:83-104.

42. Rodriguez-Iturbe B. Epidemic poststreptococcal glomerulonephritis. Kidney Int 1984; 25:129-36.

43. Kincaid-Smith P, Bennett WM, Dowling JP and Ryan GB. Acute renal failure and tubular necrosis associated with hematuria due to glomerulonephritis. Clin Nephrol 1983; 19:206-10.

44. Galle P, Mahieu P. Electron dense alteration of kidney basement membranes. Am J Med 1975; 58:749-64.

45. Sibley RK and Kim Y. Dense intramembranous deposit disease: New pathologic features. Kidney Int 1984; 25:660-70.

46. Savage COS, Winearls CG, Evans DJ, Rees AJ and Lockwood CM. Microscopic polyarteritis: presentation, pathology and prognosis. Quart J Med 1985; 56:467-83.

47. Weiss MA and Crissman JD. Segmental necrotizing glomerulonephritis: diagnostic, prognostic, and therapeutic significance. Am J Kidney Dis 1985; 6:199-211.

48. Furlong TJ, Ibels LS and Eckstein RP. The clinical spectrum of necrotizing glomerulonephritis. Medicine 1987; 66:192-201.

49. Case Records of the Massachusetts General Hospital, Case 13-1993, N Engl J Med 1993; 328:951-8.

50. Lewis EJ and Schwartz MM. Idiopathic crescentic glomerulonephritis. Sem Nephrol 1982; 2:193-213.

51. Whitworth JA, Morel-Maroger L, Mignon F and Richet G. The significance of extracapillary proliferation. Nephron 1976; 16:1-19.

52. McLeish KR, Yum MN and Luft FC. Rapidly progressive glomerulonephritis in adults: clinical and histologic cor-

relations. Clin Nephrol 1978; 10:43–50.

53. Morrin PAF. Rapidly progressive glomerulonephritis. Am J Med 1978; 65:446–60.

54. Beirne GJ, Wagnild JP, Zimmerman SW, Macken PD and Burkholder PM. Idiopathic crescentic glomerulonephritis. Medicine 1977; 56:349–81.

55. Neild GH, Cameron JS, Ogg CS, Turner DR, Williams DG, Brown CB0 et al. Rapidly progressive glomerulonephritis with extensive glomerular crescent formation. Quart J Med 1983; 52:395–416.

56. Sadjadi SA, Seelig MS, Berger AR and Milstoc M. Rapidly progressive glomerulonephritis in a patient with rheumatoid arthritis during treatment with high-dosage D-penicilla-mine. Am J Nephrol 1985; 5:212–6.

57. Ntoso KA, Tomaszewski JE, Jimenez SA and Neilson EG. Penicillamine-induced rapidly progressive glomerulone-phritis in patients with progressive systemic sclerosis: suc-cessful treatment of two patients and a review of the litera-ture. Am J Kidney Dis 1986; 8:159–63.

58. Sonsino E, Nabarra B, Kazatchkine M, Hinglais N and Kreis H. Extracapillary proliferative glomerulonephritis so-called malignant glomerulonephritis. Adv Nephrol 1972; 2:121–63.

59. Heilman RL, Offord KP, Holley KE and Velosa JA. Analysis of risk factors for patient and renal survival in crescentic glomerulonephritis. Am J Kidney Dis 1987; 9:98–107.

60. Stilmant MM, Bolton WK, Sturgill BC, GW Schmitt and Couser WG. Crescentic glomerulonephritis without immune deposits: clinicopathologic features. Kidney Int 1979; 15:184–95.

61. Bolton WK and Sturgill BC. Methylprednisolone therapy for acute crescentic rapidly progressive glomerulonephritis. Am J Nephrol 1989; 9:368–75.

62. Bruns FJ, Adler S, Fraley DS and Segel DP. Long-term follow-up of aggressively treated idiopathic rapidly pro-gressive glomerulonephritis. Am J Med 1989; 86:400–6.

63. Bhuyan UN, Dash SC, Srivastave RN, Sharma RK and Malhotra KK. Immunopathology, extent and course of glomerulonephritis with crescent formation. Clin Nephrol 1982; 18:280–5.

64. Falk RJ and Jennette JC. Anti-neutrophil cytoplasmic au-toantibodies with specificity for myeloperoxidase in patients with systemic vasculitis and idiopathic necrotizing and crescentic glomerulonephritis. N Engl J Med 1988; 318:1651–7.

65. Tervaert JWC, Goldschmeding R, Elema JD, van der Giessen M, Huitema MG, van der Hem GK et al. Autoan-tibodies against myeloid lysosomal enzymes in crescentic glomerulonephritis. Kidney Int 1990; 37:799–806.

66. D'Amico G. The commonest glomerulonephritis in the world: IgA nephropathy. Quart J Med 1987; 64:709–27.

67. Druet Ph, Bariety J, Bernard D and Lagrue G. Les glomerulopathies primitives a dépôts mésangiaux d'IgA et D'IgG. La Presse Med 1970; 78:583–7.

68. DeWerra P, Morel-Maroger L, Leroux-Robert C and Richet G. Glomerulites a depots d'IgA diffus dans le mesangium. Schweiz med Wschr 1973; 103:761–8.

69. Rodicio JL. Idiopathic IgA nephropathy. Kidney Int 1984;

25:717–29.

70. Levy M, Gonzalez-Burchard G, Broyer M, Dommergues J-P, Foulard M, Sorez J-P et al. Berger's disease in children. Medicine 1985; 64:157–80.

71. Clarkson AR, Seymour AE, Thompson AJ, Haynes WDG, Chan Y-L and Jackson B. IgA nephropathy: a syndrome of uniform morphology, diverse clinical features and uncer-tain prognosis. Clin Nephrol 1977; 8:459–71.

72. Wyatt RJ, Julian BA, Bhathena DB, Mitchell BL, Holland NH and Malluche HH. IgA nephropathy: presentation, clinical course, and prognosis in children and adults. Am J Kidney Dis 1984; 4:192–200.

73. Nicholls KM, Fairley KF, Dowling JP and Kincaid-Smith P. The clinical course of mesangial IgA associated nephropathy in adults. Quart J Med 1984; 53:227–50.

74. Abuelo JG, Esparza AR, Matarese RA, Endreny RG, Car-valho JS and Allegra SR. Crescentic IgA nephropathy. Medicine 1984; 63:396–406.

75. Welch TR, McAdams J and Berry A. Rapidly progressive IgA nephropathy. AJDC 1988; 142:789–93.

75a. Praga M, Gutierrez-Millet V, Navas JJ, Ruilope LM, Morales JM, Alcazar JM, et al. Acute worsening of renal function during episodes of macroscopic hematuria in IgA nephropathy. Kidney Int 1985; 69–74.

75b. Hill PA, Davies DJ, Kincaid-Smith P, Ryan GB. Ultra-structural changes in renal tubules associated with glomerular bleeding. Kidney Int 1989; 36:992–7.

76. Swainson CP, Robson JS, Thomson D and MacDonald MK. Mesangiocapillary glomerulonephritis: a long-term study of 40 cases. J Pathol 1983; 141:449–68.

77. Magil AP, Price JDE, Bower G, Rance CP, Huber J and Chase WH. Membranoproliferative glomerulonephritis type I: comparison of natural history in children and adults. Clin Nephrol 1979; 11:239–44.

78. Donadio JV, Slack TK, Holley KE and Ilstrup DM. Idiopathic membranoproliferative (Mesangiocapillary) glomerulonephritis. Mayo Clin Proc 1979; 54:141–50.

79. Watson AR, Poucell S, Thorner P, Arbus GS, CP Rance and Baumal R. Membranoproliferative glomerulonephritis Type I in children: correlation of clinical features with pathologic subtypes. Am J Kidney Dis 1984; 4:141–6.

80. Taguchi T and Bohle A. Evaluation of change with time of glomerular morphology in membranoproliferative glome-rulonephritis: a serial biopsy of 33 cases. Clin Nephrol 1989; 31:297–306.

81. Cameron JS, Turner DR, Heaton J, Williams DG, Ogg CG, Chantler C et al. Idiopathic mesangiocapillary glomerulonephritis. Am J Med 1983; 74:175–92.

82. Kashtan CE, Burke B, Burch G, Fisker SG and Kim YG. Dense intramembranous deposit disease: A clinical com-parison of histological subtypes. Clin Nephrol 1990; 33:1–6.

83. Bennett WM, Fassett RG, Walker RG, Fairley KF, d'Apice AJF and Kincaid-Smith P. Mesangiocapillary glomerulonephritis type II (Dense-deposit disease): clinical features of progressive disease. Am J Kidney Dis 1989; 13:469–76.

84. Habib R, Loirat C, Gubler MC and Levy M. Morphology and serum complement levels in membranoproliferative

glomerulonephritis. Adv Nephrol 1974; 4:109–35.

85. Johnson RJ, Gretch DR, Yamabe H, Hart J, Bacchi CE, Hartwell P et al. Membranoproliferative glomerulonephritis associated with hepatitis C virus infection. N Engl J Med 1993; 328:465–70.

86. Sechi LA, Pirisi M and Bartoli E. Membranoproliferative glomerulonephritis associated with hepatitis C infection with no evidence of liver disease. JAMA 1994; 271:194.

87. Sissons JGP, West RJ, Fallows J, Williams DG, Boucher BJ, Amos N et al. The complement abnormalities of lipodystrophy. N Engl J Med 1976; 294:461–5.

88. McEnerny PT, McAdams AJ and West CD. The effect of prednisone in a high-dose, alternate-day regimen on the natural history of idiopathic membranoproliferative glomerulonephritis. Medicine 1986; 64:401–24.

89. Ooi YM, Vallota EH and West CD. Classical complement pathway activation in membranoproliferative glomerulonephritis. Kidney Int 1976; 9:46–53.

90. Nissenson AR, Baraff LJ, Fine RN and Knutson DW. Poststreptococcal acute glomerulonephritis: fact and controversy. Ann Intern Med 1979; 91:76–86.

91. Melby PC, Musick WD, Luger AM and Khanna R. Poststreptococcal glomerulonephritis in the elderly. Am J Nephrol 1987; 7:235–40.

92. Colman G, Tanna A, Efstratiou A and Gaworzewska ET. The serotypes of Streptococcus pyogenes present in Britian during 1980–1990 and their association with disease. J Med Microbiol 1993; 39:165–78.

93. Tejani A and Ingulli E. Poststreptococcal glomerulonephritis. Nephron 1990; 55:1–5.

94. Sagel I, Treser G, Ty A, Yoshizawa N, Kleinberger H, Yuceoglu AM et al. Occurrence and nature of glomerular lesions after Group A streptococci infections in children. Ann Intern Med 1973; 79:493–9.

95. Dodge WF, Spargo BH, Travis LB, Srivastava RN, Carvajal HF, DeBeukelaer MM et al. Poststreptococcal glomerulonephritis. N Engl J Med 1972; 286:273–8.

96. Chugh KS, Malhotra HS, Sakhuja V, Bhusnurmath S, Singhal PC and Unni VN. Progression to end stage renal disease in post-streptococcal glomerulonephritis (PSGN) – Chandigarh study. Int'l J Artif Org 1987; 10:189–94.

97. Tewodros W, Muhe L, Daniel E, Schalen C and Kronvall G. A one-year study of streptococcal infections and their complications among Ethiopian children. Epidemiol Infect 1992; 109:211–25.

98. Rodriguez-Iturbe B, Garcia R, Rubio L, Cuenca L, Treser G and Lange K. Epidemic glomerulonephritis in Maracaibo. Evidence for progression to chronicity. Clin Nephrol 1976; 5:197–206.

99. Ludmerer KM and Kissane JM. Septic polyarthritis and acute renal failure in a 57-year-old man. Am J Med 1991; 91:293–9.

100. Pauker SG and Kopelman RI. Treating before knowing. N Engl J Med 1992; 327:1366–9.

101. Nissenson AR, Mayon-White R, Potter EV, Mayon-White V, Abidh S, Poon-King T et al. Continued absence of clinical renal disease seven to 12 years after poststreptococcal acute glomerulonephritis in Trinidad. Am J Med 1979; 67:255–62.

102. Levy M. Infections and glomerular diseases. Clin Immunol Allergy 1986; 6:255–85.

103. Bergholm A-M and Holm SE. Effect of early penicillin treatment on the development of experimental poststreptococcal glomerulonephritis. Acta Path Microbiol Immunol Scand Sect C 1983; 91:271–81.

104. Vogl W, Renke M, Mayer-Eichberger D, Schmitt H and Bohle A. Long-term prognosis for endocapillary glomerulonephritis of poststreptococcal type in children and adults. Nephron 1986; 44:58–65.

105. Lien JWK, Mathew TH and Meadows R. Acute poststreptococcal glomerulonephritis in adults: a long-term study. Quart J Med 1979; 48:99–111.

106. Druet P, Letonturier P, Contet A and Mandet C. Cryoglobulinaemia in human renal diseases. Clin exp Immunol 1973; 15:483–96.

107. Adam C, Morel-Maroger L and Richet G. Cryoglobulins in glomerulonephritis not related to systemic disease. Kidney Int 1973; 3:334–41.

108. Neugarten J and Baldwin DS. Glomerulonephritis in bacterial endocarditis. Am J Med 1984; 77:297–304.

109. Neugarten J, Gallo GR and Baldwin DS. Glomerulonephritis in bacterial endocarditis. Am J Kidney Dis 1984; 3:371–9.

110. Levy RL and Hong R. The immune nature of subacute bacterial endocarditis (SBE) nephritis. Am J Med 1973; 54:645–52.

111. Kauffmann RH, Thompson J, Valentijn RM, Daha MR and Van Es LA. The clinical implications and the pathogenetic significance of circulating immune complexes in infective endocarditis. Am J Med 1981; 71:17–25.

112. Beaufils M, Morel-Maroger L, Sraer J-D, Kanfer A, Kourilsky O and Richet G. Acute renal failure of glomerular origin during visceral abscesses. N Engl J Med 1976; 295:185–9.

113. Narchi H, Taylor R, Azmy AF, Murphy AV and Beattie TJ. Shunt nephritis. J Ped Surg 198; 23:839–41.

114. Arze RS, Rashid H, Morley R, Ward MK and Kerr DNS. Shunt nephritis: report of two cases and review of the literature. Clin Nephrol 1983; 19:48–53.

115. Noe HN and Roy S III. Shunt nephritis. J Urol 1981; 125:731–3.

116. Rifkinson-Mann S, Rifkinson N and Leong T. Shunt nephritis. J Neurosurg 1991; 74:656–9.

117. Nossent JC, Bronsveld W and Swaak AJG. Systemic lupus erythematosus. III. Observations on clinical renal involvement and follow up of renal function: Dutch experience with 110 patients studied prospectively. Ann Rheum Dis 1989; 48:810–6.

118. Baldwin DS, Gluck MC, Lowenstein J and Gallo GR. Lupus nephritis. Clinical course as related to morphologic forms and their transitions. Am J Med 1977; 62:12–30.

119. Appel GB, Silva FG, Pirani CL, Meltzer JI and Estes D. Renal involvement in systemic lupus erythematosus (SLE): a study of 56 patients emphasizing histologic classification. Medicine 1978; 57:371–410.

120. Esdaile JM, Levinton C, Federgreen W, Hayslett JP and Kashgarian M. The clinical and renal biopsy predictors of long-term outcome in lupus nephritis: a study of 87 patients

and review of the literature. Quart J Med 1989; 72:779–833.

121. Magil AB, Ballon HS and Rae A. Focal proliferative lupus nephritis. Am J Med 1982; 72:620–30.

122. Wallace DJ, Podell TE, Weiner JM, Cox MB, Klinenberg JR, Forouzesh S et al. Lupus nephritis. Experience with 230 patients in a private practice from 1950 to 1980. Am J Med 1982; 72:209–20.

123. Morel-Maroger L, Mery J-Ph, Droz D, Godin M, Verroust, Kourilsky O et al. The course of lupus nephritis: contribution of serial renal biopsies. In: Hamburger J, Crosnier J and Maxwell MH, editors. Adv Nephrol 1976; 6:79–118.

124. Striker GE, Kelly MR, Quadracci LJ and Scribner BH. The course of lupus nephritis. In: Kincaid-Smith P, Mathew TH, Becker EL, editors. Glomerulonephritis morphology, natural history, and treatment, Part II. John Wiley & Sons, New York, 1973;1141–66.

125. Banfi G, Mazzucco G, Di Belgiojoso GB, Bosisio MB, Stratta P, Confalonieri R et al. Morphological parameters in lupus nephritis: their relevance for classification and relationship with clinical and histological findings and outcome. Quart J Med 1985; 55:153–68.

126. Gonzalez-Dettoni H and Tron F. Membranous glomerulopathy in systemic lupus erythematosus. In: Grunfeld JP and Maxwell MH, editors. Adv Nephrol 1985; 14:347–64.

127. Cameron JS, Turner DR, Ogg CS, Williams DG, Lessof MH, Chantler C and Leibowitz S. Systemic lupus with nephritis: a long-term study. Quart J Med 1979; 98:1–24.

128. Clark WF, Linton AL, Cordy PE, Keown PE, Lohmann RC and Lindsay RM. Immunologic findings, thrombocytopenia and disease activity in lupus nephritis. CMA Journal 1978; 118:1391–4.

129. Hill GS, Hinglais N, Tron F and Bach J-F. Systemic lupus erythematosus. Am J Med 1978; 64:61–79.

130. Hebert LA. Diagnostic significance of hypocomplementemia. Kidney Int. 1991; 39:811–21.

131. Magil AB, Ballon HS, Chan V, Lirenman DS, Rae A and Sutton RAL. Diffuse proliferative lupus glomerulonephritis. Medicine 1984; 63:210–20.

132. Cheigh JS and Stenzel KH. End-stage renal disease in systemic lupus erythematosus. Am J Kidney Dis 1993; 21:2–8.

133. Correia P, Cameron JS, Ogg CS, Williams DG, Bewick M and Hicks JA. End-stage renal failure in systemic lupus erythematosus with nephritis. Clin Nephrol 1984; 22:293–302.

134. Coplon NS, Diskin CJ, Petersen J and Swenson RS. The long-term clinical course of systemic lupus erythematosus in end-stage renal disease. N Engl J Med 1983; 308:186–90.

135. Phadke K, Trachtman H, Nicastri A, Chen C and Tejani A. Acute renal failure as the initial manifestation of systemic lupus erythematosus in children. J Pediatr 1984; 105:38–41.

136. Bygren P, Rasmussen N, Isaksson B and Wieslander J. Anti-neutrophil cytoplasm antibodies, anti-GBM antibodies and anti-dsDNA antibodies in glomerulonephritis. Eur J Clin Invest 1992; 22:783–92.

137. Kuster S, Apenberg S, Andrassy K and Ritz E. Antineutrophil cytoplasmic antibodies in systemic lupus erythematosus. Contrib Nephrol 1992; 99:94–8.

138. Schur PH. Clinical features of SLE. In: Kelley WN, Harris ED, Ruddy Sand Clement BS, editors. Textbook of rheumatology. W.B. Saunders, Philadelphia, 1993; 1017–42.

139. Hoover LA, Hall-Craggs M and Dagher FJ. Polyarteritis nodosa involving only the main renal arteries. Am J Kidney Dis 1988; 11:66–9.

140. Templeton PA and Pais SO. Renal artery occlusion in PAN. Radiology 1985; 156:308.

141. Lie JT. Retroperitoneal polyarteritis nodosa presenting as ureteral obstruction. J Rheumatol 1992; 19:1628–31.

142. Croker BP, Lee T and Caulie Gunnells J. Clinical and pathologic features of polyarteritis nodosa and its renal-limited variant: Primary crescentic and necrotizing glomerulonephritis. Hum Pathol 1987; 18:38–44.

143. Serra A, Cameron JS, Turner DR, Hartley B, Ogg CS, Neild GH et al. Vasculitis affecting the kidney: presentation, histopathology and long-term outcome. Quart J Med 1984; 53:181–207.

144. Droz D, Noel LH, Leibowitch M and Barbanel C. Glomerulonephritis and necrotizing angiitis. Adv Nephrol 1979; 8:343–63.

145. Kanfer A, Sraer J-D, Feintuch M-J, Morel-Maroger L, Beaufils Ph and Richet G. Insuffisance rénale aiguë au cours de la périartérité noueuse. Nouv Presse Med 1976; 5:1883–8.

146. D'Agati V, Chander P, Nash M and Mancilla-Jiminez R. Idiopathic microscopic polyarteritis nodosa: ultrastructural observations on the renal vascular and glomerular lesions. Am J Kidney Dis 1986; 7:95–110.

147. Ronco P, Verroust P, Mignon F, Kourilsky O, Vanhille Ph, Meyrier A et al. Immunopathological studies of polyarteritis nodosa and Wegener's granulomatosis: a report of 43 patients with 51 renal biopsies. Quart J Med 1983; 52:212–23.

148. Kallenberg CGM and Leontine Mulder AH. Antineutrophil cytoplasmic antibodies: a still-growing class of autoantibodies in inflammatory disorders. Am J Med 1992; 93:675–82.

149. Scott DGI, Bacon PA, Elliott PJ, Tribe CR and Wallington TB. Systemic vasculitis in a district general hospital 1972–1980: clinical and laboratory features, classification and prognosis of 80 cases. Quart J Med 1982; 203:292–311.

150. Guillevin L, Huong Du LT, Godeau P, Jais P and Wechsler B. Clinical findings and prognosis of polyarteritis nodosa and Churg-Strauss angitiis: A study in 165 patients. Brit J Rheumatol 1988; 27:258–64.

151. Ewald EA, Griffin D and McCune WJ. Correlation of angiographic abnormalities with disease manifestations and disease severity in polyarteritis nodosa. J Rheumatol 1987; 14:952–6.

152. Albert DA, Rimon D and Silverstein MD. The diagnosis of polyarteritis nodosa. Arthritis Rheum 1988; 31:1117–27.

153. Hoffman GS, Kerr GS, Leavitt RY, Hallahan CW, Lebovics RS, Travis WD et al. Wegener granulomatosis: an analysis of 158 patients. Ann Intern Med 1992; 116:488–98.

154. Anderson G, Coles ET, Crane M, Douglas AC, Gibbs AR, Geddes DM et al. Wegener's granuloma. A series of 265 British cases seen between 1975 and 1985. A report by a subcommittee of the British Thoracic Society Research Com-

mittee. Quart J Med 1992; 83:427–38.

155. Pinching AJ, Lockwood CM, Pussell BA, Rees AJ, Sweny P and Evans DJ. Wegener's granulomatosis: Observations on 18 patients with severe renal disease. Quart J Med 1983; 52:435–60.

156. Appel GB, Gee B, Kashgarian M and Hayslett JP. Wegener's granulomatosis – clinical-pathologic correlations and long-term course. Am J Kidney Dis 1981; 1:27–37.

157. Grotz W, Wanner C, Keller E, Bohler J, Peter HH, Rohrbach R et al. Crescentic glomerulonephritis in Wegener's granulomatosis: morphology, therapy, outcome. Clin Nephrol 1991; 35:243–51.

158. Lombard CM, Duncan SR, Rizk NW and Colby TV. The diagnosis of Wegener's granulomatosis from transbronchial biopsy specimens. Hum Pathol 1990; 21:838–42.

159. Andrassy K, Erb A, Koderisch J, Waldherr R and Ritz E. Wegener's granulomatosis with renal involvement: patient survival and correlations between initial renal function, renal histology, therapy and renal outcome. Clin Nephrol 1991; 35:139–47.

160. Gross WL, Schmitt WH and Csernok E. ANCA and associated diseases: immunodiagnostic and pathogenic aspects. Clin Exp Immunol 1993; 91:1–12

161. Austin HA III and Balow JE. Henoch-Schonlein nephritis: prognostic features and the challenge of therapy. Am J Kidney Dis 1983; 2:512–20.

162. Faull RJ, Woodroffe AJ, Aarons I and Clarkson AR. Adult Henoch-Schonlein nephritis. Aust NZ J Med 1987; 17:396–401.

163. Fogazzi GB, Pasquali S, Moriggi M, Casanova S, Damilano I, Mihatsch MJ et al. Long-term outcome of Schonlein-Henoch nephritis in the adult. Clin Nephrol 1989; 31:60–6.

164. Roth DA, Wilz DR and Theil GB. Schonlein-Henoch syndrome in adults. Quart J Med 1985; 55:145–52.

165. Lee HS, Koh HI, Kim MJ and Rha HY. Henoch-Schonlein nephritis in adults: a clinical and morphological study. Clin Nephrol 1986; 26:125–30.

166. Piette WW and Stone MS. A cutaneous sign of a IgA-associated small dermal vessel leukocytoclastic vasculitis in adults (Henoch-Schonlein Purpura). Arch Dermatol 1989; 125:53–6.

167. Brouet J-C, Clauvel J-P, Danon F, Klein M and Seligmann M. Biologic and clinical significance of cryoglobulins. A report of 86 cases. Am J Med 1974; 57:775–88.

168. Gorevic PD, Kassab HJ, Levo Y, Kohn R, Meltzer M, Prose P et al. Mixed cryoglobulinemia: clinical aspects and long-term follow-up of 40 patients. Am J Med 1980; 69:287–308.

169. Montagnino G. Reappraisal of the clinical expression of mixed cryoglobulinemia. Springer Semin Immunopathol 1988; 10:1–19.

170. Musset L, Diemert MC, Taibi F, Thi Huong Du L, Cacoub P, Leger JM et al. Characterization of cryoglobulins by immunoblotting. Clin Chem 1992; 38; 798–802.

171. Tarantino A, De Vecchi A, Montagnino G, Imbasciati E, Mihatsch MJ, Zollinger HU et al. Renal disease in essential mixed cryoglobulinaemia. Long-term follow-up of 44 patients. Quart J Med 1981; 50:1–30.

172. Misiani R, Bellavita P, Fenili D, Borelli G, Marchesi D, Massazza M et al. Hepatitis C virus infection in patients with essential mixed cryoglobulinemia. Ann Intern Med 1992; 117:573–7.

173. D'Amico G, Colasanti G, Ferrario F and Sinico RA. Renal involvement in essential mixed cryoglobulinemia. Kidney Int 1989; 35:1004–14.

174. Cordonnier D, Vialtel P, Renversez J Ch, Chenais F, Favre M, Tournoud A et al. Renal diseases in 18 patients with mixed type II IgM-IgG cryoglobulinemia: Monoclonal lymphoid infiltration (2 cases) and membranoproliferative glomerulonephritis (14 cases). Adv Nephrol 1983; 12:177–204.

175. Maggiore Q, Bartolomeo F, L'Abbate A, Misefari V, Martorano C and Caccamo A. Glomerular localization of circulating antiglobulin activity in essential mixed cryoglobulinemia with glomerulonephritis. Kidney Int 1982; 21:387–94.

176. Agnello V, Chung RT and Kaplan LM. A role for hepatitis C virus infection in type II cryoglobulinemia. N Engl J Med 1992; 327:1490–5.

177. Weber MFA, Andrassy K, Pullig O, Koderisch J and Netzer K. Antineutrophil-cytoplasmic antibodies and antiglomerular basement membrane antibodies in Goodpasture's syndrome and in Wegener's granulomatosis. J Am Soc Nephrol 1992; 2:1227–34.

178. Jayne DRW, Marshall PD, Jones SJ and Lockwood CM. Autoantibodies to GBM and neutrophil cytoplasm in rapidly progressive glomerulonephritis. Kidney Int 1990; 37:965–70.

179. Savage COS, Pusey CD, Bowman C, Rees AJ and Lockwood CM. Antiglomerular basement membrane antibody mediated disease in the British Isles 1980–4. BMJ 1986; 292:301–4.

180. Wilson CB and Dixon FJ. Anti-glomerular basement membrane antibody-induced glomerulonephritis. Kidney Int 1973; 3:74–89.

181. Teague CA, Doak PB, Simpson IJ, Rainer SP and Herdson PB. Goodpasture's syndrome: an analysis of 29 cases. Kidney Int 1978; 13:492–504.

182. Briggs WA, Johnson JP, Teichman S, Yeager HC and Wilson CB. Antiglomerular basement membrane antibody-mediated glomerulonephritis and Goodpasture's syndrome. Medicine 1979; 58:348–61.

183. Case Records of the Massachusetts General Hospital. Case 16-1993. N Engl J Med 1993; 328:1183–90.

184. Johnson JP, Moore J Jr., Austin HA III, Balow JE, Antonovych TT and Wilson CB. Therapy of anti-glomerular basement membrane antibody disease: analysis of prognostic significance of clinical, pathologic and treatment factors. Medicine 1985; 62:219–27.

185. Urizar RE, McGoldrick D and Cerda J. Pulmonary-renal syndrome. Its clinicopathologic approach in 1991. NY State J Med 1991; 91:212–21.

186. Salant DJ. Immunopathogenesis of crescentic glomerulonephritis and lung purpura. Kidney Int 1987; 32:408–25.

187. Holdsworth S, Boyce N, Thomson NM and Atkins RC. The clinical spectrum of acute glomerulonephritis and lung haemorrhage (Goodpasture's syndrome). Quart J

Med 1985; 216:75–86.

188. Bosch X, Mirapeix E, Font J, Borellas X, Rodriguez R, Lopez-Soto A et al. Prognostic implication of anti-neutrophil cytoplasmic autoantibodies with myeloperoxidase specificity in anti-glomerular basement membrane disease. Clin Nephrol 1991; 36:107–13.

189. Cameron JS, Healy MJR and Adu D. The medical research council trial of short-term high-dose alternate day prednisolone in idiopathic membranous nephropathy with nephrotic syndrome in adults. Quart J Med 1990; 274:133–56.

190. Murphy BF, Fairley KF and Kincaid-Smith PS. Idiopathic membranous glomerulonephritis: Long-term follow-up in 139 cases. Clin Nephrol 1988; 30:175–81.

191. Donadio JV, Torres VE, Velosa JA, Wagoner RD, Holley KE, Okamura M et al. Idiopathic membranous nephropathy: the natural history of untreated patients. Kidney Int 1988; 33:708–15.

192. Zimmerman SW, Moorthy AV, Dreher WH, Friedman A and Varanasi U. Prospective trial of warfarin and dipyridamole in patients with membranoproliferative glomerulonephritis. Am J Med 1983; 75:920–7.

193. Brown CB, Cameron JS, Turner DR, Chantler C, Ogg CS, Williams DG et al. Focal segmental glomerulosclerosis with rapid decline in renal function ("malignant FSGS"). Clin Nephrol 1978; 10:51–61.

194. Detwiler RK. Collapsing glomerulopathy: a clinically and pathologically distinct variant of focal segmental glomerulosclerosis. Kidney Int 1994; 45:1416–24.

195. Korbet SM, Schwartz MM, Rosenberg BF, Sibley RK and Lewis EJ. Immunotactoid glomerulopathy. Medicine 1985; 64:228–43.

196. Alpers CE, Rennke HG, Hopper J and Biava CG. Fibrillary glomerulonephritis: an entity with unusual immunofluorescence features. Kidney Int 1987; 31:781–9.

197. Fogo A, Qureshi N and Horn RG. Morphologic and clinical features of fibrillary glomerulonephritis versus immunotactoid glomerulopathy. Am J Kidney Dis 1993; 22:367–77.

198. Jones RH, Mackay JD, Hayakawa H, Parsons V and Watkins PJ. Progression of diabetic nephropathy. Lancet 1979; 1:1105–6.

199. Goldstein DA and Massry SG. Diabetic nephropathy. Nephron 1978:20:286–96.

200. Ordonez JD and Hiatt RA. Comparison of type II and type I diabetics treated for end-stage renal disease in a large prepaid health plan population. Nephron 1989; 51:524–9.

201. Ogg CS, Cameron JS, Williams DG and Turner DR. Presentation and course of primary amyloidosis of the kidney. Clin Nephrol 1981; 15:9–13.

202. Martinez-Vea A, Garcia C, Carreras M, Revert L and Oliver JA. End-stage renal disease in systemic amyloidosis: clinical course and outcome on dialysis. Am J Nephrol 1990; 10:283–9.

203. Alpers CE, Tu W, Hopper J and Biava CG. Single light subclass (kappa chain) immunoglobulin deposition in glomerulonephritis. Hum Pathol 1985; 16:294–304.

204. Ganeval D, Noel LH, Preud'Homme JL, Droz D and Grunfeld JP. Light-chain deposition disease: Its relation with AL-type amyloidosis. Kidney Int 1984; 26:1–9.

205. Heilman RL, Velosa JA, Holley KE, Offord KP and Kyle RA. Long-term follow-up and response to chemotherapy in patients with light-chain deposition disease. Am J Kidney Dis 1992; 20:34–41.

206. Buxbaum JN, Chuba, JV, Hellman GC, Solomon A and Gallo GR. Monoclonal immunoglobulin deposition disease: light chain and light and heavy deposition diseases and their relation to light chain analysis. Ann Intern Med 1990; 112:455–64.

207. Grishman E, Churg J and Porush JG. Glomerular morphology in nephrotic heroin addicts. Lab Invest 1976; 35:415–24.

208. Cunningham EE, Brentjens JR, Zielezny MA, Andres GA and Venuto RC. Heroin nephropathy. A clinicopathologic and epidemiologic study. Am J Med 1980; 68:47–53.

209. Langs C, Gallo GR, Schacht RG, Sidhu G and Baldwin DS. Rapid renal failure in AIDS-associated focal glomerulosclerosis. Arch Intern Med 1990; 150:287–92.

210. Bourgoignie, JJ. Renal complications of human immunodeficiency virus type 1. Kidney Int 1990; 37:1571–84.

211. Nochy D, Glotz D, Dosquet P, Pruna A, Lemoine R, Guettier C et al. Renal lesions associated with human immunodeficiency virus infection: North American vs. European experience. Adv Nephrol 1993; 22:269–86.

212. Carbone L, D'Agati V, Cheng J and Appel GB. Course and prognosis of human immunodeficiency virus-associated nephropathy. Am J Med 1989; 87:389–95.

213. Rao TKS. Human immunodeficiency virus (HIV) associated nephropathy. Annu Rev Med 1991; 42:391–401.

214. Smith JD and Hayslett JP. Reversible renal failure in the nephrotic syndrome. Am J Kidney Dis 1992; 19:201–13.

215. Yamauchi H and Hopper J. Hypovolemic shock and hypotension as a complication in the nephrotic syndrome. Ann Intern Med 1964; 60:242–54.

216. Crowley JP, Matarese RA, Quevado SF and Garella S. Fibrinolytic therapy for bilateral renal vein thrombosis. Arch Intern Med 1984; 144:159–60.

217. Rowe JM, Rasmussen RL, Mader SL, Dimarco PL, Cockett ATK and Marder VJ. Successful thrombolytic therapy in two patients with renal vein thrombosis. Am J Med 1984; 77:1111–4.

218. Gertz MA, Chin-Yang L, Shirahama T and Kyle RA. Utility of subcutaneous fat aspiration for the diagnosis of systemic amyloidosis (immunoglobulin light chain). Arch Intern Med 1988; 148:929.

219. Sungur C, Sungur A, Ruacan S, Arik N, Yasavul U, Turgan C et al. Diagnostic value of bone marrow biopsy in patients with renal disease secondary to familial Mediterranean fever. Kidney Int 1993; 44:834–6.

220. Maschio G, Oldrizzi L and Rugiu C. Is there a "point of no return" in progressive renal disease? J Am Soc Nephrol 1991; 2:832–40.

221. Klahr S, Schreiner G and Ichikawa I. Mechanisms of disease. N Engl J Med 1988; 318:1657–66.

12. Tubular causes of renal failure

DOUGLAS SHEMIN

INTRODUCTION

Tubular causes of acute renal failure may be broadly divided into two pathophysiologic categories: syndromes of *acute tubular cell necrosis (ATN)*, and syndromes of *tubular obstruction* with secondary tubular cell damage (Table 12.1). The first category encompasses a wide variety of processes, including tubular cell necrosis due to ischemia, exogenous toxins or the endogenous proteins, myoglobin and hemoglobin. In the second category, intratubular obstruction may be caused by immunoglobulin light chains, uric acid, or by a variety of exogenous toxins, such as ethylene glycol metabolites, rifampin, methotrexate, and sulfonamide antibiotics.

ACUTE TUBULAR NECROSIS

General Features

While there are many causes of ATN, certain general diagnostic principles apply. All patients have a distinct rise in BUN and Scr. *Hyperkalemia and a normal anion gap metabolic acidosis*, reflecting decreased renal tubular secretion of potassium and hydrogen, are common. Typically, urine output is in the nonoliguric range; oliguria is not unusual, but anuria is rare. The urinalysis may show *renal tubular cells, granular casts, and tubular cell casts*, but nephrotic or nephritic findings, such as heavy proteinuria, significant hematuria (>100 RBC/hpf), or red blood cell casts, are rare. Patients with tubular renal failure usually have urine sodium concentrations above 20 mEq/L, reflecting impaired tubular reabsorptive capacity. Typically, administration of isotonic fluid does not improve

Table 12.1. Tubular causes of renal failure

Acute tubular necrosis	*Tubular obstruction*
Ischemia	Myeloma kidney
Exogenous toxins	Ig light chains
Aminoglycosides	Tumor lysis syndrome
Other drugs and chemicals	Uric acid/phosphate
Pigments	Miscellaneous etiologies
Myoglobin	Oxalic acid
Hemoglobin	Other substances

renal function or urine output; in fact, when given fluid, patients may develop volume overload. Histologic study on renal biopsy shows *necrosis of tubular cells*, obstruction of the tubular lumen by *cellular debris*, and normal glomeruli and blood vessels.

Pathophysiology. Although the disease processes causing ATN do not directly affect glomerular function, they may decrease GFR by three mechanisms. First, necrosed and sloughed tubular cells may *obstruct the tubular lumen* and oppose glomerular filtration (Figure 12.1). Second, tubular fluid may *reenter capillaries after filtration* via damaged and permeable tubular cells. Third, in a process termed tubuloglomerular feedback, impaired proximal tubular reabsorption of sodium leads to increased distal delivery, triggering *glomerular hypoperfusion*.

Acute Tubular Necrosis Due to Ischemia

Definition

Renal hypoperfusion accounts for about half of all cases of acute renal failure in hospitalized patients [1–3]. A reduction in renal perfusion may cause a continuum of renal functional abnormalities: if the reduction is mild or of short duration, prerenal azotemia results, and renal function generally normalizes with correction of volume depletion or renal blood flow. If the ischemic insult is severe or

J.G. Abuelo (ed.), Renal Failure, 117–130.
© 1995 *Kluwer Academic Publishers.*

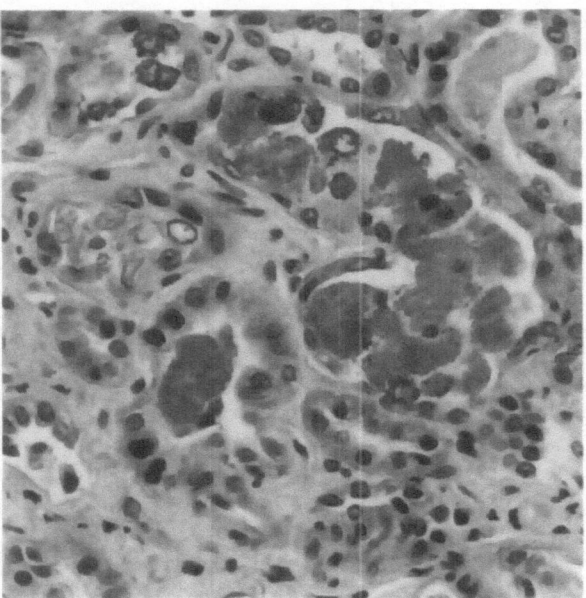

Fig. 12.1. Renal biopsy from a patient with ischemic ATN. It shows tubules with exfoliation of necrotic cells and debris in the form of large pigmented granular casts. (Courtesy of Dr. Alfredo Esparza.)

long lasting, ATN occurs and restoration of renal perfusion will not immediately reverse the renal failure.

Causes

Ischemic ATN occurs in three clinical circumstances (Table 12.2): *hypotension* resulting from renal or gastrointestinal fluid loss, hemorrhage, extensive burns, severe myocardial dysfunction or septic shock, *surgical interruption of aortic blood flow*, or *acute renal vasoconstriction*, which may occur in sepsis and endotoxemia [4] or liver failure [5].

Clinical picture

Patients with ischemic ATN have varying presentations depending upon the etiology. With a deficit in intravascular volume, there is a *history of hemorrhage, vomiting or diarrhea, or excess diuresis*, and physical examination shows orthostatic hypotension, tachycardia, flat neck veins, dry mucous membranes, and decreased skin turgor. Cardiogenic shock may be caused by acute myocardial infarction, acute valvular dysfunction due to a ruptured papillary muscle or endocarditis, or a viral or ischemic cardiomyopathy. Patients will have clinical evidence of *left ventricular dysfunction*, with

Table 12.2. Causes of ischemic ATN

Hypotensive states
  Hypovolemia
  Cardiogenic shock
  Septic shock
Surgical interruption of perfusion
Renal vasoconstriction
  Sepsis
  Liver failure

hypotension, jugular venous distension, pulmonary edema, and an S3 gallop. The risks of renal failure are greatest with systolic blood pressures below 80 mmHg [6]. A surgical interruption of aortic blood flow occurs with *cardiac, aortic, or renal vascular surgery*, and the risk of renal failure varies directly with ischemia time. Acute renal failure is likely if suprarenal aortic cross-clamping time exceeds 50 minutes [7] or if cardiopulmonary bypass time exceeds 160 minutes [8]. With renal vasoconstriction due to sepsis, patients have fever, hypotension, tachycardia, leukocytosis, and bacteremia, especially with *gram negative organisms*. However, in some septic individuals, the blood pressure, temperature, and white cell count may be normal [9]. Both oliguric and nonoliguric states have been reported [2, 3]. ATN in various types of cirrhosis and liver failure may occur as a consequence of the hepatorenal syndrome, with superimposed effective volume depletion and decreased renal perfusion [10].

Patients with ischemic ATN manifest common laboratory findings. The urine sediment usually shows granular casts and other elements typical of tubular necrosis (see above). Urine tests reflect impaired tubular water and sodium reabsorption, with the urine specific gravity about 1.010, the urine sodium concentration above 20 mEq/L and the urinary fractional excretion of sodium greater than 1.0 percent [11]. The BUN/Scr ratio is generally not greater than 15 or 20 (0.60 or 0.80 in SI units), since the urea and creatinine clearances decline at proportionate rates.

Pathology. Renal biopsies show *patchy* tubular epithelial cell necrosis, with *distal* tubular segments primarily involved; this tends to differentiate ischemic from toxic tubular injury, which is characterized by a more diffuse pattern, involving proximal segments [12].

Diagnosis

The diagnosis of ischemic acute tubular necrosis is one of exclusion. Reversible prerenal and postrenal causes should be ruled out by history, physical examination, and in selected cases by bladder catheterization and renal ultrasound. Tubular nephrotoxins should be identified. If none of these factors is present, and there is evidence of volume depletion, hypotension, or bacterial sepsis, then ischemic ATN is a likely diagnosis. Typical urine tests and urine sediment are supportive evidence. Many patients with renal hypoperfusion are critically ill and receive multiple nephrotoxic agents; frequently, decreased renal perfusion is only one of a number of factors contributing to acute renal failure.

> *Pitfalls.* The blood pressure may fall, precipitate ischemic tubular necrosis and then return to normal by the time azotemia is noted. The physician may not learn of this transient ischemia, unless he examines the previous blood pressure records. Patients with ATN due to sepsis or liver failure may not have hypotension (systolic blood pressure less than 100 to 110 mmHg). Urine sodium content may be misleading. ATN with a FENa less than 1% can occur, especially with cardiac surgery, liver failure, myoglobinuria, burns, and sepsis [13].

Acute Tubular Renal Failure Due to Exogenous Toxins

Definition

ATN may occur as a result of exposure to a variety of drugs and toxins. Because several nephrotoxic drugs are often administered simultaneously or in the setting of multiorgan involvement, hemodynamic instability, and infection, all causes of tubular ischemia, it may be difficult to attribute acute renal failure to one tubular insult.

Causes (Table 12.3)

The *aminoglycoside antibiotics*, gentamicin, tobramycin, netilmicin, streptomycin, kanamycin, and amikacin cause tubular toxicity, with specific proximal tubular effects. They lead to renal failure in five to ten percent of all patients treated [14], and are implicated as one of the four leading causes of acute renal failure in hospitalized patients [1, 15].

Other antibiotics cause ATN in rare cases. The first generation *cephalosporins* cephaloridine and cephalothin, no longer in current use, were noted to induce ATN in early reports. The antifungal agent,

Table 12.3. Exogenous tubular toxins

Aminoglycosides
Amphotericin B
Pentamidine
Foscarnet
Cisplatin
Heavy metals
Other drugs and chemicals (see Appendix)

---

amphotericin B, produces tubular toxicity in a majority of patients treated [16, 17]. The antiprotozoal agent, *pentamidine*, used to treat pneumocystis infections in human immunodeficiency virus disease, and the antiviral agent, *foscarnet*, are also nephrotoxic [18, 19].

Among antineoplastic chemotherapeutic agents, *cisplatin* is the most common tubular toxin, leading to renal failure in about 20 % of cases [20]; its analogue carboplatin is less nephrotoxic, but tubular damage and azotemia have been reported [21]. Besides platinum, other *heavy metals*, including mercury, cadmium, and arsenic, have been infrequently associated with tubular toxicity. Other drugs and chemicals induce ATN in rare cases (see appendix).

Clinical picture

Aminoglycosides. Nephrotoxicity will not generally develop until seven to ten days after initiation of therapy. High urine sodium concentrations and a nonoliguric state, reflecting decreased tubular reabsorption of sodium and water, are characteristic. Renal losses may cause hypokalemia and hypomagnesemia [14, 22]. Risk factors for nephrotoxicity include liver disease with *hyperbilirubinemia* [23, 24], *septic shock* [24], and an *elevated trough level* of the drug (greater than 2.0 mg/L (4.2 μmol/L) in the case of gentamicin and tobramycin), although renal failure may occur with therapeutic levels [24].

Amphotericin B. Nephrotoxicity may develop after one or two days of therapy [17, 25], and can occur after doses as low as 20 mg. However, renal failure usually occurs after one week of treatment [26], and its incidence rises markedly with a *daily dose greater than 0.5 mg/kg* [25]. Patients are nonoliguric and frequently hypokalemic and hypomagnesemic due to urinary losses. Although not usually necessary for a diagnosis, renal biopsies show tubular necrosis with interstitial and intratubular calcifications [17, 27].

Pentamidine. Renal failure occurs after seven to ten days of therapy. It is typically associated with severe *hyperkalemia* and *type IV renal tubular acidosis*, with low levels of renin and aldosterone [18]. Life threatening hyperkalemia may be present with only modest levels of azotemia [28].

Foscarnet. Nephrotoxicity may develop within five days of initiation of therapy, but mostly occurs after 14 days of therapy [19, 29]. The urine sediment is inactive; low grade proteinuria is sometimes a feature [19, 29]. Renal biopsy shows proximal tubular necrosis with a normal interstitium [19].

Cisplatin. This drug accumulates in renal tissue within one hour of intravenous administration [30] and clinical nephrotoxicity develops immediately after an initial dose. Patients are typically nonoliguric; indeed, impairment of proximal tubular sodium reabsorption tends to cause *polyuria and orthostatic hypotension* [31]. Renal magnesium and potassium wasting, causing *hypokalemia*, *hypomagnesemia*, and *hypocalcemia*, is common [30, 31]. As in other causes of nephrotoxic ATN, a renal biopsy is generally not mandatory for a diagnosis, but light microscopy shows tubular cell degeneration and interstitial edema, electron microscopy shows degeneration of intracellular mitochondria and brush border microvilli, and glomeruli are normal [32].

> Chronic nephrotoxicity may also occur. With multiple courses of therapy GFR may slowly worsen for up to two years and produce irreversible renal failure [33, 34].

Diagnosis
The diagnosis of nephrotoxic ATN should be made in patients who develop acute azotemia immediately after exposure in the cases of cisplatin, or after seven to ten days of exposure to pentamidine, amphotericin, or aminoglycosides. A nonoliguric state, a normal extracellular volume, a urine sodium content and sediment compatible with ATN, and lack of evidence for other causes of renal failure, support the diagnosis.

Acute Tubular Necrosis Due to Myoglobin and Hemoglobin Pigments

Definition
Renal failure due to a high intratubular concentration of the endogenous pigments, *myoglobin* or *hemoglobin*, is another common cause of ATN. Myoglobin and hemoglobin are structurally similar. Myoglobin is present in skeletal, cardiac, and smooth muscle tissue and hemoglobin is present in erythrocytes. Muscle injury, or *rhabdomyolysis*, releases myoglobin into the plasma. When the amount of myoglobin overwhelms the ability of plasma proteins to bind it, the free myoglobin level increases, myoglobin is readily filtered, and *myoglobinuria* results. The higher molecular weight of hemoglobin, and its binding to haptoglobin normally prevent its glomerular filtration, so that nephrotoxic levels of *hemoglobinuria* only occur with *massive intravascular hemolysis* and extremely elevated free hemoglobin levels [35].

> *Pathophysiology.* The mechanism of injury in myoglobinuria or hemoglobinuria is probably not via a direct toxic or obstructive effect on the tubule. Infusions of myoglobin or hemoglobin do not reliably cause renal failure. Concomitant renal ischemia, decreased renal tubular flow from volume depletion, and aciduria with production of nephrotoxic metabolites of myoglobin and hemoglobin at a low urine pH are exacerbating factors [36].

Causes

Myoglobinuric ATN. Rhabdomyolysis and myoglobinuria occur in conditions associated with skeletal muscle damage (Table 12.4). Wartime crush injuries led to the first reported cases [37]. The most common causes now are prolonged *seizures*, and *muscle compression* during alcohol and narcotic induced stupor, especially in the settings of hypophosphatemia and hypokalemia [38]. The illicit drugs, *cocaine* and *"crack"*, can cause the syndrome even in the absence of immobility and muscle compression [39]. Exhaustive exercise, especially in heat [40], pheochromocytoma [41], hyperosmolar coma [42], the hypolipidemic drug, lovastatin, especially with the concomitant use of cyclosporine A [43] or gemfibrozil [44], and overdoses of the sympathetic agonists, theophylline and terbutaline [45, 46] have all been implicated.

Table 12.4. Causes of myoglobinuric ATN

Nontraumatic injury	Drugs and toxins
Heat stroke/exhaustion	"Crack"/cocaine
β-Agonist Excess	Alcohol
β-agonist overdose	Heroin/methadone
Amphetamines	Lovastatin
Pheochromocytoma	Gemfibrozil
Infectious agents	Muscle injury
Viral influenza	Muscle compression
Coxsackie virus	Exhaustive exercise
Electrolyte abnormalities	Prolonged seizures
Hypokalemia	High voltage electric shock
Hypophosphatemia	*Traumatic injury*
Hyperosmolar state	Crush injury

Hemoglobinuric ATN. Hemoglobinuria occurred much more commonly in the past, usually after hemolytic *blood transfusion reactions* [36]. Currently, hemoglobinuric ATN is rare. Causes include inadvertent intravenous or intravesical administration of hypotonic fluids, such as water, glycerol, and glycine, [47] and exposure to a number of chemicals or gases [48]. Cases reported from outside the United States have included poisonous snakebite [49], *P. falciparum* malaria [50], and the hemoglobinopathy, glucose-6-phosphate dehydrogenase deficiency, in the setting of favism or other ingestions [51].

Clinical picture

Myoglobinuric ATN. Myoglobinuric renal failure occurs predominately in males [38, 52, 53]; it is unclear whether this is due to a greater incidence of alcohol and narcotic use in men or whether increased muscle mass produces higher levels of myoglobinuria after rhabdomyolysis. Patients with rhabdomyolysis and myoglobinuric ATN always manifest *acute muscle injury.* Muscles in the extremities, thorax and abdomen may be edematous and tender, and signs of compartment syndrome, with compression of nerves and vessels in an edematous extremity, may be present [52]. The muscle enzymes *creatine phosphokinase (CPK)* and aldolase are always elevated. The CPK ranges from 500 IU/L to greater than 100,000 IU/L, but is most commonly >16,000 IU/L [40, 53], and the degree of CPK elevation roughly correlates with the risk of and the severity of renal failure [53]. Serum levels of other intracellular substances (lactate

dehydrogenase, aminotransferases, potassium, uric acid, phosphorus) are generally elevated. Because creatine and creatinine are released from muscle cells, the Scr may be disproportionately elevated compared to the BUN [54], and the serum creatinine usually rises more rapidly than in other etiologies of acute renal failure; elevations by increments of >2.5 mg/dL/day are usual. The fractional excretion of sodium may be lower than 1% [55]. The *urine myoglobin level* is transiently elevated.

> Myoglobin reacts with the orthotoluidine test strip on a urinalysis dipstick, and a positive urine dipstick for blood is a more sensitive test for urine myoglobin than the spectrophotometric urine assay performed in most laboratories [35]. A patient with rhabdomyolysis and myoglobinuria will typically have a positive urine dipstick for blood, but no erythrocytes on examination of the sediment. Simultaneously, the spectrophotometric urine assay for myoglobin is often negative. Very high levels of myoglobin impart a reddish-brown tinge to the urine.

Urine pH tends to be maximally acidic (pH <5.5), which enhances the risk of renal failure [53]. *Hypocalcemia* is common, and is a result of decreased renal hydroxylation of vitamin D, increased calcium uptake into injured muscle cells, and release of phosphate from muscle leading to calcium-phosphate deposition [56].

Hemoglobinuric ATN. This results from massive hemolysis, and patients invariably demonstrate anemia with spherocytes, red cell fragments, and elevated lactate dehydrogenase especially, fractions 1 and 2. The reticulocyte count and the total and indirect bilirubin are increased, and haptoglobin is decreased. The urine is red or reddish-brown, and as in myoglobinuria, intact red blood cells are not seen in the urine sediment examination, but the dipstick orthotoluidine test is positive for blood. Patients with hemoglobinuric ATN have pink serum, reflecting the free hemoglobin. In contrast, in myoglobinuric ATN, the serum is clear because the kidneys filter myoglobin from serum unless oligoanuria is present [35].

Diagnosis
The diagnosis of myoglobinuric ATN should be suspected in patients with acute muscle injury when the urine dipstick orthotoluidine reaction is positive

and there are no red cells in the urine sediment. CPK and aldolase levels should be ordered; a CPK of greater than 16,000 IU/L strongly suggests the diagnosis, but any CPK over 500 IU/L is compatible. A urine myoglobin assay should be ordered. A positive test supports the diagnosis, but a negative result is not helpful. The clinical findings associated with rhabdomyolysis are unique enough that a diagnosis can generally be made by a history, physical examination, and laboratory studies; a renal biopsy is typically not necessary.

The rarer diagnosis of hemoglobinuric ATN should be made in patients with evidence of massive hemolysis, especially when the urine dipstick is positive for blood, and there are no red cells in the urine sediment. Haptoglobin, lactic dehydrogenase, total and indirect bilirubin, reticulocyte count, and a serum free hemoglobin should be ordered. The haptoglobin will be low and the other tests will always be high. In most cases, the diagnosis can be made on clinical grounds, without a renal biopsy.

Pitfalls. The urine dipstick test for heme pigments may be negative in occasional cases of myoglobinuric ATN due to the transiency of myoglobin release [38]. In other cases, because of a concomitant urologic cause, the urine sediment may contain erythrocytes, rendering the positive dipstick test for heme less useful.

TUBULAR OBSTRUCTION

Intratubular precipitation of a variety of endogenous and exogenous substances may cause obstruction and renal failure.

Tubular Obstruction Due to Light Chains (Myeloma Kidney)

Definition

Immunoglobulin light chains often cause acute renal failure by tubular obstruction in *multiple myeloma*. (Chapter 11 discusses the glomerular lesions seen in myeloma: amyloidosis and light chain deposition disease; this section considers tubular involvement.) Immunoglobulin light chains, also called Bence-Jones proteins, are synthesized by plasma cells and have either a kappa or lambda structural configuration. Normally, these light chains are freely filtered by the glomerulus, then

reabsorbed and catabolized by proximal tubular cells [57]. When, in myeloproliferative disorders, production of light chains exceeds the resorptive capacity of the proximal tubules, light chains are excreted in the urine and acute renal failure occurs by two mechanisms. High intratubular concentrations of light chains form inspissated casts, either alone or in conjunction with Tamm-Horsfall protein, which is synthesized in the distal nephron [58; 59]; these casts then block urine flow. Light chains may also have an acute tubular toxic effect [60]. This entity is called *myeloma kidney* or *cast nephropathy*.

Pathology. The renal biopsy typically shows *intratubular proteinaceous casts* surrounded by giant cells; the tubular epithelium is frequently degenerated or necrotic (Figure 12.2). Extratubular abnormalities, such as an increase in glomerular mesangial matrix, glomerular amyloid, and nephrocalcinosis, may also be seen [58].

Causes

While the usual cause of renal failure due to tubular obstruction by light chains is *multiple myeloma* [57, 59], rare cases have been reported with lymphoma and Waldenstrom macroglobulinemia. About a third of patients with Waldenstrom macroglobulinemia have light chains in the urine but they rarely cause tubular obstruction [57].

Pathogenesis. Not all light chains are nephrotoxic. In one study, injection of equal amounts of light chains from different myeloma patients into mice caused renal failure in some animals [61], but the nephrotoxic characteristics of light chains have not been identified. The quantitative amount of light chains in the urine [58] or their isoelectric point [60] does not correlate with renal failure, and kappa and lambda light chains occur in myeloma kidney patients in roughly equal proportion [58, 62, 63].

Other mechanisms may contribute to renal failure in multiple myeloma, including volume depletion, sepsis, hypercalcemia, amyloidosis, the use of nephrotoxic drugs, and urinary obstruction [57–60, 62, 63], but tubular obstruction by Bence-Jones proteins is the leading one.

Clinical picture

Patients with acute renal failure due to myeloma kidney have typical features of multiple myeloma. Patients are generally middle-aged or elderly, and few are under 50 years old. Physical examination

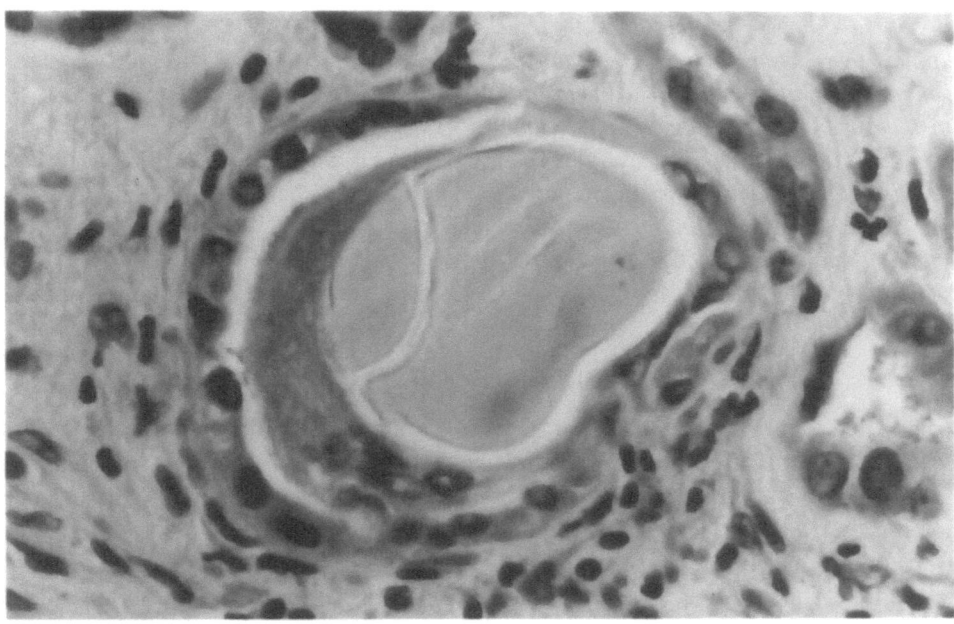

Fig. 12.2. Renal biopsy from a patient with multiple myeloma and cast nephropathy. It shows a large homogeneous cast surrounded by a multinucleated giant cell histiocyte. The epithelial cells lining the tubule show mild degenerative changes. (Courtesy of Dr. Alfredo Esparza.)

may show *pallor* and local *bone or back tenderness.* Anemia with rouleaux formation is common. *Hypercalcemia,* and a *low or negative anion gap,* due to high concentrations of cationic paraproteins are typical laboratory abnormalities. Light chains produce proximal tubular damage and one may observe the *Fanconi syndrome,* with glycosuria, phosphaturia, aminoaciduria, hypokalemia, and renal tubular acidosis. *Osteopenia* and *lytic bone lesions* can be seen on radiographs [59, 64]. Occasionally, the patient may be otherwise asymptomatic from myeloma, and renal failure will be the presenting complaint. A *monoclonal paraprotein in the serum or urine* and infiltration of the bone marrow by *plasma cells* are pathognomonic of multiple myeloma. Some myelomas produce only light chains; these are cleared from the blood by the kidneys and can only be detected in the urine, unless renal failure develops. Although heavy chains do not cause renal failure, IgD myeloma and IgA myeloma feature renal failure more commonly (60% and 33% respectively) than IgG myeloma, which has a renal failure risk of 14% [59]. The urine dipstick protein test, which is relatively specific for albumin, may be negative, but light chains in the urine will react strongly in the *sulfosalicylic acid*

test for protein or the *toluene-sulfonic acid* test for Bence-Jones protein. A urine protein to creatinine ratio will also detect light chains in the urine. In one study, a majority of myeloma patients with renal failure had visible myeloma casts, with giant cells, on urine cytology [65].

Diagnosis
The diagnosis of renal failure due to myeloma kidney should be suspected in patients with signs suggestive of multiple myeloma: infection, bone pain, and anemia with rouleaux formation. Given the high incidence of the disease in the elderly, it is reasonable to consider it in patients over the age of 60 with unexplained renal failure, even in the absence of symptoms.

A urine sulfosalicylic acid or other non-dipstick protein test, urine protein electrophoresis, and serum protein electrophoresis can be used. Immunofixation electrophoresis can be used to characterize any monoclonal protein found on protein electrophoresis. A bone marrow biopsy, typically showing plasmacytosis, is the definitive diagnostic test for myeloma, and it is indicated if a monoclonal protein is detected. Serum viscosity, uric acid, and calcium should be ordered to investigate potential contributing nephrotoxic effects.

A renal biopsy is not necessary to make the diagnosis of myeloma kidney or to dictate treatment. It may be helpful if the clinical findings are atypical or if the bone marrow biopsy or electrophoretic studies are inconclusive or conflicting. If significant urinary albumin excretion is noted, for example, the renal biopsy could diagnose amyloidosis associated with myeloma. Renal histologic findings are also helpful in predicting outcome [58, 66].

Tubular Obstruction Due to Tumor Lysis Syndrome

Definition

Tumor lysis syndrome occurs as a result of therapy for *neoplastic disorders*, especially when neoplasms are *rapidly proliferating* and the therapy causes massive *tumor cell destruction*. The lysis of tumor releases intracellular nucleic acids, uric acid, phosphate, and potassium into the extracellular space, leading to hyperuricemia, hyperphosphatemia, and hyperkalemia, and in turn to hyperuricosuria and hyperphosphaturia. *Uric acid*, particularly in the presence of low urine flow and pH, precipitates and obstructs renal tubules [67]. In some cases, increased intratubular *xanthine*, a uric acid precursor [68] or *phosphate* [69–71] can also produce tubular obstruction.

Causes

The prototypic diseases associated with tumor lysis syndrome are *non-Hodgkin's lymphomas* of high or intermediate grade histology. In particular, the syndrome has been reported in *Burkitt lymphoma*, which is a rapidly growing bulky abdominal tumor, invariably fatal without treatment, and very responsive to induction chemotherapy [67]. The syndrome may also occur with treatment of different types of leukemia, and, less commonly, solid tumors (Table 12.5).

Tumor lysis syndrome may follow a wide variety of cytotoxic chemotherapeutic agents [67, 70, 71, 73–77, 79–82]; it has also been reported after radiation therapy [78], interferon [83], tamoxifen [84], and high dose glucocorticoids [85]. The syndrome tends to occur with *induction*, rather than maintenance, chemotherapy and with the use of *multiple*, rather than single chemotherapeutic agents [67, 71]. In rare cases, hematopoietic tumors may proliferate so rapidly that they produce tumor lysis syndrome even without treatment [86, 87].

Table 12.5. Neoplasms that cause tumor lysis syndrome

Leukemias	*Solid tumors*
Acute lymphoblastic [72]	Breast carcinoma [76]
Chronic lymphocytic [73]	Merkel cell cancer [77]
Acute myelomonocytic [74]	Medulloblastoma [78]
Chronic myelogenous [75]	Bronchogenic carcinoma [79]

Lymphomas (67, 80)
Burkitt's
Other Non-Hodgkin's
Lymphosarcoma (68)

Clinical picture

Tumor lysis syndrome typically occurs in patients with lymphoproliferative malignancies. Physical examination and imaging studies generally reveal bulky tumor masses, adenopathy, and hepatosplenomegaly. Hyperuricemia and azotemia preceding administration of chemotherapy increases the risk for acute renal failure [67, 71], as does a markedly elevated pre-therapy lactate dehydrogenase level [71, 80].

Tumor lysis syndrome typically occurs 24 to 48 hours after chemotherapy with a clinically evident decrease in tumor size and adenopathy, and progressive azotemia and oliguria. Laboratory studies show *hyperuricemia*, often with levels above 20 mg/dL (1200 μmol/L) [78, 83, 85], and *hyperphosphatemia*, with levels above 10 mg/dL (3.23 mmol/L) [67, 71]. Hyperkalemia may be out of proportion to the degree of renal failure, reflecting efflux of potassium from cells. Levels of greater than 9.0 mEq/L, with ventricular tachycardia and cardiac arrest, have been reported [81, 82]. *Hypocalcemia* can be severe, although tetany and cardiac toxicity are rare [67, 71, 80]. Hypocalcemia is primarily due to hyperphosphatemia with precipitation of calcium phosphate salts; decreased renal calcitriol synthesis may also play a role [88]. Urine phosphate excretion is markedly increased [71], with phosphate crystals visible on examination of the sediment; sheets of uric acid crystals may also be seen (Figure 5.1C) [83, 89].

Although laboratory abnormalities associated with tumor lysis (hyperphosphatemia, hyperkalemia, hyperuricemia, hypocalcemia) are common, azotemia occurs in less than ten percent of patients at risk [80], probably due to preventive therapy with intravenous fluids and xanthine oxidase inhibitors (see Chapter 16).

Diagnosis

The diagnosis of the tumor lysis syndrome should be suspected when a lymphoproliferative or other neoplastic process responds dramatically to chemotherapy with shrinkage of tumor mass and a rise in serum levels of uric acid, phosphate, and potassium. Suspicion is increased by finding phosphate or uric acid crystals in the urine sediment.

In the differential diagnosis are leukemic or lymphomatous infiltration of the kidneys [90], and acute urinary obstruction by retroperitoneal tumor or adenopathy. These entities tend to produce renal failure before, rather than after, chemotherapy, but an ultrasound should be ordered to exclude them.

In most cases, the diagnosis can be made by history, physical examination, and serum and urine studies, and a diagnostic renal biopsy is not necessary.

Intratubular Obstruction Due to Miscellaneous Etiologies

Definition

A number of other substances, primarily drugs and toxins, can also cause acute renal failure by blocking flow of filtrate within the tubular lumen.

Causes (see Table 12.6)

The kidneys normally excrete small amounts of *oxalic acid* derived from the diet and from the metabolism of ascorbic and amino acids. Excess urinary oxalic acid leads to tubular obstruction in a variety of contexts. Very high doses of ascorbic acid may cause intratubular oxalate crystals and renal failure [91]. Oxalic acid is a byproduct of ethylene glycol, the active ingredient in commercial antifreeze, and acute renal failure due to intratubular oxalate crystals is a common consequence of ethylene glycol ingestion [92]. Patients with jejunoileal bypass operations for obesity [93] or malabsorption and steatorrhea [94] exhibit increased gastrointestinal oxalate absorption and increased urinary oxalate concentrations. They may have tubular precipitation of oxalate with acute renal failure. Primary oxaluric syndromes are autosomal recessive enzyme defects characterized by excess synthesis of oxalate, systemic oxalate deposition, and hyperoxaluria with intratubular and interstitial precipitation; renal failure is progressive and occurs before adulthood [95].

Table 12.6. Miscellaneous causes of renal failure due to tubular obstruction

Oxalic acid	Sulfonamides
Ascorbic acid overdose	Acyclovir
Ethylene glycol	Triamterene
Intestinal bypass surgery	Rifampin
Malabsorption	Acetazolamide
Primary oxaluria	Methotrexate

In rare cases sulfonamide antibiotics [96, 97], acyclovir [98], methotrexate [99], triamterene [100], rifampin [101], and acetazolamide [102] have been shown to cause renal failure by intratubular obstruction.

Clinical picture

The clinical presentation of acute renal failure due to intratubular obstruction by oxalate varies according to the cause. Patients take *ethylene glycol* for an inebriating effect or in suicide attempts. Initially, they are lethargic or intoxicated, and may develop cardiopulmonary failure. A high anion gap metabolic acidosis, with a high serum osmolality and a high osmolal gap (see below), are characteristic, and ethylene glycol will be present in serum sent for toxicological analysis. Oliguria and azotemia do not usually occur until 24 hours after ingestion. Urinalysis often shows calcium oxalate crystals (Figure 5.1D). Renal biopsies are seldom indicated, but if done, calcium oxalate crystals are seen obstructing renal tubules and inside proximal tubular cells (Figure 12.3) [91, 103, 104].

Patients with *hyperoxaluric renal failure due to malabsorption* have chronic diarrhea and steatorrhea. Flank pain and calcium oxalate nephrolithiasis are often features, and renal ultrasonography may show parenchymal calcification. Renal biopsy also shows intratubular and intracellular calcium oxalate crystals [94]. Hyperoxaluric renal failure following *jejunoileal bypass* surgery demonstrates similar findings [93]. Now that alternative treatments for morbid obesity are preferred, this entity rarely occurs.

Sulfonamide induced acute renal failure has been described with sulfamethoxazole [96] and sulfadiazine [97]; oliguria, hematuria, and urinary crystals, with a "shocks of wheat" configuration have been reported [96, 97]. Although sulfonamide use in the acquired immunodeficiency syndrome may be increasing the incidence of this entity [97], it remains rare.

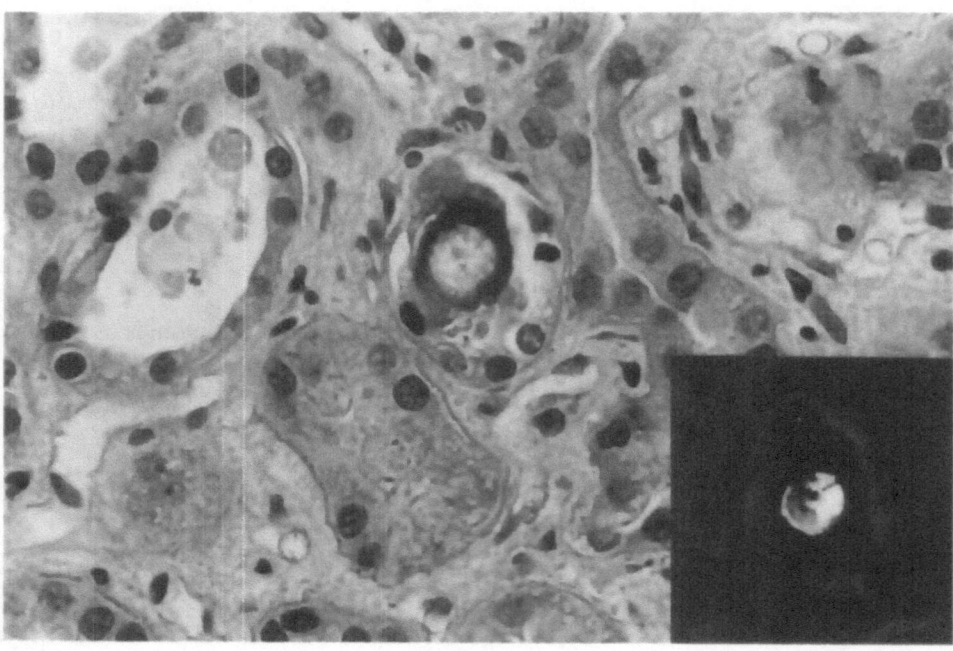

Fig. 12.3. Isolated calcium oxalate crystal in a loop of Henle, showing central radiating stria. Inset: the crystal is birefringent under polarized light. (Courtesy of Dr. Alfredo Esparza.)

Methotrexate is known to cause acute renal failure with tubular necrosis and intratubular methotrexate deposits on biopsy [99]. In one early study, methotrexate-induced renal failure was reported in 38% of patients [105]. A later, larger series reported renal failure only in 3% and only in patients who received concomitant nephrotoxins such as nonsteroidal anti-inflammatory agents or radiocontrast dye [106]. Volume depletion and acidosis are also contributing factors [98]. Patients have toxic methotrexate levels (above 1 micromole/L) [106], along with bone marrow suppression, mucositis, and dermatitis.

Acyclovir, especially at high doses with volume depletion, may precipitate inside tubules and cause azotemia [98].

Rifampin causes renal failure in rare cases. This typically occurs during long term therapy for tuberculosis. Patients have polyclonal light chains in the urine, without a serum monoclonal protein spike or any other evidence of multiple myeloma. Renal biopsy shows tubular proteinaceous casts with histologic staining for kappa and lambda chains [101]. Rifampin may also produce azotemia by triggering an acute interstitial nephritis (see Chapter 13).

Acetazolamide rarely causes renal failure, but one reported case had anuria, hypertension, no ultrasonographic evidence of urinary obstruction, and a renal biopsy which showed intratubular obstruction by Tamm-Horsfall protein without tubular atrophy or interstitial disease [102].

Triamterene crystal deposition has been reported as a cause of renal failure in one case [100].

Diagnosis

The diagnosis of acute renal failure due to ethylene glycol and intratubular oxalate deposition should be suspected in lethargic or obtunded patients with histories of depression or substance abuse, especially if a high anion gap metabolic acidosis and urinary oxalate crystals are present. The detection of ethylene glycol in the serum confirms the diagnosis, but this assay may not be universally or immediately available. Other diagnostic tests can support the diagnosis and may justify initiation of therapy while awaiting the ethylene glycol level. The serum osmolality should be ordered; it is almost always elevated. The osmolal gap (the measured serum osmolarity minus the combined osmolarity of serum sodium, glucose, and urea nitrogen) should be calculated (see formulas). A gap of greater than 10 mmol/kg supports the diagnosis. If the diagnosis is still in doubt, the patient's urine should be exposed to a Wood's lamp. Fluorescein is added to some commercial ethylene glycol preparations, and if those preparations have been ingested, the urine will fluoresce [107]. Clinical and laboratory findings in ethylene glycol associated renal failure are sufficiently unique that a renal biopsy is not necessary for a diagnosis.

$$\text{osmolal gap} = \text{measured plasma osmolarity} - [(Na \times 2) + \frac{BUN(mg/dL)}{2.8} + \frac{glucose(mg/dL)}{18}].$$

In SI units:

$$\text{osmolal gap} = \text{measured plasma osmolarity} - [(Na \times 2) + BUN(mmol/L) + glucose(mmol/L)]$$

Table 12.7. Clinical clues to tubular causes of renal failure

Condition	Clues
Ischemic ATN	Hypotension, volume depletion, sepsis, cardiogenic shock, aortic or cardiac surgery
Nephrotoxic ATN	Use of aminoglycosides, cisplatin or amphotericin B
Myoglobinuric ATN	Muscle injury, ↑ CPK, exercise, heat exhaustion, substance abuse, dipstick hematuria without RBC's in urine
Hemoglobinuric ATN	Hemolysis, dipstick hematuria without RBC's in urine
Myeloma kidney	Bone pain, severe anemia, ↑ Ca, old age
Tumor lysis syndrome	Rx of lymphoproliferative disorder, ↑ serum uric acid or phosphate
Intratubular obstruction	
Oxalate	↑ Osmolal & anion gaps, Ca oxalate crystals in urine, malabsorption
Drugs	Sulfonamides, acyclovir, etc.

CPK – creatine phosphokinase, Rx – therapy.

The diagnosis of renal failure due to an acquired hyperoxaluric syndrome should be suspected in patients with gastrointestinal disease or a jejunoileal bypass, especially if malabsorption and steatorrhea are present, and the urinalysis shows oxalate crystals. A renal ultrasound should be ordered; it may show parenchymal calcification or hydronephrosis from calculi. 24 hour urinary excretion of oxalate should be ordered; a value of greater than 100 mg/24 hours supports the diagnosis.

The diagnosis of acute renal failure due to sulfonamides, methotrexate, acyclovir, rifampin, triamterene, or acetazolamide should be considered in patients receiving one of these drugs who have no other potential causes for renal failure. Given the rarity of these entities and the fact that many patients have multisystem illness, a renal biopsy may be necessary for diagnosis if cessation of the drug is not followed by improvement in renal function.

CONCLUSION

The tubular causes of renal failure discussed in this chapter have characteristic historical features, physical signs, urinalyses and laboratory findings. Table 12.7 summarizes the clinical clues that should prompt an evaluation for one of the tubular renal diseases.

REFERENCES

1. Hou SH, Bushinsky DA, Wish JB et al. Hospital-acquired renal insufficiency: a prospective study. Am J Med 1983; 74:243–8.
2. Dixon BS and Anderson RJ. Nonoliguric acute renal failure. Am J Kidney Dis 1985; 6:71–80.
3. Anderson RJ, Linas SL, Berns AS et al. Nonoliguric acute renal failure. New Engl J Med 1977; 296:1134–8.
4. Zager RA. Endotoxemia, renal hypoperfusion and fever: interactive risk factors for aminoglycoside and sepsis-associated acute renal failure. Am J Kidney Dis 1992; 20:223–30.
5. Mandal AK, Lansing M and Fahmy A. Acute tubular necrosis in hepatorenal syndrome: an electron microscopy study. Am J Kidney Dis 1982; 2:363–74.
6. Badr KF and Ichikawa I. Prerenal failure: a deleterious shift from renal compensation to decompensation. N Engl J Med 1988; 319:623–9.
7. Myers BD, Miller DC, Mehigan JT et al. Nature of the renal injury following total renal ischemia in man. J Clin Invest 1984; 73:329–41.
8. Hilberman M, Myers BD, Carrie G et al. Acute renal failure following cardiac surgery. J Thorac Cardiovasc Surg 1979; 77:880–8.
9. Rayner BL, Willcox PA and Pascoe MD. Acute renal failure in community-acquired bacteremia. Nephron 1990; 54:32–5.
10. Wilkinson SP, Hirst D, Day DW et al. Spectrum of renal tubular damage in renal failure secondary to cirrhosis and fulminant hepatic failure. J Clin Path 1978; 31:101–7.
11. Miller TR, Anderson RJ, Linas SL et al. Urinary diagnostic indices in acute renal failure: a prospective study. Ann Intern Med 1978; 89:47–50.

12. Levinsky NG. Pathophysiology of acute renal failure. N Engl J Med 1977; 296:1453–8.

13. Zarich S, Fang LST and Diamond JR. Fractional excretion of sodium: exceptions to its diagnostic value. Arch Intern Med 1985; 145:108–2.

14. Appel GB. Aminoglycoside nephrotoxicity. Am J Med 1990; 88(S3c):16S–20S.

15. Shusterman N, Strom BL, Murray TG et al. Risk factors and outcome of hospital-acquired acute renal failure. Am J Med 1987; 83:65–71

16. Appel GB and Neu HC. The nephrotoxicity of antimicrobial agents. N Engl J Med 1977; 296:663–70, 722–7, 784–7.

17. Butler WT, Bennett JE, Alling DW et al. Nephrotoxicity of amphotericin B. Ann Intern Med 1964; 61:175–87.

18. Lachaal M and Venuto RC. Nephrotoxicity and hyperkalemia in patients with acquired immunodeficiency syndrome treated with pentamidine. Am J Med 1989; 87:260–3

19. Deray G, Martinez F, Katlama C et al. Foscarnet nephrotoxicity: mechanism, incidence, and prevention. Am J Nephrol 1989; 9:316–21.

20. Erlanger H and Cutler RE. Cisplatin nephrotoxicity. Dial Transplant 1992; 21:559–66.

21. McDonald BR, Kirmani S, Vasquez M et al. Acute renal failure associated with the use of intraperitoneal carboplatin: a report of two cases and review of the literature. Am J Med 1991; 90:386–91.

22. Humes HD. Aminoglycoside nephrotoxicity. Kidney Int 1988; 33:900–11.

23. Moore RD, Smith CR, Lipsky JJ et al. Risk factors for nephrotoxicity in patients treated with aminoglycosides. Ann Intern Med 1984; 100:352–7.

24. Boucher BA, Coffey BC, Kuhl DA et al. Algorithm for assessing renal dysfunction risk in critically ill trauma patients receiving aminoglycosides. Am J Surg 1990; 160:473–80.

25. Fisher MA, Talbot GH. Maislin G et al. Risk factors for amphotericin B associated nephrotoxicity. Am J Med 1989; 87:547–52.

26. Stamm AM, Diasio RB, Dismukes WE et al. Toxicity of amphotericin B plus flucytosine in 194 patients with cryptococcal meningitis. Am J Med 1987; 83:230–42.

27. Sacks P and Fellner SK. Recurrent reversible acute renal failure from amphotericin. Arch Intern Med 1987; 147:593–5.

28. Peltz S and Hashimi S. Pentamidine-induced severe hyperkalemia. Am J Med 1989; 87:698–9.

29. Cacoub P, Deray G, Baumelou A et al. Acute renal failure induced by foscarnet: 4 cases. Clin Nephrol 1988; 29:315–88.

30. Blachley JD and Hill JB. Renal and electrolyte disturbances associated with cisplatin. Ann Intern Med 1981; 95:628–32.

31. Hutchison F, Perez EA, Gandara DR et al. Renal salt wasting in patients treated with cisplatin. Ann Intern Med 1988; 108:21–5.

32. Madias NE and Harrington JT. Platinum nephrotoxicity. Am J Med 1978; 65:307–14.

33. Fjeldborg P, Sorenson J and Helkjaer PE. The long-term effect of cisplatin on renal function. Cancer 1986; 58:2214–7.

34. Guinee DG, Van Zee B van Houghton DC. Clinically silent progressive renal tubulointerstitial disease during cisplatin chemotherapy. Cancer 1993; 71:4050–4.

35. Hamilton RW, Hopkins MB and Shihabi ZK. Myoglobinuria, hemoglobinuria, and acute renal failure. Clin Chem 1989; 35:1713–20.

36. Zager RA and Gamelin LM. Pathogenetic mechanisms in experimental hemoglobinuric acute renal failure. Am J Physiol 1989; 256:F446–F455.

37. Bywaters EG. 50 years on: the crush syndrome. BMJ 1990; 301:1412–5.

38. Gabow PA, Kaehny WD and Kelleher SP. The spectrum of rhabdomyolysis. Medicine 1982; 61:141–50.

39. Roth D, Alarcon FJ, Fernandez JA et al. Acute rhabdomyolysis associated with cocaine intoxication. N Engl J Med 1988; 319:673–7.

40. Shieh S-D, Lin Y-F, Lu K-C et al. Role of creatine phosphokinase in predicting acute renal failure in hypocalcemic exertional heat stroke. Am J Nephrol 1992; 12:252–8.

41. Shemin D, Cohn P and Zipin SB. Pheochromocytoma presenting as rhabdomyolysis and acute myoglobinuric renal failure. Arch Intern Med 1990; 150:2384–5.

42. Singhal PC, Abramovici M and Venkatesan J. Rhabdomyolysis in the hyperosmolal state. Am J Med 1990; 88:9–12.

43. Corpier CL, Jones PH, Suki WN et al. Rhabdomyolysis and renal injury with lovastatin use. JAMA 1988; 260:239–41.

44. Pierce LR, Wyskowski DK and Gross TP. Myopathy and rhabdomyolysis associated with lovastatin-gemfibrozil combination therapy. JAMA 1990; 264: 71–5.

45. MacDonald JB, Jones HM and Cowas RA. Rhabdomyolysis and acute renal failure after theophylline overdose. Lancet 1985; 1:932–3.

46. Blake PG and Ryan F. Rhabdomyolysis and acute renal failure after terbutaline overdose. Nephron 1989; 53:76–7.

47. Hagnevik K, Gordon E, Lins LE et al. Glycerol-induced haemolysis with haemoglobinuria and acute renal failure. Lancet 1974; 1:75–7.

48. Abuelo JG. Renal failure caused by chemicals, foods, plants, animal venoms, and misuse of drugs. Arch Intern Med 1990; 150:505–10.

49. Chugh KS, Pal Y, Chakravarty RN et al. Acute renal failure following poisonous snakebite. Am J Kidney Dis 1984; 4:30–8.

50. Sitprija V. Nephropathy in falciparum malaria. Kidney Int 1988; 34:867–77.

51. Symvoulidis A, Voidclaris S, Mountokalakis T et al. Acute renal failure in G-6-PD deficiency. Lancet 1972; 2:819–20.

52. Koffler A, Friedler RM and Massry SG. Acute renal failure due to nontraumatic rhabdomyolysis. Ann Intern Med 1976; 85:23–8.

53. Ward MM. Factors predictive of acute renal failure in rhabdomyolysis. Arch Intern Med 1988; 148:1553–7.

54. Honda N. Acute renal failure and rhabdomyolysis. Kidney Int 1983; 23:888–98.

55. Corwin HL, Schreiber MJ and Fang LS. Low fractional excretion of sodium: occurrence with hemoglobinuric and myoglobinuric acute renal failure. Arch Intern Med 1984; 144:981–2.

56. Llach F, Felsenfeld AJ and Haussler MR. The pathophysiology of altered calcium metabolism in rhabdomyolysis-induced renal failure. N Engl J Med 1981; 305:117–23.

57. Fang LST. Light chain nephropathy. Kidney Int 1985; 27:582–92.

58. Rota S, Mougenot B, de Mayer-Brasseur M et al. Multiple myeloma and severe renal failure: a clinicopathologic study of outcome and prognosis in 34 patients. Medicine 1987; 66:126–37.

59. Smolens P. The kidney in dysproteinemic states. AKF Nephrology Letter 1987; 4:27–42.

60. Iggo N and Parsons V. Renal disease in multiple myeloma: current perspectives. Nephron 1990; 56:229–33.

61. Solomon A, Weiss DT and Kattine A. Nephrotoxic potential of Bence Jones proteins. N Engl J Med 1991; 324:1845–51.

62. Alexanian R, Barlogie B and Dixon D. Renal failure in multiple myeloma. Arch Intern Med 1990; 150:1693–5.

63. Cohen DJ, Sherman WH, Osserman EF et al. Acute renal failure in patients with multiple myeloma. Am J Med 1984; 76:247–56.

64. Kyle RA. Multiple myeloma: review of 869 cases. Mayo Clin Proc 1975; 50:29–39.

65. Cheson BD, De Bellis CC, Schumann GB et al. The urinary myeloma cast. Am J Clin Path 1985; 83:421–5.

66. Pozzi C, Pasquali S and Donini U. Prognostic factors and effectiveness of treatment in acute renal failure due to multiple myeloma: a review of 50 cases. Clin Nephrol 1987; 28:1–9.

67. Cohen LF, Balow JE, Magrath IT et al. Acute tumor lysis syndrome: a review of 37 patients with Burkitt's lymphoma. Am J Med 1980; 68:486–91.

68. Band PR, Silverberg DS, Henderson JF et al. Xanthine nephropathy in a patient with lymphosarcoma treated with allopurinol. N Engl J Med 1970; 283:354–7.

69. Zager RA. Hyperphosphatemia: a factor that provokes severe experimental acute renal failure. J Lab Clin Med 1982; 100:230–9.

70. Monballyu J, Zachee P, Verberckmoes R et al. Transient acute renal failure due to tumor-lysis induced severe phosphate load in a patient with Burkitt lymphoma. Clin Nephrol 1984; 22:47–50.

71. Tsokos GC, Balow JE, Spiegel RJ et al. Renal and metabolic complications of undifferentiated and lymphoblastic lymphomas. Medicine 1981; 60:218–29.

72. Loosveld OJL, Schouten HC, Gaillard CA et al. Acute tumor lysis syndrome in a patient with acute lymphoblastic leukemia after a single dose of prednisone. Br J Haematol 1991; 77:122–3.

73. List AF, Kummet TD, Adams JD et al. Tumor lysis syndrome complicating treatment of chronic lymphocytic leukemia with fludarabine phosphate. Am J Med 1990; 89:388–90.

74. Dombret H, Hunnault M, Faucher C et al. Acute lysis pneumopathy after chemotherapy for acute myelomocytic leukemia with abnormal marrow eosinophils. Cancer 1992; 69:1356–61.

75. Przepiorka D and Gonzales-Chambers A. Acute tumor lysis syndrome in a patient with chronic myelogenous leukemia in blast crisis: role of high dose ara C. Bone Marrow Transplant 1990; 6:281–2.

76. Stark ME, Dyer MCD and Coonley CJ. Fatal acute tumor lysis syndrome with metastatic breast carcinoma. Cancer 1987; 60:762–4.

77. Dirix LY, Prove A, Becquart D et al. Tumor lysis syndrome in a patient with metastatic Merkel cell carcinoma. Cancer 1991; 67:2207–10.

78. Tomlinson GC and Solberg LA. Acute tumor lysis syndrome with metastatic medulloblastoma. Cancer 1984; 53:1783–5.

79. Vogelzang NJ, Nelimark RA and Nath KA. Tumor lysis syndrome after induction chemotherapy of small-cell bronchogenic carcinoma. JAMA 1983; 249:513–4.

80. Hande KR and Garrow GC. Acute tumor lysis syndrome in patients with high-grade non-Hodgkin's lymphoma. Am J Med 1993; 94:133–9.

81. Vogler WR, Morris JG and Winton EF. Acute tumor lysis in T-cell leukemia induced by amsacrine. Arch Intern Med 1983; 143:165–6.

82. Thomas MR, Robinson WA, Mughal TI et al. Tumor lysis syndrome following VP-16-213 in chronic myeloid leukemia in blast crisis. Am J Hematol 1984; 16:185–8.

83. Fer MF, Bottino GC, Sherwin SA et al. Atypical tumor lysis syndrome in a patient with T cell lymphoma treated with recombinant leukocyte interferon. Am J Med 1984; 77:953–6.

84. Cech P, Block JB, Cone LA et al. Tumor lysis syndrome after tamoxifen flare. N Engl J Med 1986; 315:263–4.

85. Sparano J, Ramirez M and Wiernik PH. Increasing recognition of corticosteroid-induced tumor lysis syndrome in non-Hodgkin lymphoma. Cancer 1990; 65:1072–3.

86. Kanwar YS and Manaligod JR. Leukemic urate nephropathy. Arch Path 1975; 99:467–72.

87. Khan A, Sinks LF, Silhaug M et al. Acute lymphocytic leukemia mimicking renal failure. Ca–Cancer Jl for Clinicians 1979; 29:319–20.

88. Dunlay RW, Camp MA, Allon M et al. Calcitriol in prolonged hypocalcemia in the tumor lysis syndrome. Ann Intern Med 1989; 110:162–4.

89. Haller C and Dhadly M. The tumor lysis syndrome. Ann Intern Med 1991; 114:808–9.

90. Lundberg WB, Cadman ED, Finch SC et al. Renal failure secondary to leukemic infiltration of the kidneys. Am J Med 1977; 62:638–42.

91. Lawton JM, Conway LT, Crosson JT et al. Acute oxalate nephropathy after massive ascorbic acid administration. Arch Intern Med 1985; 145:950–1.

92. Verrilli MR, Deyling CL, Pippenger CE et al. Fatal ethylene glycol intoxication. Cleve Clin J Med 1987; 54:289–95.

93. Ehlers SM, Posalaky Z, Strate RG et al. Acute reversible renal failure following jejunoileal bypass for morbid obesity: a clinical and pathological study of a case. Surgery 1977; 82:629–34.

94. Wharton R, D'Agati V, Magun AM et al. Acute deterioration of renal function associated with enteric hyperoxaluria. Clin Nephrol 1990; 34:116–21.

95. Williams HE. Oxalic acid and the hyperoxaluric syndromes. Kidney Int 1978; 13:410–7.

96. Buchanan N. Sulphamethoxazole, hypoalbuminemia, crystalluria, and renal failure. BMJ 1978; 2:178.
97. Sahai J, Heimberger T, Collins K et al. Sulfadiazine-induced crystalluria in a patient with the acquired immunodeficiency syndrome: a reminder. Am J Med 1988; 84:791–2.
98. Sawyer MH, Webb DE, Balow JE et al. Acyclovir-induced renal failure. Am J Med 1988; 84:1067–71.
99. Garnick MB and Mayer RB. Acute renal failure associated with neoplastic disease and its treatment. Sem Oncol 1978; 5:155–65.
100. Roy LF, Villeneuve J-P, Dumont A et al. Irreversible renal failure associated with triamterene. Am J Nephrol 1991; 11:486–8.
101. Soffer O, Nassar VH, Campbell WG et al. Light chain cast nephropathy and acute renal failure associated with rifampin therapy. Am J Med 1987; 82:1052–6.
102. Rossert J, Rondeau E, Jondeau G et al. Tamm Horsfall protein accumulation in glomeruli during acetazolamide-induced renal failure. Am J Nephrol 1989; 9:56–7.
103. Curtin L, Kraner J, Wine H et al. Complete recovery after massive ethylene glycol ingestion. Arch Intern Med 1992; 152:1311–3.
104. Collins JM, Hennes DM, Holzgang CR et al. Recovery after prolonged oliguria due to ethylene glycol intoxication. Arch Intern Med 1970; 125:1059–62.
105. Condit PT, Changes RE and Joel W. Renal toxicity of methotrexate. Cancer 1969; 23:126–31.
106. Maiche AG, Lappalainen K and Teerenhovi L. Renal insufficiency in patients treated with high dose methotrexate. Acta Oncol 1988; 27:73–4.
107. Winter ML, Ellis MD and Snodgrass WR. Urine fluorescence using a Wood's lamp to detect the antifreeze additive sodium fluorescein: a qualitative adjunctive test in suspected ethylene glycol ingestions. Ann Emerg Med 1990; 19:663–7.

13. Interstitial causes of renal failure

AARON SPITAL

There are three major interstitial disorders causing renal failure: acute interstitial nephritis, chronic interstitial nephritis and neoplastic infiltration of the interstitium (Table 13.1). This chapter will discuss these disorders except for noninfectious causes of chronic interstitial nephritis, which are covered in Chapter 7.

ACUTE INTERSTITIAL NEPHRITIS

General Comments

Definition
Acute interstitial nephritis may be defined as an acute inflammatory process of the renal tubules and interstitium [1–5]. Although this histological pattern may accompany glomerulonephritis [2, 6], the following discussion will be limited to cases in which interstitial inflammation is the primary lesion. This process is usually caused by drugs, less commonly by certain infections or systemic diseases, and rarely by an idiopathic process. The pathogenesis is often uncertain, but in most cases immunological mechanisms appear to be involved [7]. Clinically, this disorder often presents as unexplained acute renal failure, though milder cases may manifest only asymptomatic urinary abnormalities [4].

The importance of being familiar with acute interstitial nephritis is that when it is recognized and properly treated it is frequently reversible; on the other hand, if not recognized and not treated, it may progress to end stage renal disease [8]. Therefore, when evaluating unexplained renal failure, this diagnostic possibility must always be kept in mind.

Table 13.1. Interstitial causes of renal failure

Acute interstitial nephritis
  Drugs
  Infections
  Systemic diseases
  Idiopathic

Chronic interstitial nephritis
  Infections
  Analgesics and other drugs
  Multiple myeloma
  Calcium nephropathy
  Lead nephropathy
  Oxalate nephropathy
  Obstructive uropathy
  Reflux nephropathy (chronic pyelonephritis)

Neoplastic interstitial infiltration
  Lymphoma
  Leukemia
  Solid tumor

Frequency
The incidence of acute interstitial nephritis is not known, but it is not rare. Acute interstitial nephritis has been estimated to account for as many as 8–14% of cases of acute renal failure investigated by renal biopsy and 1–8% of all cases of acute renal failure in general [2, 9, 10]. These figures probably underestimate the true incidence of the disease, since many mild cases may never be diagnosed.

Clinical manifestations
Since there are no pathognomonic clinical findings or laboratory tests, a definitive diagnosis can be made only by histological evaluation of renal tissue [11]. Nonetheless, there may be important clues in the clinical presentation which suggest the diagnosis. Some of these are characteristic of a specific cause; for example, a hypersensitivity reac-

J.G. Abuelo (ed.), Renal Failure, 131–141.
© 1995 *Kluwer Academic Publishers.*

tion is seen frequently in drug-induced disease, but less commonly with other etiologies. (These relatively specific clues will be discussed more fully below under the individual causes.) Other clues are more general and may be seen with acute interstitial nephritis of any cause.

The general manifestations are fairly predictable when one considers the inflammatory nature of the process and the functions of the primary target of attack: the tubulo-interstitium of the kidney. As a result of inflammation and swelling, renal size is normal or large, and a few patients experience flank discomfort [1, 2, 10]. Since the glomeruli are usually spared, proteinuria is generally mild and tubular in origin [4, 5]. In the urinary sediment one may see red blood cells, white blood cells and renal tubular epithelial cells as well as white blood cell, tubular cell and granular casts. Red blood cell casts are rare and suggest glomerulonephritis [7]. Since the proximal tubule is the major site for reabsorption of glucose, uric acid, phosphorus, bicarbonate, and amino acids, severe injury to this segment can lead to inappropriate renal losses of all of these substances; this is known as the Fanconi syndrome [1, 4, 5]. Normoglycemic glycosuria, easily detected with a dipstick on routine urinalysis, is an important (and sometimes the only) clue to the presence of proximal tubular dysfunction. When such dysfunction is severe, relatively or frankly low serum levels of uric acid and phosphorus may be seen. Injury to the distal tubules may result in sodium wasting, impaired concentrating ability and metabolic acidosis and hyperkalemia out of proportion to the degree of renal failure [4, 5].

Drug-Induced Acute Interstitial Nephritis

Causes

Nearly 100 drugs have been reported to cause acute interstitial nephritis (Table 13.2) [2]. However, most cases are due to agents belonging to two major classes: the beta-lactam antibiotics (which include penicillins and cephalosporins) and the nonsteroidal anti-inflammatory drugs (NSAIDs) [2, 3]. Because the clinical presentation of interstitial nephritis can vary with the class of the offending agent, the most important ones will be discussed separately.

Beta-lactam antibiotics

Clinical Picture. Virtually any penicillin and many of the cephalosporins can cause acute interstitial nephritis. Patients of all ages and both sexes can be affected, though there is a male predominance [6]. In one large series, the mean duration of drug therapy prior to the onset of clinical renal disease was 11 days (range 6–29 days) [12]. However, some patients have developed renal involvement within two to three days of beginning therapy. Although the development of nephritis is said not to be dose dependent, most patients have been on large doses of these antibiotics for at least several days [1].

Many cases are accompanied by a hypersensitivity reaction which classically includes the triad of fever (which is especially significant when it develops after fever caused by infection subsides), a maculopapular skin rash and eosinophilia [1–7, 9–12]. (It is this reaction which led to the designa-

Table 13.2. Major drugs causing acute interstitial nephritis [2, 6]

Antibiotics	NSAIDS
Beta-lactams	Almost all NSAIDs have been implicated
Penicillins	*Anticonvulsants*
Cephalosporins	Carbamazepine
Rifampin	Phenytoin
Sulfonamides	Valproic acid
Ciprofloxacin	*Other drugs*
Erythromycin	Allopurinol
Vancomycin	Alpha-interferon
Diuretics	Captopril
Chlorthalidone	Cimetidine
Furosemide	Interleukin-2
Thiazides	Omeprazole
Triamterene	Sulfinpyrazone

tion *"allergic" interstitial nephritis*, though the immunopathogenesis remains uncertain.) Occasional patients may also experience arthralgias or flank pain. Severe cases manifest sudden deterioration in renal function, which may be oliguric or nonoliguric. Some patients require dialysis. Blood pressure is frequently normal and edema is often absent [10, 11]. The urinalysis usually reveals minimal proteinuria, sterile pyuria and hematuria. Gross hematuria, white cell and granular casts may be seen as well. The kidneys will be normal in size or enlarged.

Diagnosis

Beta-lactam induced interstitial nephritis should be considered in any patient who develops unexplained renal failure while taking any drug in this class. Suspicion should be greatly increased by the simultaneous appearance of any of the components of a hypersensitivity reaction. The presence of hematuria, pyuria and mild proteinuria further supports the diagnosis. Serum IgE levels may be elevated, but only in about half of reported cases [2, 9]. Most patients will demonstrate eosinophiluria in a stained urinary sediment and the predictive value of this finding likely increases as the degree of eosinophiluria increases [1, 2, 4, 12, 13]. Hansel's stain may be more sensitive for detecting urinary eosinophils than is Wright's stain [13]. Gallium scanning frequently demonstrates intense renal uptake in acute interstitial nephritis [9, 14], but unfortunately is nonspecific [1, 2, 4, 9]. Nevertheless, gallium scans may be useful to support the diagnosis when biopsy is contraindicated and to separate patients with acute interstitial nephritis from those with acute tubular necrosis [9]. While occasional patients may have a low fractional excretion of sodium [9], urinary indices are generally not helpful as they usually resemble those found in acute tubular necrosis [2, 9, 15]. Ultimately, a definitive diagnosis requires renal biopsy. However, biopsy may not be necessary in typical cases which respond rapidly to withdrawal of the suspected causative agent with improvement in renal function.

Pitfalls. (1) Although this condition usually is seen after several days of high dose antibiotic therapy, it can also present after a few doses of antibiotic prophylaxis [1]. (2) Not all patients develop signs of a hypersensitivity reaction and fewer than one third manifest the full classic triad [1]. Therefore,

the absence of such a reaction does not exclude the diagnosis. (3) Similarly, eosinophiluria, though common, is neither universal nor specific [1–3, 5, 7, 9]. (4) Although usually indicative of glomerulonephritis, red blood cell casts may be seen rarely in isolated interstitial nephritis [16].

NSAIDs

Causes. Fenoprofen is the most common cause of this syndrome, but it has been seen with virtually all NSAIDs [2, 17–20].

Clinical Picture. The presentation of acute interstitial nephritis secondary to NSAIDs differs in several respects from the classical picture seen with beta-lactam antibiotics (Table 13.3) [1, 2, 17–20]. First, most affected patients are elderly females. Second, the duration of exposure prior to the development of nephritis is notably longer in cases of NSAID-induced disease, the mean being several months. Third, evidence of a systemic hypersensitivity reaction, such as fever, skin rash, eosinophilia and eosinophiluria, is usually absent, occurring in fewer than 20% of cases. Fourth, in contrast to almost all other causes of acute interstitial nephritis, nephrotic range proteinuria is seen frequently, perhaps in as many as 75% of cases; diffuse fusion of foot processes appears to be responsible. While this unusual pattern of interstitial nephritis and minimal change disease can be seen rarely with other drugs [20–23], NSAIDs, are by far the most common cause. Finally, in contrast to nephritis induced by antibiotics, in cases caused by NSAIDs, edema is the most common presenting symptom and the fractional excretion of sodium is often low, probably because of the associated heavy proteinuria [17].

As with other causes of acute interstitial nephritis, most patients will also have variable degrees of renal insufficiency. The urinalysis will be typical of acute interstitial nephritis, except for the presence of heavy proteinuria.

Diagnosis

Acute interstitial nephritis must be considered in all patients taking NSAIDs who develop unexplained renal insufficiency, especially in association with heavy proteinuria. Unfortunately, no risk factors have been identified which help pinpoint susceptible individuals. Though most patients have been elderly,

Table 13.3. Contrasting clinical features of Beta-lactam and NSAID-induced acute interstitial nephritis

	Beta-lactams	NSAIDs
Age	Any	Older
Sex	Male predominance	Female predominance
Duration of exposure	Days to weeks	Months
Hypersensitivity reaction	Common	Unusual
Nephrotic syndrome	Rare	Frequent
Presentation	Renal failure	Edema
FENa	>1%	<1%

this may simply reflect a population with a high rate of NSAID consumption [1]. Similarly, there are no confirmatory tests. Indeed, in contrast to beta-lactam associated disease, eosinophiluria and eosinophilia are frequently absent in cases caused by NSAIDs [2, 17, 19, 20]. However, the fractional excretion of sodium is often less than 1%, and this may be a clue to the diagnosis [17]. As with all types of acute interstitial nephritis, a definitive diagnosis requires renal biopsy. However, biopsy is not necessary if renal function improves rapidly after cessation of the drug [17].

> *Pitfalls.* The absence of a systemic hypersensitivity reaction is to be expected and should not be used to exclude the diagnosis. Furthermore, while most cases manifest heavy proteinuria, several patients have been described with isolated interstitial nephritis and only mild proteinuria [17, 19, 20].

Rifampin

Rifampin-induced acute interstitial nephritis often presents in a unique way [1, 2, 24, 24a]. Most cases have appeared after intermittent or discontinuous therapy. Within hours of reintroducing the drug after a drug-free interval, patients may develop systemic symptoms, including fever, chills, myalgias, arthralgias, nausea and vomiting. Many will complain of flank pain and experience the abrupt onset of oliguric renal failure. Thrombo-

cytopenia, hemolysis, or hepatitis may be seen. Rash, eosinophilia and eosinophiluria are unusual. The urinalysis frequently reveals hematuria. Many of these patients have high levels of circulating anti-rifampin antibodies, which may be of pathogenic significance [1, 2, 24].

Rarely, rifampin-induced acute interstitial nephritis may develop during continuous drug therapy [22, 25]. In contrast to those receiving discontinuous therapy, these patients do not have an explosive presentation. Rather, they present with the insidious onset of nonoliguric renal failure, often associated with a variety of renal tubular functional defects. Heavy proteinuria has also been described [22].

Diuretics

On rare occasion, diuretics can cause acute interstitial nephritis. These cases are often associated with typical signs of hypersensitivity such as fever, skin rash and eosinophilia [1,2,26–28]. Thiazides, triamterene or furosemide have been implicated in most cases and many patients have underlying glomerular disease.

Allopurinol

Allopurinol is another drug that can cause acute interstitial nephritis [1, 2, 29, 30]. There is often systemic involvement which may include fever, exfoliative dermatitis, cutaneous vasculitis, and hepatitis. Although this syndrome has been reported in a patient with previously normal renal function, renal insufficiency appears to be a risk factor, perhaps because of reduced clearance of drug metabolites [1].

Other drugs

A number of other commonly used drugs have been incriminated as potential causes of acute interstitial nephritis (Table 13.2). These include [1, 2, 9, 31–34, 34a, 34b, 34c]: many nonbeta-lactam antibiotics, such as sulfonamides, ciprofloxacin, erythromycin and rarely vancomycin; anticonvulsants; cimetidine; ranitidine; captopril; omeprazole; and interleukin-2. On the other hand, some classes of drugs have yet to be incriminated, such as beta-blockers and calcium channel blockers. Nevertheless, the list of possible causative agents continues to grow. Therefore the clinician should always consider the possibility of drug-induced interstitial nephritis in all medicated patients with unexplained acute renal failure, regardless of the therapeutic agents employed.

Acute Interstitial Nephritis Associated with Infections

Definition

Acute interstitial nephritis occasionally occurs during the course of a variety of bacterial, viral, and parasitic infections, in the absence of another identifiable cause [1–4, 6]. In some infections, such as acute pyelonephritis, direct microbial tissue invasion is responsible. In other cases there may be no evidence of the intact pathogen in the kidney [4]. These latter cases are probably mediated by immunological mechanisms. While clinically significant interstitial nephritis due to infection is uncommon, asymptomatic renal involvement occurs more frequently [35, 36].

Causes

Streptococcal infections have long been known to be associated with acute interstitial nephritis. A recent report confirmed that such infections are still an important cause of this condition, at least in children [37]. Other infectious diseases which have been implicated as causing acute interstitial nephritis include leptospirosis, legionnaires' disease, infectious mononucleosis, toxoplasmosis and mycoplasma pneumonia [2, 6, 35–41] (Table 13.4). In Asia and Europe, infections with the Hantavirus group is another important cause [42]. Finally, although renal function is usually well preserved in acute pyelonephritis, on rare occasion acute renal failure due to interstitial nephritis may occur; interestingly, almost all of these cases are caused by *E. coli* [43–45].

Table 13.4. Infectious causes of acute interstitial nephritis [2,6]

Bacteria	Viruses
Diphtheria	Epstein-Barr virus
Streptococci	Cytomegalovirus
Legionella	Hantaan virus
Leptospira	Measles
Brucella	*Other*
E. Coli (Pyelonephritis)	Toxoplasma
Yersinia	Mycoplasma
	Rickettsii

Clinical Picture. This entity should be suspected in all infected patients who present with unexplained renal failure, especially in the absence of hypotension and nephrotoxic drugs. The urinalysis will be typical of that seen with other causes of acute interstitial nephritis and, when present, normoglycemic glycosuria provides an important clue [37]. However, the clinical picture will likely be dominated by signs and symptoms of the underlying infectious disease.

Diagnosis

There are no specific laboratory finding which can confirm the diagnosis. Even when renal dysfunction appears during the course of acute pyelonephritis, other causes of renal failure, such as acute tubular necrosis secondary to sepsis, must be considered. Ultimately, the diagnosis of interstitial nephritis can only be established by renal biopsy. However, as the histological appearance is etiologically nonspecific, even this does not prove that the associated infection is responsible. Therefore, one must be careful not to overlook other potentially treatable causes of interstitial nephritis, especially drug-induced disease.

Pitfalls. (1) On occasion, the presentation of the underlying infectious process may be atypical. For example, several patients with acute renal failure secondary to acute pyelonephritis have presented without flank pain or high fever [44, 45]. (2) When renal disease complicates the course of streptococcal pharyngeal or skin infections, one must consider acute interstitial nephritis in addition to classic post-streptococcal glomerulonephritis [37]. The presence of red blood cell casts and depressed complement levels points toward the latter diagnosis, since they are usually absent in the former.

Acute Interstitial Nephritis Caused by Systemic Disease

Certain idiopathic immunologic disorders may occasionally cause acute interstitial nephritis (Table 13.5).

Sarcoidosis

While renal granulomas are not uncommon in autopsy series of patients with sarcoidosis, these lesions rarely cause renal failure [46–49]. Diminished renal function in patients with sarcoidosis is usually due to disordered calcium metabolism, which may cause hypercalcemia, nephrocalcinosis,

Table 13.5. Systemic diseases that cause interstitial nephritis

---

Sarcoidosis
Sjogren's syndrome
Systemic lupus erythematosus
Primary biliary cirrhosis

---

nephrolithiasis and volume depletion (see Chapter 10) [47, 49–51]. However, a few patients have developed renal failure secondary to noncaseating granulomatous interstitial nephritis [46–51].

Clinical Picture. These patients present with unexplained renal failure, which can be rapidly progressive and severe [48]. While other manifestations of sarcoidosis are usually apparent, isolated renal failure has sometimes led to the diagnosis of the underlying disease [48, 50]. Despite the tendency for renal failure to reduce serum calcium levels, in this condition the serum calcium is usually normal or slightly increased [48]. As expected for an interstitial process, the urinalysis may show minimal proteinuria, mild hematuria and pyuria. Evidence of tubular dysfunction, such as normoglycemic glycosuria has been described [48, 51].

Diagnosis
Interstitial nephritis should be suspected in all patients with sarcoidosis and unexplained renal failure, particularly in the absence of hypercalcemia and nephrolithiasis. The diagnosis is supported by typical urinary findings and if present, evidence of tubular dysfunction. Determination of angiotensin-converting enzyme activity is of little or no value in establishing the diagnosis [48]. Ultimately, definitive diagnosis rests upon the demonstration of granulomatous interstitial nephritis on renal biopsy. However, it should be noted that even this histologic appearance is not specific and may develop in response to drugs, tuberculosis, vasculitis, cancer and can even be seen as an idiopathic process [49, 52].

Sjogren's Syndrome
Lymphocytic infiltration of the renal interstitium appears to be common in this condition, and is similar in appearance to what is seen in the salivary and lacrimal glands [46, 53–55]. Perhaps as a result of this infiltrative process, renal tubular function is commonly abnormal. Patients may demonstrate nephrogenic diabetes insipidus, distal renal tubular acidosis and, less commonly, proximal tubular dysfunction [46, 53–55]. These tubular defects are usually not clinically significant. Rarely, interstitial involvement can be severe, resulting in an active inflammatory process and renal failure [53, 54].

Diagnosis
This process should be considered in all patients with Sjogren's syndrome and unexplained renal failure, especially when proteinuria is mild and tubular dysfunction is prominent. A renal biopsy is needed to confirm the diagnosis.

Systemic Lupus Erythematosus. Glomerular involvement in lupus nephritis is often accompanied by an active interstitial nephritis, associated with deposition of immunoglobulins and complement along the tubular basement membranes and small blood vessels [6, 46]. In fact, rare patients have been described with acute renal failure attributed primarily to acute interstitial nephritis, rather than to glomerular disease [2, 6, 46, 56]. Presumably, in these cases the immunological attack is primarily directed at the interstitium. Of interest, one report suggested that isolated interstitial nephritis in SLE might actually be a manifestation of concurrent Sjogren's syndrome [57].

Diagnosis. *This rare disorder should be considered in patients with systemic lupus and renal failure when proteinuria is mild. However, a definitive diagnosis can be made only with a renal biopsy.*

Primary Biliary Cirrhosis. Several recent reports have suggested that renal failure due to interstitial nephritis may also be seen during the course of primary biliary cirrhosis [58, 59]. This is not surprising in view of the known association between this disease and renal tubular acidosis.

Idiopathic Acute Interstitial Nephritis

Definition
This unusual disorder may be defined as acute interstitial nephritis which develops in the absence of an identifiable underlying cause [60–62]. While the pathogenesis of this condition is unknown, cell-mediated immune mechanisms are thought to play a role in most cases [61–63].

Clinical Picture. Although both sexes and all ages may be affected, females predominate [2, 62, 63]. Most patients present with a prodrome of nonspecific constitutional symptoms and a few experience flank or abdominal pain [62]. Unlike the classic drug-induced allergic interstitial nephritis, signs of hypersensitivity, such as fever, skin rash and eosinophilia, are usually absent. Renal function is variable, but severe renal failure is frequent. Nonetheless, most patients are nonoliguric and blood pressure is often normal [62]. The urinalysis is typical of interstitial nephritis and usually shows mild proteinuria and occasional white blood cells, red blood cells and granular casts. As with secondary forms of the disease, evidence of tubular dysfunction, particularly normoglycemic glycosuria, is an important clue to the diagnosis [61, 62, 64].

Idiopathic acute interstitial nephritis is frequently associated with unilateral or bilateral anterior uveitis, which may develop before, during or after the appearance of renal disease [62–66]. Indeed, when renal function is not markedly abnormal, uveitis may be an important clue to an underlying acute interstitial nephritis. Rarely, bone marrow and lymph node granulomas may also be seen [67].

Diagnosis
Idiopathic acute interstitial nephritis should be considered in any patient who presents with unexplained acute renal failure, constitutional symptoms and a urinalysis typical of interstitial disease in the absence of drug exposure or an underlying systemic or infectious disease. The presence of uveitis should increase the index of suspicion, though it is important to remember that uveitis and interstitial nephritis can be seen in several systemic diseases, including sarcoidosis [5]. As in other types of acute interstitial nephritis, renal gallium scanning may be positive but is nonspecific [63]. Therefore gallium scans are only recommended for patients with a compatible clinical presentation, but in whom renal biopsy is contraindicated. Although renal biopsy can confirm the presence of active interstitial inflammation, one still needs to carefully exclude known causes including unsuspected drugs, infection and systemic disease.

CHRONIC INTERSTITIAL NEPHRITIS ASSOCIATED WITH INFECTION

Xanthogranulomatous pyelonephritis and renal malacoplakia
Xanthogranulomatous pyelonephritis and renal malacoplakia are two rare inflammatory con-

ditions of the kidney related to chronic urinary tract infection [68–75]. Both are believed to result from an unusual inflammatory response to incomplete intracellular bacterial killing. These conditions are seen most often in middle-aged to elderly women. Both can present with constitutional symptoms, fever, flank pain and pyuria.

Xanthogranulomatous pyelonephritis is seen primarily in patients with a history of urological disease [68–70]. It is almost always unilateral and imaging studies usually reveal an enlarged nonfunctioning kidney. Renal calculi are frequent and are often of the staghorn type [68–71]. Most cases appear to be associated with *E. coli* or *P. mirabilis* infection, though other pathogens may be found [68–70]. Since this disorder is unilateral, renal failure is unusual [69, 70].

Diagnosis. *This disorder should be suspected in older women with a history of previous urinary tract infections or renal stone disease who present with nonspecific constitutional symptoms, fever, flank pain, pyuria and a positive urine culture. Although radiological investigations are helpful, a definitive diagnosis requires histological demonstration of large foamy lipid-laden macrophages (xanthoma cells) in the kidney [68, 70].*

Renal Malacoplakia is typically associated with *E. coli* urinary infections in immunocompromised hosts. It is often bilateral and can cause acute renal failure [68, 72–77]. The kidneys are frequently enlarged. Malacoplakia also has a unique histological marker, the Michaelis-Gutmann body, which is seen in the cytoplasm of foamy histocytes known as von Hansemann cells.

Diagnosis. *This disorder should be suspected in older immunocompromised women who present with fever, flank pain, pyuria, a positive urine culture, bilaterally enlarged kidneys and renal failure. A renal biopsy is necessary for diagnosis [73].*

Tuberculosis. On rare occasion, tuberculosis may cause a diffuse granulomatous interstitial nephritis, which can progress to end stage renal disease [78]. This process differs from the more typical pattern of renal tuberculosis, i.e., obstructive uropathy or massive caseous destruction of the renal parenchyma. These patients often have accompanying extrarenal disease.

Diagnosis. *This rare complication should be suspected in patients with tuberculosis and unexplained renal failure. Interestingly, a search for acid fast bacilli in the urine may be negative, and the demonstration of tubercle bacilli on renal biopsy may be required to make the diagnosis [78].*

NEOPLASTIC INTERSTITIAL
INFILTRATION

Definition
This unusual syndrome is caused by massive infiltration of the kidneys by tumor cells, most commonly in patients with hematological malignancies [2, 79–83]. It is worth emphasizing that in these settings renal infiltration by malignant cells is actually quite common, but renal failure is rare. When renal failure does occur, the pathogenesis is unclear, but may involve tubular compression and intrarenal obstruction [80].

Causes
Most cases are caused by diffuse histiocytic lymphoma, although this process may also be seen with other types of lymphoma and leukemia (Table 13.6) [79–82]. Rarely, a similar syndrome may occur secondary to renal metastases from a nonhematological malignancy [84].

Clinical Picture. The typical patient presents with systemic signs and symptoms of the underlying malignancy and unexplained renal failure. Most patients have aggressive and extensive disease [79]. However, in several cases the malignant process had not been previously diagnosed. In fact, on occasion this syndrome of renal failure secondary to neoplastic infiltration will be the presenting feature of lymphoma [83]. Renal failure is often severe and sometimes oliguric [80]. Urinalysis findings are nonspecific and proteinuria is almost always mild [83].

Diagnosis
An important clue to the diagnosis is the combination of renal failure and bilaterally enlarged, nonobstructed kidneys (evaluated by ultrasonography or CT scanning) [79, 80, 83]. A renal biopsy showing diffuse infiltration of tumor cells will support the diagnosis and is important in planning therapy. However, because infiltration is common, while renal failure is not, even histological proof of infiltration does not prove that it is responsible for the renal disease. Therefore, it is important to exclude other causes of acute renal failure, particularly those that occur with increased frequency in such patients. These include: prerenal azotemia secondary to nausea and vomiting, urinary tract obstruction, paraproteinemia and "myeloma kidney", uric acid nephropathy, hypercalcemia, and renal toxicity secondary to chemotherapy [83]. Only after excluding these possibilities and observing an improvement in renal function following appropriate cancer therapy, can the diagnosis of acute renal failure secondary to neoplastic infiltration be assured.

CONCLUSION

Many of the conditions discussed in this chapter have characteristic clinical features. When present, these clues should point the physician toward the correct diagnosis and indicate the need for appropriate confirmatory studies. The most useful clinical clues are reviewed on Table 13.7.

Table 13.6. Malignancies that may cause renal failure by interstitial infiltration

Lymphoma	Leukemia
Non-Hodgkin's lymphoma	Acute lymphoblastic
Histiocytic	Chronic granulocytic
Lymphocytic	
Lymphoblastic	*Solid tumor*
Burkitt's	Adenocarcinoma of lung
Reticulum cell sarcoma	
Hodgkin's lymphoma	

REFERENCES

1. Appel GB and Kunis CL. Acute tubulo-interstitial nephritis. In: Cotran RS, Brenner BM and Stein JH, editors. Tubulo-interstitial nephropathies. Churchill Livingstone, New York, 1983;151–85.
2. Grunfeld JP, Kleinknecht D and Droz D. Acute interstitial nephritis. In: Schrier RW and Gottschalk C, editors. Diseases of the kidney. Little, Brown and Company, Boston, 1993;1331–53.
3. Revert L and Montoliu J. Acute interstitial nephritis. Semin Nephrol 1988; 8:82–8.
4. Toto RD. Review: acute tubulointerstitial nephritis. Am J Med Sci 1990; 299:392–410.
5. Ten RM, Torres VE, Milliner DS, Schwab TR, Holley KE and Gleich GJ. Acute interstitial nephritis: immunologic and clinical aspects. Mayo Clin Proc 1988; 63:921–30.

Table 13.7. Clinical clues to interstitial causes of renal failure

Condition	Clue
Acute interstitial nephritis	Drugs: antibiotics, NSAIDs, anticonvulsants, diuretics, allopurinol, cimetidine
	Sarcoidosis, Sjogren's syndrome, systemic infection
	Fever, rash, eosinophilia, uveitis
	Normoglycemic glycosuria, other tubular dysfunction
Chronic interstitial nephritis associated with infection	
Xanthogranulomatous pyelonephritis	Fever, flank pain, pyuria, UTI, one enlarged nonfunctioning kidney
Renal malacoplakia	Fever, flank pain, pyuria, *E. coli* UTI, bilaterally enlarged kidneys
Tuberculosis	Unexplained renal failure during tuberculosis
Neoplastic interstitial infiltration	Bilaterally enlarged nonobstructed kidneys

UTI – urinary tract infection.

6. Cameron JS. Immunologically mediated interstitial nephritis: primary and secondary. Adv Nephrol 1989; 18:207–48.
7. Neilson EG. Pathogenesis and therapy of interstitial nephritis. Kidney Int 1989; 35:1257–70.
8. Frommer P, Uldall R, Fay WP and Deveber GA. A case of acute interstitial nephritis successfully treated after delayed diagnosis. Can Med Assoc J 1979; 121:585–91.
9. Linton AL, Clark WF, Driedger AA, Turnbull DI and Lindsay RM. Acute interstitial nephritis due to drugs. Ann Intern Med 1980; 93:735–41.
10. Pusey CD, Saltissi D, Bloodworth L, Rainford DJ and Christie JL. Drug associated acute interstitial nephritis: clinical and pathological features and the response to high dose steroid therapy. Q J Med 1983; 52:194–211.
11. Buysen JGM, Houthoff HJ, Krediet RT and Arisz L. Acute interstitial nephritis: a clinical and morphological study in 27 patients. Nephrol Dial Transplant 1990; 5:94–9.
12. Galpin JE, Shinaberger JH, Stanley TM, Blumenkrantz MJ, Bayer AS, Friedman GS et al. Acute interstitial nephritis due to methicillin. Am J Med 1978; 65:756–65.
13. Nolan CR, Anger MS and Kelleher SP. Eosinophiluria-a new method of detection and definition of the clinical spectrum. N Engl J Med 1986; 315:1516–9.
14. Shibasaki T, Ishimoto F, Sakai O, Kensuke J and Aizawa S. Clinical characterization of drug-induced allergic nephritis. Am J Nephrol 1991; 11:174–80.
15. Lins RL, Verpooten GA, DeClerck DS and DeBroe ME. Urinary indices in acute interstitial nephritis. Clin Nephrol 1986; 26:131–3.
16. Sigala JF, Biava CG and Hulter HN. Red blood cell casts in acute interstitial nephritis. Arch Intern Med 1978; 138:1419–21.
17. Abraham PA and Keane WF. Glomerular and interstitial disease induced by nonsteroidal anti-inflammatory drugs. Am J Nephrol 1984; 4:1–6.
18. Brezin JH, Katz SM, Schwartz AB and Chinitz JL. Reversible renal failure and nephrotic syndrome associated with nonsteroidal anti-inflammatory drugs. N Engl J Med 1979; 301:1271–3.
19. Levin ML. Patterns of tubulo-interstitial damage associated with nonsteroidal anti-inflammatory drugs. Semin Nephrol 1988; 8:55–61.
20. Porile JL, Bakris GL and Garella S. Acute interstitial nephritis with glomerulopathy due to nonsteroidal anti-inflammatory agents: a review of its clinical spectrum and effects of steroid therapy. J Clin Pharmacol 1990; 30:468–75.
21. Averbuch SD, Austin HA, Sherwin SA, Antonovych T, Bunn PA and Longo DL. Acute interstitial nephritis with the nephrotic syndrome following recombinant leukocyte A interferon therapy for mycosis fungoides. N Engl J Med 1984; 310:32–5.
22. Neugarten J, Gallo GR and Baldwin DS. Rifampin-induced nephrotic syndrome and acute interstitial nephritis. Am J Nephrol 1983; 3:38–42.
23. Rennke HG, Roos PC and Wall SG. Drug-induced interstitial nephritis with heavy glomerular proteinuria. N Engl J Med 1980; 302:691–2.
24. Davis CE, Carpenter JL, Ognibene AJ and McAllister CK. Rifampin-induced acute renal failure. South Med J 1986; 79:1012–5.
24a Pelaez E, Rodriguez JC, Cigarran S and Pereira A. Acute renal failure caused by two single doses of rifampicin with a year of interval. Nephron 1993; 64:152.
25. Quinn BP and Wall BM. Nephrogenic diabetes insipidus and tubulointerstitial nephritis during continuous therapy with rifampin. Am J Kidney Dis 1989; 14:217–20.
26. Bailey RR, Lynn KL, Drennan CJ and Turner GAL. Triamterene-induced acute interstitial nephritis. Lancet 1982; 1:226.
27. Case Records of the Massachusetts General Hospital (Case 42–1983). N Engl J Med 1983; 309:970–8.
28. Lyons H, Pinn VW, Cortell S, Cohen JJ and Harrington, JT. Allergic interstitial nephritis causing reversible renal failure in four patients with idiopathic nephrotic syndrome. N Engl J Med 1973; 288:124–8.
29. Gelbart DR, Weinstein AB and Fajardo LF. Allopurinol-induced interstitial nephritis. Ann Intern Med 1977; 86:196–8.
30. Magner P, Sweet J and Bear RA. Granulomatous interstitial

nephritis associated with allopurinol therapy. Can Med Assoc J 1986; 135:496-7.

31. Allon M, Lopez EJ and Min KW. Acute renal failure due to ciprofloxacin. Arch Intern Med 1990; 150:2187-9.

32. Bergman MM, Glew RH and Ebert TH. Acute interstitial nephritis associated with vancomycin therapy. Arch Intern Med 1988; 148: 2139-40.

33. Kaye WA, Passero MA, Solomon RJ and Johnson LA. Cimetidine-induced interstitial nephritis with response to prednisone therapy. Arch Intern Med 1983; 143:811-2.

34. Smith WR, Neill J, Cushman WC and Butkus DE. Captopril-associated acute interstitial nephritis. Am J Nephrol 1989; 9:230-5.

34a Christensen PB, Albertsen KE and Jensen P. Renal failure after omeprazole. Lancet 1993; 341:55.

34b Diekman MJM, Vlasveld LT, Krediet RT, Rankin EM and Arisz L. Acute interstitial nephritis during continuous intravenous administration of low-dose interleukin-2. Nephron 1992; 60:122-3.

34c Gaughan WJ, Sheth VR, Francos GC, Michael HJ and Burke JF. Ranitidine-induced acute interstitial nephritis with epithelial cell foot process fusion. Am J Kidney Dis 1993; 22:337-40.

35. Arm JP, Rainford DJ and Turk EP. Acute renal failure and infectious mononucleosis. J Infect 1984; 9:293-7.

36. Lee S and Kjellstrand CM. Renal disease in infectious mononucleosis. Clin Nephrol 1978; 9:236-40.

37. Ellis D, Fried WA, Yunis EJ and, Blau EB. Acute interstitial nephritis in children: a report of 13 cases and review of the literature. Pediatrics 1981; 67:862-70.

38. Krane NK, Roland P and Herrera G. Morning report at Charity Hospital: acute renal failure in a jaundiced patient. Am J Med Sci 1989; 297:394-8.

39. Winearls CG, Chan L, Coghlan JD, Ledingham JGG and Oliver DO. Acute renal failure due to leptospirosis: clinical features and outcome in six cases. Q J Med 1984; 212:487-95.

40. Poulter N, Gabriel R, Porter KA, Bartlett C, Kershaw M, McKendrick GDW et al. Acute interstitial nephritis complicating legionaires' disease. Clin Nephrol 1981; 15:216-20.

41. Kopolovic J, Pinkus G and Rosen S. Interstitial nephritis in infectious mononucleosis. Am J Kidney Dis 1988; 12:76-7.

42. Bruno P, Hassell LH, Brown J, Tanner W and Lau A. The protean manifestations of hemorrhagic fever with renal syndrome. Ann Intern Med 1990; 113:385-91.

43. Jones BF, Nanra RS and White KH. Acute renal failure due to acute pyelonephritis. Am J Nephrol 1991; 11:257-9.

44. Jones SR. Acute renal failure in adults with uncomplicated acute pyelonephritis: case reports and review. Clin Infect Dis 1992; 14:243-6.

45. Thompson C, Verani R, Evanoff G and Weinman E. Suppurative bacterial pyelonephritis as a cause of acute renal failure. Am J Kidney Dis 1986; 8:271-3.

46. Benabe JE and Martinez-Maldonado M. Tubulo-interstitial nephritis associated with systemic disease and electrolyte abnormalities. Semin Nephrol 1988; 8:29-40.

47. Casella FJ and Allon M. The kidney in sarcoidosis. J Am Soc Nephrol 1993; 3:1555-62.

48. Hannedouche T, Grateau G, Noel LH, Godin M, Fillastre JP, Grunfeld JP et al. Renal granulomatous sarcoidosis: report of six cases. Nephrol Dial Transplant 1990; 5:18-24.

49. Mignon F, Mery JP, Mougenot B, Ronco P, Roland J and Morel-Maroger L. Granulomatous interstitial nephritis. Adv Nephrol 1984; 13:219-45.

50. Korzets Z, Schneider M, Taragan R, Bernheim J and Bernheim J. Acute renal failure due to sarcoid granulomatous infiltration of the renal parenchyma. Am J Kidney Dis 1985; 6:250-3.

51. Singer DRJ and Evans DJ. Renal impairment in sarcoidosis: granulomatous nephritis as an isolated cause (two case reports and review of the literature). Clin Nephrol 1986; 26:250-6.

52. Schwarz A, Krause PH, Keller F, Offermann G and Mihatsch, MJ. Granulomatous interstitial nephritis after nonsteroidal anti-inflammatory drugs. Am J Nephrol 1988; 8:410-6.

53. Emlen W, Steigerwald JC and Arend WP. Rheumatoid arthritis, Sjogren's syndrome, and dermatomyositis-polymyositis. In: Schrier RW and Gottschalk C, editors. Diseases of the kidney. Little, Brown and Company, Boston, 1993;2049-61.

54. Rayadurg J and Koch AE. Renal insufficiency from interstitial nephritis in primary Sjogren's syndrome. J Rheumatol 1990; 17:1714-8.

55. Shiozawa S, Shiozawa K, Shimizu S, Nakada M, Isobe T and Fujita T. Clinical studies of renal disease in Sjogren's syndrome. Ann Rheum Dis 1987; 46:768-72.

56. Tron F, Ganeval D and Droz D. Immunologically-mediated acute renal failure of nonglomerular origin in the course of systemic lupus erythematosus (SLE). Am J Med 1979; 67:529-32.

57. Graninger WB, Steinberg AD, Meron G and Smolen JS. Interstitial nephritis in patients with systemic lupus erythematosus: a manifestation of concomitant Sjogren's syndrome? Clin Exp Rheumatol 1991; 9:41-5.

58. Kamouchi M, Tsuji T, Hirakata H, Okamura K, Ishitsuka T, Murai K et al. Tubulointerstitial disorders in the kidney associated with primary biliary cirrhosis (PBC). Clin Nephrol 1991; 35:134-5.

59. Macdougall IC, Isles CG, Whitworth JA, More IAR and MacSween RNM. Interstitial nephritis and primary biliary cirrhosis: a new association? Clin Nephrol 1987; 27:36-40.

60. Chazan JA, Garella S and Esparza A. Acute interstitial nephritis: a distinct clinico-pathological entity? Nephron 1972; 9:10-26.

61. Enriquez R, Gonzalez C, Cabezuelo JB, Lacueva J, Ruiz JA, Tovar JV et al. Relapsing steroid-responsive idiopathic acute interstitial nephritis. Nephron 1993; 63:462-5.

62. Spital A, Panner BJ and Sterns RH. Acute idiopathic tubulointerstitial nephritis: report of two cases and review of the literature. Am J Kidney Dis 1987; 9:71-8.

63. Hirano K, Tomino Y, Mikami H, Ota K, Aikawa Y, Shirato I et al. A case of acute tubulointerstitial nephritis and uveitis syndrome with a dramatic response to corticosteroid therapy. Am J Nephrol 1989; 9:499-503.

64. Lessard M and Smith JD. Fanconi syndrome with uveitis in an adult woman. Am J Kidney Dis 1989; 13:158-9.

65. Cacoub P, Deray G, LeHoang P, Baumelou A, Beaufils H,

DeGroc F et al. Idiopathic acute interstitial nephritis associated with anterior uveitis in adults. Clin Nephrol 1989; 31:307–10.

66. Salu P, Stempels N, Vanden Houte K and Verbeelen D. Acute tubulointerstitial nephritis and uveitis syndrome in the elderly. Br J Ophthalmol 1990; 74:53–5.

67. Dobrin RS, Vernier RL and Fish AJ. Acute eosinophilic interstitial nephritis and renal failure with bone marrow-lymph node granulomas and anterior uveitis. Am J Med 1975; 59:325–33.

68. Ronald AR and Nicolle LE. Infections of the upper urinary tract. In: Schrier RW and Gottschalk C, editors. Diseases of the kidney. Little, Brown and Company, Boston, 1993;973–1006.

69. Chuang CK, Lai MK, Chang PL, Huang MH, Chu SH, Wu CJ et al. Xanthogranulomatous pyelonephritis: experience in 36 cases. J Urol 1992; 147:333–6.

70. Goodman M, Curry T and Russell T. Xanthogranulomatous pyelonephritis (XGP): a local disease with systemic manifestations. Medicine 1979; 58:171–81.

71. Parker MD and Clark RL. Evolving concepts in the diagnosis of xanthogranulomatous pyelonephritis. Urol Radiol 1989; 11:7–15.

72. Cadnapaphornchai P, Rosenberg BF, Taher S, Prosnitz EH and McDonald FD. Renal parenchymal malakoplakia: an unusual cause of renal failure. N Engl J Med 1978; 299:1110–3.

73. Dobyan DC, Truong LD and Eknoyan G. Renal malacoplakia reappraised. Am J Kidney Dis 1993; 22:243–52.

74. Esparza AR, McKay DB, Cronan JJ and Chazan JA. Renal parenchymal malakoplakia: histologic spectrum and its relationship to megalocytic interstitial nephritis and xanthogranulomatous pyelonephritis. Am J Surg Pathol 1989; 13:225–36.

75. Hurwitz G, Reimund E, Moparty KR and Hellstrom WJG. Bilateral renal parenchymal malacoplakia: a case report. J Urol 1992; 147:115–7.

76. Ling BN, Delaney VB and Campbell WG. Acute renal failure due to bilateral renal parenchymal malacoplakia. Am J Kidney Dis 1989; 13:430–3.

77. Long JP and Althausen AF. Malacoplakia: A 25-year experience with a review of the literature. J Urol 1989; 141:1328–31.

78. Mallinson WJW, Fuller RW, Levison DA, Baker LRI and Cattell WR. Diffuse interstitial renal tuberculosis-an unusual cause of renal failure. Q J Med 1981; 50:137–48.

79. Flombaum CD. Acute renal failure and dialysis in cancer patients. Crit Care Clin 1988; 4:61–79.

80. Glicklich D, Sung MW and Frey M. Renal failure due to lymphomatous infiltration of the kidneys: report of three new cases and review of the literature. Cancer 1986; 58:748–53.

81. Harris KPG, Hattersley JM, Feehally J and Walls J. Acute renal failure associated with haematological malignancies: a review of 10 years experience. Eur J Haematol 1991; 47:119–21.

82. Lundberg WB, Cadman ED, Finch SC and Capizzi RL. Renal failure secondary to leukemic infiltration of the kidneys. Am J Med 1977; 62:636–42.

83. Truong LD, Soroka S, Sheth AV, Kessler M, Mattioli C and Suki W. Primary renal lymphoma presenting as acute renal failure. Am J Kidney Dis 1987; 9:502–6.

84. Clinicopathologic conference. Renal failure and death in a 60-year-old man with lung cancer. Am J Med 1987; 82:257–63.

PART FOUR

The differential diagnosis

14. Review of diagnostic practices

J. GARY ABUELO

The diagnosis of renal failure begins with the initial data collection, which is a medical history, physical examination, Scr, BUN, serum electrolyte concentrations, urinalysis, and investigation of any extrarenal diseases or symptoms. With just this information, the cause of the renal failure will be suspected or obvious in perhaps half of patients, although some physicians with more experience in this area will be better at diagnosing unusual conditions.

THE OBVIOUS DIAGNOSIS

The physician makes the obvious diagnosis by recognizing the typical features of the condition, and if needed by doing a test or two to confirm the diagnosis or to exclude clinically similar etiologies. The confirmatory test is often the response of renal failure to treatment. Even if urinary obstruction is not suspected it should be excluded with a renal sonogram, unless one expects a rapid fall in Scr with treatment or is certain of the cause, as in typical ischemic ATN. The most common obvious etiologies are recapitulated on Table 14.1.

The history, physical examination and laboratory testing make up the clinical picture that the physician must recognize. Of all these elements, the urinalysis is perhaps the most useful and most undervalued as a diagnostic tool. Although already covered in Chapter 5, Initial Laboratory Studies, the various urinary findings are listed on Table 14.2 with their associated renal diagnoses.

ADDITIONAL LABORATORY INVESTIGATION

If the physician does not suspect or have a diagnosis based on the initial information, further laboratory investigation, as outlined in Chapter 6, is in order (Table 6.1). It should include a renal sonogram, general screening tests like a chest X-ray and complete blood count, and tests to further evaluate any abnormal initial findings, such as protein electrophoresis in an elderly patient with proteinuria (Table 6.2). In certain cases, this new information will point towards a diagnosis not previously suspected.

Certain extrarenal problems like fever, malignancy, or severe anemia are common in azotemic patients. They may suggest causes for the renal failure, and lead the physician to carry out key diagnostic tests. These extrarenal problems are listed on Table 14.3 with the renal disorders that may be associated with them.

CONCLUSION

The diagnosis of renal failure is based on information gathering, syndrome recognition, and confirmatory testing. Although some conditions require a high level of sophistication to be correctly identified, this process succeeds in the majority of azotemic patients.

J.G. Abuelo (ed.), Renal Failure, 145–148.
© 1995 *Kluwer Academic Publishers.*

Table 14.1. Obvious causes of renal failure

Cause	Characteristics	Similar conditions	Confirmation
False renal failure	↑ Scr, normal BUN, UA normal	None	D/C cimetidine, cefoxitin, trimethoprim → ↓ Scr, Rx ketosis → ↓ Scr
Chronic renal failure	Slow ↑ Scr	Obstruction, ↑ Ca, myeloma/L.C.D.D., analgesic nephropathy	US, calcium level. protein studies normal
Prerenal renal failure	↓ BP, BUN:Scr ≥ 1 : 20, UA: S.G. > 1.015	ATN	U_{Na}, U_{Cl} <20 mEq/L, ↑ BP → ↓ Scr
Postrenal renal failure	Urinary tract pain, difficult voiding	Renal embolism	Urethral catheter or US, urinary drainage → ↓ Scr
Hepatorenal syndrome	Severe liver disease, low normal BP	Prerenal azotemia, ATN	U_{Na}, U_{Cl} <20 mEq/L, R/O hypovolemia, US
Vasomotor disturbance	Contrast media, drugs	Atheroembolic disease	Peak Scr day 3–5 after contrast, D/C ACE inhibitor or NSAID → ↓ Scr
Atheroembolic disease	Atherosclerosis, arterial manipulation, ischemic toes	Nephrosclerosis, GN, renal artery stenosis, malignant hypertension	Eosinophilia, US normal
Malignant hypertension	Diastolic BP >130 mmHg, headaches, severe retinopathy	GN	↓ BP → ↓ Scr , US normal
Ischemic ATN	Hypotension, UA: S.G. ~ 1.010, muddy granular casts	Prerenal azotemia	U_{Na}, U_{Cl} > 20 mEq/L, ↑ BP → ↓ Scr 1–4 weeks
Tumor lysis syndrome	Rx → tumor lysis	Obstruction, nephrotoxic chemotherapy	↑↑ uric acid, PO_4
Allergic interstitial nephritis	β-lactam antibiotic, fever, rash, eosinophilia	ATN due to sepsis, GN due to infection, collagen disease	D/C drug → ↓ Scr, US normal

Abbreviations: BP – blood pressure, D/C – discontinue, L.C.D.D. – light chain deposition disease, R/O – rule out, Rx – treatment, US – renal sonogram.

Table 14.2. Causes of renal failure associated with certain urinalysis findings

Specific gravity > 1.015 Prerenal renal failure Hepatorenal syndrome Vasomotor disturbance 2° sepsis	*Red cells* <5/high power field Prerenal renal failure Vasomotor disturbances Excludes GN
Protein: (−) to trace (<200 mg/day) Prerenal renal failure Postrenal renal failure Vasomotor disturbances Renal scleroderma crisis Renal artery stenosis	*Red cells* > 50–100/high power field GN Postrenal renal failure Atheroembolic disease Malignant hypertension Hemolytic uremic syndrome Thrombotic thrombocytopenic purpura Acute cortical necrosis Renal infarction Acute interstitial nephritis Polycystic kidney disease

Protein: (−) to 2+ (<1 g/day)
ATN
Acute interstitial nephritis
Neoplastic interstitial infiltration
Prerenal azotemia with transient proteinuria
    Congestive heart failure
    Sepsis
    Pancreatitis
    Burns
	Red cell casts
	GN
	Rarely in:
	    Atheroembolic disease
	    Malignant hypertension
	    Hemolytic uremic syndrome
	    Thrombotic thrombocytopenic purpura
	    Acute cortical necrosis
	    Renal infarction
	    Diabetic nephropathy
	    Allergic interstitial nephritis

Protein: 3+ to 4+ (>2.5 g/day)
GN
Nephrotic diseases
Some cases of:
    Atheroembolic disease
    Malignant hypertension
    Hemolytic uremic syndrome
    Thrombotic thrombocytopenic purpura
    Acute cortical necrosis
    Renal artery stenosis
    Renal infarction
    Myeloma kidney
	White cells > 5/high power field
	Acute pyelonephritis
	Acute interstitial nephritis
	Postrenal renal failure
	Atheroembolic disease
	Renal infarction
	GN

Table 14.3. Causes of renal failure associated with common extrarenal problems

---

Liver disease
Prerenal azotemia & C.P.C. 2° to C.H.F.
Hepatorenal syndrome
Biliary infections/sepsis (see below)
ATN 2° to shock
ATN & jaundice 2° to hemolysis (see anemia)
Hornet stings
GN 2° to:
   Collagen vascular disease
   Hepatic abscess
   Cirrhosis
   Essential mixed cryoglobulinemia
   Polyarteritis nodosa (HB+)
Nephrotoxic ATN*
   Acetaminophen overdose
   Toxic mushrooms
   Copper, thallium, phosphorous
   Carbon tetrachloride, chlorinated solvents
Interstitial nephritis
   Leptospirosis
   Sarcoidosis
   Biliary cirrhosis
   Azathioprine and other drugs
Polycystic disease of the liver and kidney

Infection/sepsis
Vasomotor disturbance
Acute cortical necrosis
GN
Ischemic ATN
Myoglobinuric ATN
Antibiotic nephrotoxicity*
Acute interstitial nephritis
Xanthogranulomatous pyelonephritis
Renal malacoplakia
Renal tuberculosis

Malignancy
Obstructive uropathy
Hypercalcemia
Hemolytic uremic syndrome
Glomerulonephritis
Amyloidosis
Light chain deposition disease
Myeloma kidney
Tumor lysis syndrome
Neoplastic infiltration
Radiation nephritis
Nephrotoxic drugs*
   Cisplatin
   Carboplatin
   Ifosfamide
   Interleukin-2
   Methotrexate
   Mitomycin-C
   Nitrosoureas
   Plicamycin
   Streptozocin

Lung disease
Infection/sepsis (see below)
Malignancy (see below)
P.E. 2° to renal vein thrombosis
ATN 2° to diquat/paraquat herbicides*
Interstitial nephritis 2° to sarcoidosis
Scleroderma
GN 2° to:
   Collagen vascular disease
   Goodpasture's syndrome
   Right-sided endocarditis

Fever
Infection/Sepsis (see below)
Malignancy (see below)
Renal infarction
GN 2° to collagen vascular disease
Drug-induced acute interstitial nephritis
Atheroembolic renal disease (rare)

Central nervous system disease
False renal failure 2° to isopropyl alcohol
Malignancy (see below)
Hypercalcemia
Hepatorenal syndrome (hepatic coma)
Thrombotic thrombocytopenic purpura
Malignant hypertension
GN 2° to collagen vascular disease
Eclampsia
Tubular obstruction 2° ethylene glycol
Nephrotoxic ATN*
   Toluene and other solvents
   Lead
   Water hemlock
Myoglobinuria ATN*
   Alcohol
   Other mood-altering drugs

Severe anemia
Prerenal azotemia 2° to blood loss
Ischemic ATN 2° to blood loss
Microangiopathic hemolytic anemia
   Scleroderma
   Malignant hypertension
   Hemolytic uremic syndrome
   Thrombotic thrombocytopenic purpura
   Sepsis with intravascular coagulation
GN
   Collagen vascular disease
   Goodpasture's syndrome
Hemoglobinuric ATN
   Transfusion reaction
   Hypotonic fluids
   Arthropod stings & snake bites*
   Chemicals*
Multiple myeloma
   Amyloidosis
   Light chain deposition disease
   Myeloma kidney

---

* See Appendix.
Abbreviations: C.H.F. – congestive heart failure, C.P.C. – chronic passive congestion, P.E. – pulmonary embolus.

15. The undiagnosed patient

J. GARY ABUELO

Only the occasional azotemic individual cannot be diagnosed by syndrome recognition. These challenging patients usually present without many of the characteristic features of their diseases. The *Pitfalls* sections in Part III of this book describe many such atypical situations. In extreme cases renal failure occurs "out of the blue" without prior symptoms, physical findings, significant urinary abnormalities or specific changes on renal sonography. Since the physician has no indication in which direction to proceed in the evaluation of these cases, broad scale but selective testing must be carried out. This involves conducting definitive diagnostic tests for all possible etiologies, even though the usual hallmarks are absent and the tests may be invasive. If any evidence, however slim, points to a cause, the physician should first look for that condition.

CHRONIC RENAL FAILURE

The difficulty in recognizing this condition occurs in the patient who comes to medical attention with a stable elevation in Scr. While the diagnosis may be confirmed by repeating the Scr periodically over the ensuing months, this approach may allow potentially treatable conditions like acute interstitial nephritis to progress to a fibrotic and irreversible stage. Therefore, a *renal biopsy* is needed, more to identify reversible diseases than to diagnose chronic renal failure.

PRERENAL RENAL FAILURE

Prerenal azotemia may occur without many of its typical features, i.e. without a suggestive history, hypotension, a high BUN to Scr ratio, or a concentrated salt-poor urine. In rare cases, none of these hallmarks are present. The diagnosis is made by observing a fall in Scr after intravenous or oral *volume expansion*. Such a trial of volume expansion should be carried out unless the patient is hypertensive in the recumbent and upright position or exhibits clear-cut hypervolemia on physical examination.

POSTRENAL RENAL FAILURE

Rarely obstructed patients do not have hydronephrosis. Also, occasionally hydronephrosis detected by ultrasound is of unclear functional significance. Grade I hydronephrosis, residual hydronephrosis and hydronephrosis in pregnancy were three examples of this given in Chapter 9. A *urologist* should be consulted to help evaluate these undiagnosed patients. Possible investigative techniques include diuretic renography, visualization of the urinary tract with pyelography, and a trial of urinary drainage.

LARGE VESSEL DISEASES

Patients with renal artery stenosis, renal infarction and renal vein thrombosis may offer few clues to the underlying process. These conditions will all be diagnosed by *renal arteriography* with additional studies of the venous phase of the injection. Thus, angiography should be considered in the undiagnosed patient.

J.G. Abuelo (ed.), Renal Failure, 149–150.
© 1995 *Kluwer Academic Publishers.*

SMALL VESSEL, GLOMERULAR, TUBULAR & INTERSTITIAL CAUSES

From time to time patients with these disorders have such nonspecific manifestations that no particular etiology stands out, and a *renal biopsy* is needed for diagnosis. A good example is the patient with idiopathic crescentic nephritis and anuria as the only symptom.

CONCLUSION

The evaluation of the undiagnosed patient requires investigation for hypovolemia with a fluid "challenge", arterial and venous patency with angiography, parenchymal disease with a renal biopsy, and urinary obstruction with urologic evaluation or a trial of urinary drainage. Figure 15.1 is a schematic representation of the diagnostic approach just described.

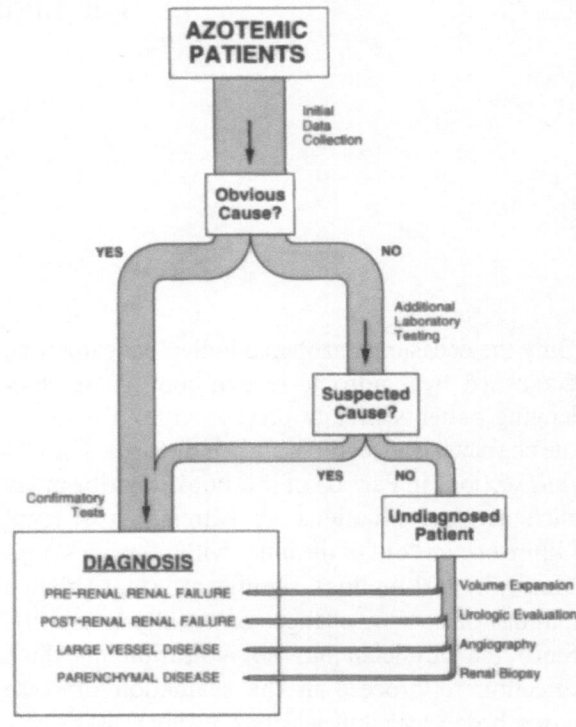

Fig. 15. Algorithm for diagnosing patients with renal failure.

PART FIVE

Management of Renal Failure

16. General management of the patient with acute renal failure

REX L. MAHNENSMITH

Acute renal failure is broadly defined as a rapid deterioration in renal function sufficient to cause accumulation of nitrogenous wastes in the body fluids. Uremia and attendant complications such as pericarditis, encephalopathy, convulsions, and bleeding are the principal threats. With acute renal failure, however, other renally excreted substances accumulate as well. These include potassium, sodium, acids, water, and phosphorus. The build-up of these substances contributes importantly to the morbidity of this clinical event and must become a focus of management along with uremic complications.

INITIAL MANAGEMENT

Role of Accurate Etiologic Diagnosis

Accurate etiologic diagnosis is the first clinical challenge, for one's initial therapeutic interventions should intend to halt or ameliorate the injuring process and prevent further progression of renal insufficiency. Any delay may leave the patient with prolonged or even permanent renal injury. Initial evaluation of a patient exhibiting rising BUN and Scr should include a search for prerenal, intrarenal, and postrenal processes. The search should be systematic, for more than one condition may be affecting kidney function. Yet, even upon first recognition of kidney failure, untoward consequences of acute renal failure can be present, such as hyperkalemia, fluid overload, or metabolic acidosis, and therapeutic interventions aimed at these eventualities may require immediate attention. In the long run, however, elucidation of the initiating factors for acute renal insufficiency is crucial, as etiologically focused therapeutic in-

terventions may be the most effective means to treat the emergent complications of renal failure (Table 16.1).

MANAGEMENT OF THE CONSEQUENCES OF ACUTE RENAL FAILURE

The consequences of acute renal failure arise simply from the failure of the kidney to excrete and regulate. Knowing that the kidney is responsible for maintaining fluid and electrolyte balance through regulated excretion of water, sodium, potassium, various acids, calcium, phosphorus, magnesium, and nitrogenous wastes allows one to anticipate excess retention and the ensuing consequences (Table 16.2). During the established phase of acute renal failure, accumulation of these substances has additional consequences (Table 16.3). Management requires surveillance, anticipation, prevention, and specific interventions to preempt or counteract untoward eventualities (Table 16.1).

Maintaining Fluid and Electrolyte Balance

Water
Water balance is normally defended by the kidneys as a function of effective plasma osmolality through hypothalamic production and release of vasopressin. Because sodium and its attendant anions constitute the bulk of osmotically active solute in the extracellular fluid, overall water balance is governed in relation to the plasma sodium concentration. Thus, properly ordered water homeostasis will be reflected as a normal plasma sodium concentration, whereas disturbed water homeostasis will be reflected as an abnormal serum

J.G. Abuelo (ed.), Renal Failure, 153–168.
© 1995 *Kluwer Academic Publishers.*

Table 16.1. Management priorities in acute renal failure

Initiation phase	Maintenance phase
Search for and correct prerenal and postrenal factors	Monitor blood chemistries, fluid intake and output, daily weight
Search for and treat acute complications of renal failure, e.g.	Match fluid intake to output plus insensible losses
Hyperkalemia	Limit potassium, sodium, and phosphorus intakes, as guided by
Hyponatremia	laboratory
Acidosis	Correct acidosis
Pulmonary edema	Provide phosphorus binders for phosphorus > 6 mg/dl (1.9
Optimize cardiac output and renal blood flow	mmol/L)
Discontinue nephrotoxic medications and agents which may	Initiate nutritional support early
hemodynamically decrease GFR, e.g.	Initiate dialysis before uremic complications emerge
ACE inhibitors	Dose drugs appropriate for their clearance
NSAIDs	
Establish diagnosis and initiate specific treatment	

Table 16.2. Biochemical problems in acute renal failure

Retention of:	Consequence
Nitrogen wastes	Azotemia, uremia
Acid	Acidosis
Potassium	Hyperkalemia
Sodium	Volume overload
Water	Hyponatremia
Phosphorus	Hypocalcemia

Table 16.3. Consequences of acute renal failure

Clinical problem	Etiology
Hypertension	Na & H_2O overload
Encephalopathy	Uremia, hyponatremia
Convulsions	Uremia, hypocalcemia, hyponatremia
Cardiac failure	Na & H_2O overload, acidosis, uremia
Cardiac arrhythmias	Hyperkalemia, hypocalcemia, acidosis
Pericarditis	Uremic serositis
Bleeding	Uremic platelet dysfunction, acidosis
Infection	Uremic leukocyte dysfunction, acidosis
Malnutrition	Uremic catabolic state, uremic anorexia

sodium concentration. A water surplus will manifest as hyponatremia, and a relative water deficit in the plasma will manifest as hypernatremia [1].

Failure to excrete water in the face of ongoing water intake is the usual water problem associated with acute renal failure. Hyponatremia is the con-

sequence. This complication derives etiologically from impaired glomerular filtration of blood, since adequate filtration is the first requisite toward renal water excretion. The quantity of water intake in excess of renal capacity for water excretion determines the degree of hyponatremia. Sources of sodium-free water include hypotonic intravenous fluids, most oral beverages and enteral nutrition formulas, and release of water from catabolic breakdown of muscle and adipose tissue.

Acute evolution of hyponatremia (fall in serum sodium concentration of more than 20 mEq/L over 48 hours) is more hazardous than a slow evolution of hyponatremia. The morbid consequence of acute hyponatremia is cell swelling as retained water distributes in both extracellular and intracellular compartments [2, 3]. Cell edema is most problematic in the brain, where expansion of tissue is constrained by the rigid skull. Evolution of brain edema thus results in heightened intracranial pressure, which compromises whole brain blood flow and leads to ischemia. Pressure herniation through the foramen magnum is a late and fatal outcome. If serum sodium concentration falls rapidly below 120 mEq/L, brain edema will be critical and changes in sensorium will be seen. Convulsions and death are usually imminent [4, 5].

Acutely evolving hyponatremia must be corrected quickly. Dialysis is the only maneuver that can correct hyponatremia in the oliguric patient with acute renal failure, although the two or three hours that it may take to mobilize a dialysis team may be too long. Thus, intravenous administration of hypertonic NaCl may be a lifesaving intervention, although this carries the hazard in the oliguric patient of precipitating a volume overload problem, such as pulmonary edema or severe hypertension. Hypertonic saline will reduce cerebral edema by raising effective plasma osmolality which will draw water out of cells, but since hyponatemia in the setting of acute renal failure results from total water overload, the truly effective therapy is to remove the excess water with dialysis. Accordingly, in the context of acutely evolving hyponatremia to levels less than 120 mEq/L with CNS changes, both hypertonic saline and emergent dialysis should be ordered. Hypertonic saline will mitigate cerebral edema while dialysis arrangements are underway. The goal with hypertonic saline is to raise the serum sodium concentration above 120 mEq/L over 2–4 hours. The quantity of *3% saline* required to achieve this depends upon the present serum sodium concentration and the patient's body weight [1, 2]. This may be calculated from the following formula:

Na deficit = (Desired Plasma [Na] − Measured Plasma [Na]) × Vol of Distribution of Na.

The volume of distribution of Na is actually Total Body Water or about 60% of weight (kg), which is contrary to physiologic predictions [6]. Therefore, the formula becomes:

Na deficit = (Desired Plasma [Na] − Measured Plasma [Na]) × Total Body Water.

Thus, if a patient's plasma [Na] is 110 mEq/L and Desired Plasma [Na] is 120 mEq/L, and if that patient weighs 70 kg,

the Na deficit = $(120 - 110) \times 42$ L = 10×42 = 420 mEq.

Since one liter of 3% saline contains 513 mEq of Na, this person would require 800 ml, assuming there were no ongoing losses of Na or water. In the context of acutely symptomatic hyponatremia and acute renal failure, administration of 3% saline is not a substitute for emergent hemodialysis. Once hemodialysis is commenced, infusion of 3% saline may be discontinued.

When hyponatremia evolves slowly, brain cells are able to discharge electrolytes and organic osmolytes from the cell interior and reduce overall cell tonicity [2]. This adaptation mitigates water influx into brain cells and minimizes cell edema. Thus, brain edema and threats of ischemia and

pressure herniation are not the principal threats of chronic hyponatremia. Brain electrolyte depletion is. If hyponatremia evolves slowly, major changes in mental status may not be seen even with serum sodium concentrations below 110 mEq/L, yet if such a profound hyponatremia evolved acutely, brain edema would be severe and the patient would be threatened with brain death [3]. Brain electrolyte depletion can alter neural cell functions. Lethargy, disorientation, memory impairments, and incoordination are common symptoms and signs of chronic hyponatremia.

A major hazard exists with iatrogenic attempts to correct chronic hyponatremia. Since electrolyte content of brain cells is adaptively reduced to maintain neural cell volume near-normal, rapid increments in effective extracellular osmolality (such as might occur from rapid infusion of normal or hypertonic saline) will likely result in proportional water movement out of brain cells, causing abrupt shrinkage. Abrupt changes of this nature have been associated with myelinolysis and permanent brain damage, even death [2, 3]. Thus, correction of chronic hyponatremia should be undertaken slowly simply by reducing sodium-free water intake. One's goal is to raise serum sodium concentration no faster than 10 to 12 mEq/L per 24 hours.

Ultimately, the best strategy for water management in the patient with acute renal failure is prevention of water overload. Evolution of hyponatremia must be anticipated in the oliguric patient who is able to drink or is receiving parenteral nutrition or frequent intravenous medication. In a first consideration, fluid intake should match losses in volume. Secondly, administered fluid should contain some sodium. Intravenous fluids and parenteral nutrition formulas should contain at least 35 mEq/L, more (up to 154 mEq/L) if serum sodium concentrations persist below 130 mEq/L. Thirdly, regular surveillance of serum sodium concentration is essential. If serum sodium concentration is falling, assessment and revision of fluid orders is indicated. If declines persist despite proper limitation of sodium-free fluid, dialysis will be necessary.

Sodium and volume
Intravascular volume overload is a second major concern for the patient with acute renal failure. Continued intake of sodium and water or the

necessary administration of blood products in the face of reduced renal excretory capacity inevitably leads to edema, congestive heart failure, and hypertension. Daily monitoring of body weights and fluid balance coupled to appropriate ordering of fluid inputs to match fluid losses can preclude volume overload states. Volume overload in the oliguric patient can be treated successfully only with some form of dialysis. In the non-oliguric patient with acute renal failure, the kidneys may retain some degree of diuretic responsiveness, so loop diuretics can be employed to achieve additional fluid removal [7].

Since daily fluid intake necessary to provide adequate nutrition often exceeds urine output and insensible losses, dialytic or diuretic support of fluid balance becomes strategically important to allow nutritional support to proceed. This is quite acceptable. Fluid restriction should not be ordered at the expense of necessary amino acid and calorie inputs.

A common pitfall in fluid management of the patient with acute renal failure is to use 5% Dextrose in water to give medications and keep intravenous lines open in an attempt to preclude sodium overload and its attendant complications. This prescription, however, runs the high risk of water intoxication with hyponatremia. Some sodium is essential for the patient with acute renal failure. Its input should be tailored to match ongoing losses. If fluid input cannot be reduced below output despite high-dose loop diuretic therapy, then dialysis will be necessary to manage sodium and water overload problems.

Potassium

Of all the electrolyte abnormalities associated with acute renal failure, hyperkalemia probably presents the most immediate threat. Whereas the body may tolerate deviations in serum sodium concentration of 10 to 12 mEq/L with little consequence, deviations of 2 or 2.5 mEq/L in serum potassium concentration can have mortal consequences. The ultimate threat of hyperkalemia is cardiac failure and arrest, which can occur when the serum potassium concentration reaches 6.5 mEq/L or higher. Less severe elevations in serum potassium concentration may cause reduced cardiac contractility or heart block. Severity of hyperkalemia can be judged by electrocardiographic (EKG) changes, which include peaked T-waves, prolongation of the P-R interval,

loss of P-waves, and widening of the QRS complex [8]. Loss of P waves and widening of the QRS complex indicate imminent cardiac standstill. When such EKG changes are present, emergent therapy is indicated.

Initial therapy for severe hyperkalemia associated with EKG changes is *calcium gluconate* 2 grams intravenously (Table 16.4). Intravenous calcium will stabilize cardiac membranes and temporarily counteract the depolarizing effects of hyperkalemia. While immediate in onset, which can be judged by a rapid change toward normal of the altered EKG, the salutory effects of calcium in this context are short-lived, and other therapies which lower the serum potassium concentration must follow.

Glucose plus insulin lowers serum potassium concentration by moving potassium from the extracellular to the intracellular compartment rather than removing it from the body. Therapy may be initiated with a 50 ml bolus of 50% glucose plus 5 or 10 units of regular insulin intravenously, followed by a drip infusion of 10% glucose with 20 units regular insulin per liter at a rate of 50 ml per hour (which will deliver 5 grams glucose plus 1 unit insulin per hour). Such therapy can be maintained for several hours while other means to remove potassium from the body, such as dialysis, are being mobilized. Intravenous sodium bicarbonate therapy also can lower serum potassium levels if an acidemia exists. As acidemia corrects, potassium will move intracellularly. The degree of potassium movement is not substantial with sodium bicarbonate therapy and depends upon the nature of the acidosis. Potassium shifts from cell to extracellular fluid with organic acidoses are minimal, whereas potassium movement with hyperchloremic acidoses are more substantial [9]. Therefore, sodium bicarbonate therapy in the context of a hyperchloremic acidosis will have a larger impact on hyperkalemia than with organic acidoses. Beta agonist agents are also effective against hyperkalemia. These drugs promote tissue uptake of potassium. Nebulized inhalation of 10 mg albuterol can lower plasma potassium concentrations by 0.5–1.0 mEq/L.

Ultimately, enteral administration of a cation-exchange resin such as *sodium polystyrene sulfonate (Kayexalate)* or dialytic therapy must be used to remove potassium from the body. Hemodialysis is

Table 16.4. Specific therapies for treatment of hyperkalemia

Urgency	Treatment	Dose	Time for effect
Emergent	Calcium	20 ml 10% Ca gluconate i.v. over 5 min, repeat q 15–20 min as needed	5 minutes
Urgent	Insulin & glucose	50 ml 50% dextrose plus 5 to 10 units regular insulin i.v., then 10% dextrose plus 20 units regular insulin/L at 50 to 100 ml/hour	15 minutes
Urgent	Bicarbonate	50 to 100 mEq NaHCO$_3$ i.v. over 5 min	15 minutes
Urgent	Albuterol	10 mg by nebulized inhalation over 15 minutes	15–30 minutes
Urgent	Hemodialysis	0 or 1 mEq/L K dialysate	30 minutes
Less urgent	Exchange resins	Sodium polystyrene sulfonate 30 gm orally in 100 ml 20% sorbitol or 60 gm rectally in 200 ml water	2 hours
Less urgent	Peritoneal dialysis	0 mEq/L K dialysate	4 hours
Less urgent	Loop diuretic	*i.v. furosemide Scr mg/dl (mmol/L)* 20–40 mg <1.2 (<106) 60–120 mg 1.2–2.5 (106–221) Up to 400 mg 2.5–5.0 (221–442) Not effective >5.0 (>442)	

more efficient, but the resin is more quickly available. It is usually appropriate to administer 60 g of resin in water rectally as arrangements for dialysis are being made. The resin may be repeated in four hours. The resin acts by exchanging sodium for potassium across the colonic mucosa. In general, one gram of resin will remove one mEq of potassium, providing the resin has had sufficient contact with the colonic mucosa. As a general rule of thumb, 50 g resin will lower the serum potassium concentration by 0.5 mEq/L. This resin may be administered orally as well in doses of 25 to 50 g every four hours as necessary. However, onset of action is slower with this route, and the resin must be combined with sorbitol as a purgative to assure its complete passage through the bowel.

After the immediate threat of hyperkalemia has passed, it is important that measures be taken to prevent hyperkalemia from re-emerging as a serious threat. These include an appropriate dietary restriction, avoidance of intravenous potassium, an appropriate dialysis program, and if the patient has only partial renal insufficiency or is in the early diuretic phase of recovery, avoidance of medications that interfere with renal excretion of potassium, such as potassium-sparing diuretics, angiotensin converting enzyme inhibitors, and non-steroidal anti-inflammatory drugs. A loop diuretic may increase renal potassium excretion. It is important for the clinician to realize that catabolic breakdown of tissue or ongoing hemolysis can cause significant potassium release. If hyperkalemia persists despite effective measures to prevent or treat it, including dialysis, then tissue release of potassium should be suspected and managed.

Acid-base balance

Due to the loss of renal excretory capacity in the face of ongoing production of nonvolatile acids from metabolism, metabolic acidosis is a near-universal occurrence in acute renal failure. In the hypercatabolic patient, endogenous acid production is markedly increased and substantial anion-gap acidoses will be encountered. A normal anion-gap acidosis may also co-exist due to failure of the injured kidney to manufacture ammonia and synthesize adequate amounts of new bicarbonate. Harmful effects of acidosis include nausea and anorexia, cerebral dysfunction, cardiac depression and propensity to arrhythmias, impaired intermediary metabolism, impaired platelet and leukocyte function, and impaired tissue repair [10]. Acidosis can also contribute to the occurrence of hyperkalemia.

Metabolic acidosis in acute renal failure should be treated with either oral *sodium bicarbonate or citrate*, intravenous bicarbonate, or dialysis. The administration of sodium bicarbonate in normal saline tends to produce hypernatremia. Two or three ampules of sodium bicarbonate added to 5 percent dextrose in water (100 or 150 mEq $NaHCO_3$/L) is the preferred intravenous bicarbonate solution. If the patient is receiving total parenteral nutrition, then alkali is provided by acetate in the formula. In the average resting adult, daily acid production is approximately 1 mEq per kg per day, so this amount of alkali per day would ordinarily suffice to maintain acid-base balance. However, most patients with acute renal failure are catabolic, so daily acid production is often two- to three-fold this amount, which must be matched by daily alkali administration. In many cases, hypervolemia is a contraindication to the use of sodium bicarbonate. Acidosis which cannot be managed with daily administration of alkali is an indication for dialysis, which is typically initiated for serum bicarbonate levels less than 10 to 12 mEq/L or arterial pH less than 7.10.

Mixed acid-base disturbances are not uncommon in the setting of acute renal failure, and their occurrence will depend on the patient's co-morbid problems. Examples include respiratory acidosis from chronic obstructive airways disease or acute respiratory embarrassment, metabolic alkalosis from continuous nasogastric suction, or a respiratory alkalosis from sepsis or head trauma. Acid-base disturbances should be assessed comprehensively with a careful history and physical examination, arterial blood gas measurements, and plasma bicarbonate assays. If mixed disturbances are recognized, therapy should be directed concomitantly at each process.

Calcium and phosphorus

Since phosphorus is retained by the kidney when GFR falls below 25 to 30 cc per minute, hyperphosphatemia is expected in acute renal failure. Retained phosphorus combines with calcium and precipitates out of solution when the plasma cal-

cium × phosphorus product exceeds 70 (5.7 in SI units). Hypocalcemia thus evolves as hyperphosphatemia emerges. Low levels of 1,25-dihydroxycholecalciferol and blunted action of parathyroid hormone also contribute. Thus, the hazards of hyperphosphatemia are hypocalcemia and tissue calcification. Dangers of hypocalcemia in the acute setting include myoclonus, tetany, convulsions, and cardiac dysfunction.

Phosphorus-free nutrition and magnesium-free *phosphate-binding antacids* (e.g. aluminum hydroxide, calcium carbonate, or calcium acetate) should be prescribed to preclude elevations in serum phosphorus above 6 mg/dl (1.9 mmol/L). Aluminum hydroxide is the preferred phosphate-binder if phosphate levels are already severely elevated and the calcium × phosphate product is near or exceeds 70 (5.7 in SI units), because administration of exogenous calcium in these settings will contribute to soft tissue calcification. Aluminum hydroxide is usually administered as a liquid starting with a dose of 30 ml three or four times per day. Dosage should be titrated to reduce the serum phosphorus concentration to values less than 6 mg/dl. Once the serum phosphorus level falls below 6 mg/dl, then calcium carbonate or calcium acetate may be used. Calcium carbonate is formulated as either a tablet or liquid, while calcium acetate is presently formulated only as a tablet. In tablet form, most patients will require at least 1000 mg of elemental calcium three or four times per day to maintain effective phosphorus control. As a liquid, the usual dose is 30 ml three or four times per day. Once again, one must titrate the dose to maintain serum phosphorus concentrations below 6 mg/dl (1.9 mmol/L) and calcium concentrations between 9.5 to 10.0 mg/dl (2.4 to 2.5 mmol/L) (corrected for serum albumin concentration). If the person is able to eat, then the phosphate-binder should be administered with the food. However, even in the absence of oral or intravenous phosphorus intake, serum phosphorus levels often rise owing to cell release from catabolism and acidosis. Phosphate-binding antacids are still beneficial in this context, as they will bind biliary-excreted intestinal phosphorus. Correction of acidosis can also lower serum phosphorus concentrations.

Administration of calcium is indicated for hypocalcemia-associated tetany or cardiac dysfunction, but should be withheld if the patient is asymptomatic and hyperphosphatemia is significant. When serum phosphorus is lowered below 6 mg/dl (1.9 mmol/L), then oral calcium can be commenced, as described above. If phosphorus is not lowered, administration of calcium will result in further soft tissue crystallization with calcium-phosphate salts.

Use of Drugs in Acute Renal Failure

Many but not all drugs require dosage modifications in the setting of acute renal failure. The major factor in this decision is whether the drug is eliminated by the liver or kidney. For those medications for which the kidney serves as the chief route of elimination, the dose interval must be extended or the milligram dosage reduced to avoid major drug toxicity. Precise guidelines for dosage modifications in renal failure exist for each class of drug and must be consulted [11, 12]. The physician also must know whether a given drug is removed by dialysis and to what extent. This information is usually included in the same resource that the physician consults regarding route of elimination and dose-modification recommendations.

Commonly used drugs which must have dosage modifications include *digoxin, allopurinol, aminoglycoside antibiotics, certain penicillin and cephalosporin antibiotics, vancomycin, sulfonamides, procainamide, ACE inhibitors, H-2 blockers, oral hypoglycemics,* and *certain chemotherapeutic agents.*

Insulin metabolism and clearance is also kidney function-dependent. As renal function declines, exogenous insulin lingers longer, so insulin doses require downward adjustment according to the regular monitoring of serum glucoses.

Extreme care must be taken with *narcotic analgesics.* Most analgesics are metabolized and excreted hepatically, so the concern is not drug accumulation but exaggerated actions. Thus, narcotic analgesics can magnify or compound uremia-associated mental changes. Meperidine is a special concern [12]. This drug is metabolized to normeperidine, which has less analgesic but more convulsant propensity than its parent compound, meperidine. It accumulates rapidly with multiple doses in renal failure and can cause myoclonus and convulsions. For this reason, meperidine should be avoided. Other concerns include constipation,

reduction in appetite, and slowing of respiration. Plasma protein binding of many drugs is reduced in uremia [12, 13]. This increases their availability and may necessitate an alteration in dosage. *Phenytoin* is one drug whose protein-binding is reduced, making unbound drug levels higher than expected. However, the rate of hydroxylation of phenytoin to an inactive metabolite is increased in renal failure, so this offsets the plasma protein binding issue and makes dosage alterations generally unnecessary. Plasma protein binding of *theophylline* compounds and *sodium valproate* is similarly altered. Dosage modifications are usually not required for these compounds, but one should aim for plasma levels in the lower therapeutic ranges to avoid toxicity [12].

Drugs with nephrotoxic potential should be avoided if at all possible in the setting of acute renal failure. These include aminoglycosides, amphotericin B, nonsteroidal anti-inflammatory drugs, ACE inhibitors, and radiocontrast agents. At times, circumstances or clinical threats mandate employment of one of these agents, and in such cases, risk versus benefit must be thoughtfully considered.

Diet and Nutrition

Acute uremia is a catabolic condition, regardless of its cause [14]. Associated co-morbid conditions compound the catabolic state of the patient in the grip of acute renal failure. Tissue catabolism releases potassium, phosphorus, water, and acids into the extracellular fluid and heightens generation of nitrogenous waste. Hypercatabolism also delays wound healing, impairs response to infection, and weakens mucosal-epithelial barriers, such as gastric mucosa.

This catabolic state may be mitigated by the provision of adequate calories and protein. The optimal ratio of calories to protein and the overall requirement has not yet been precisely defined, but general guidelines exist [13, 14]. First of all, nutrition should be implemented in the earliest days of acute renal failure. One should not wait for nutritional complications to arise. Secondly, the calorie-to-nitrogen ratio should probably exceed 300 Kcal-to-1g N. Insufficient calories in relation to protein leads to excess nitrogenous waste generation which will aggravate uremia [13]. The Harris-

Benedict equations can be used to calculate energy requirements. It is generally held that calorie requirements for patients with acute renal failure are approximately 35 to 40 kcal/kg/day, and at least 30 or 35% of this should be as lipid. Extremely hypercatabolic patients, such as those with burns, sepsis, or multiple trauma, require more [14]. Care should be exercised not to supply excess calories, as these will generate excess carbon dioxide, which may tax the respiratory system, and may also promote development of a fatty liver, which may impair its function.

Protein requirements are approximately 0.8 to 1.2 gm/kg/day [14]. Burn patients and patients on rapid exchange peritoneal dialysis may require more. One must be aware that excess protein may fuel ureagenesis and aggravate the uremic state. The best gauge of protein requirement in an oliguric patient is the urea nitrogen appearance rate after dialysis. If this is more than 30 to 40 mg/dl (11 to 14 mmol/L) per day, then protein feeding is excessive for the patient's anabolic capability [14].

It is now recognized that enteral feeding is superior to parenteral feeding [15, 16]. Parenteral nutrition lacks a number of semi-essential amino acids, notably cysteine and glutamine, and has been shown to be associated with broad-spectrum immune suppression. On the other hand, enteral nutrition stimulates splanchnic blood flow and hormone secretion, and these hormones plus intestinal luminal nutrients are directly trophic to stomach and intestinal mucosa, thus supporting mucosal integrity. Thus, to the extent possible, patients should receive enteral nutrition, even if it is inadequate in amount. Should enteral nutrition be insufficient to meet caloric needs, or impossible to give, then parenteral nutrition must be supplied.

Finally, trace elements and vitamins should be administered daily, particularly water soluble vitamins which are lost with all forms of dialysis [14]. Minerals such as potassium, calcium, magnesium, and phosphorus should be administered according to serum levels to avoid either surfeits or deficits.

Uremic Manifestations

Uremic complications arise in proportion to the abruptness and severity of renal failure and the degree of catabolism. *Anorexia*, *nausea*, and *vomiting* are often the earliest manifestations of uremia, and signal a need to commence dialytic therapy. Symptomatic therapy with prochlorperazine or metoclopramide is helpful, but mitigation of azotemia is the appropriate intervention. *Pruritis* is another annoying but non-threatening manifestation of uremia. In the acute setting, pruritis is not as frequent an issue as it is in the chronic setting, but symptomatic relief with antihistamines can be comforting.

Pericarditis

Pericarditis is a feared and threatening uremic complication of renal failure. This problem is manifest either as chest pain or a pericardial rub, but asymptomatic pericardial effusions are often discovered, indicating that insidious serosal inflammation frequently complicates uremia. The primary hazard of pericarditis is pericardial tamponade, which is a medical emergency. Pericardial tamponade should be expected when pulsus paradoxus greater than 10 mmHg is noted or when hypotension supervenes during dialysis despite fluid overload.

When pericarditis is diagnosed by physical exam, an echocardiogram should be done to assess for pericardial effusion. The size of any documented effusion should be monitored every three or four days by repeat echocardiography or when hypotension or pulsus paradoxus emerges, which would suggest tamponade [17, 18].

The emergence of pericarditis is an indication for repeated vigorous dialysis [17–19]. Daily hemodialysis or rapid exchange peritoneal dialysis is usually necessary to attenuate uremia sufficiently to lessen pericardial inflammation and the associated effusion. Care should be taken to limit heparin use, since the pericardium has a propensity to bleed in this setting. Bleeding into the pericardial sac can transform a relatively innocuous pericardial effusion into a threatening tamponade. Indomethacin can limit pain associated with pericarditis, but does not alter the natural course of uremic pericarditis [18, 20] In fact, in the setting of ARF, nonsteroidal anti-inflammatory drugs are relatively contraindicated due to their propensity to cause gastric irritation, platelet dysfunction, and intra-renal vasoconstriction.

If the pericardial effusion grows or remains moderate to large in size despite intensive dialysis for 10 to 14 days, or if cardiac tamponade is demonstrated, guided pericardiocentesis is necessary, followed either by 2–3 days of soft-catheter drainage or a subxiphoid pericardiotomy [17, 18, 21, 22]. Instillation of a corticosteroid preparation into the pericardial sac is advocated by some authors, but there are no controlled studies to firmly recommend this course [22–25]. Some clinicians advocate immediate sub-xiphoid pericardiotomy rather than pericardiocentesis as the safest and surest means to treat a moderate-to-large sized refractory effusion or tamponade [17, 21, 26–28]. Pericardiectomy is probably unnecessarily extensive in the setting of renal failure and carries more morbidity than pericardiotomy.

Bleeding

Bleeding problems are frequent in the setting of acute renal failure and represent another direct complication of uremia. Platelets from uremic patients are dysfunctional, so clot formation is impaired [29]. Gastrointestinal bleeding is the most frequent site of bleeding and may account for up to 20% of deaths in the setting of acute renal failure [30]. The common need for nasogastric tubes and the compromised integrity of gastrointestinal mucosa certainly contribute to this problem. Comorbid conditions such as sepsis, liver injury, trauma or surgical procedures also predispose to bleeding.

Management of bleeding must be comprehensive. Invasive punctures should be minimized. Nasogastric tubes should not be left in unnecessarily, as they promote erosions. Prophylactic antacids and use of sulcralfate and H-2 blockers may help. Limitation of heparin is indicated, and the physician should monitor coagulation functions since vitamin K-dependent factors may become depleted if broad spectrum antibiotics are in use. Commencement of dialysis, or increasing the frequency or adequacy of dialysis can improve platelet dysfunction from uremia. If bleeding is overt or if an invasive procedure is pending, the administration of *deamino-arginine vasopressin* (DDAVP) intravenously (0.3 micrograms/kg) can improve platelet-endothelial interactions and enhance clot formation [31]. DDAVP unfortunately can be administered only 2 or 3 times before tachyphylaxis develops. Similarly, *conjugated estrogens* (e.g. 50 mg conjugated estrogen per day orally or 0.6 mg/kg per day intravenously) or estrogen-progesterone compounds can also improve uremic platelet dysfunction, but their onset of action is a matter of days, not hours like with DDAVP [32]. Cryoprecipitate and hypertransfusion are older yet still effective management options to improve uremic bleeding, but run the risk of transfusion-associated complications.

Anemia

Anemia evolves in acute renal failure for many reasons. Blood-letting for tests is frequent. Blood loss from occult GI bleeding or with dialysis can be substantial over time. Additionally, red blood cell survival is reduced in uremia, while red blood production is concurrently compromised. Erythropoietin production falls within two weeks of acute renal injury and remains low until renal recovery is near-complete. The erythron's response to erythropoietin is also blunted owing to catabolism, inflammation, nutritional inadequacy, and concurrent infections. Administration of *erythropoietin* has become routine to patients with chronic renal failure, but its use in the setting of acute renal failure has not been well studied. It is clear that even supraphysiologic levels of erythropoietin do not always result in an adequate erythropoietic response in patients who are acutely ill [33]. Transfusion support is often necessary and should be undertaken as needed to maintain adequate delivery of oxygen to tissues. Erythropoietin may be useful in the stable patient with prolonged acute renal failure.

Hypertension and heart failure

Finally, hypertension and cardiac failure are frequent consequences of acute renal failure and derive largely from sodium and water overload. Accordingly, high blood pressure in this context is best managed with volume reduction by limitation of sodium and fluid input and either dialysis or aggressive diuretic therapy, if the kidneys still retain some diuretic responsiveness. Dietary sodium should be limited to 88 mEq per day (no added salt diet). It should be noted that the thiazide-class diuretics have little natriuretic effect when the GFR is less than 30–40 ml/min; only loop diuretics such as *furosemide* or *bumetanide* or the thiazide-like compound *metolazone* can exert a natriuretic effect in low GFR contexts [7]. Even the loop diuretics must be given at relatively high doses to achieve natriuresis in acute renal failure. Furosemide 100 mg intravenously is a standard beginning dose. If insufficient diuresis is achieved within 2 hours, then the dose should be increased to 200 mg intravenously. The maximum recommended single dose of furosemide is 500 mg, but accumulative dosing should not exceed 1000 mg per 24 hours. Continuous intravenous infusion of furosemide (from 10 to 60 mg per hour) may be more effective than bolus administration. For refractory cases, metolazone 5–10 mg orally may be combined with high dose intravenous furosemide to achieve and sustain a diuresis. Metolazone may be repeated every 12 hours. The addition of *dopamine* 1–3 mg/kg/min to high dose furosemide can also achieve diuresis in patients refractory to furosemide alone [34].

The employment of diuretics alone or in combination with dopamine should be cautious and guided by therapeutic objectives. Achieving a non-oliguric state with acute renal failure may aid management of hypertension and problems associated with congestive heart failure, but excessive diuresis may also reduce cardiac output and systemic blood pressure, resulting in reduced organ blood flows and a new insult to the kidneys. Hence, one must have clear intentions and goals when employing diuretics in the context of acute renal failure and be aware of the pitfalls and hazards of overdiuresis.

Dialysis

Indications for dialysis in a patient with acute renal failure are listed in Table 16.5. While the evolution of any of these in a patient with acute renal failure may compel dialytic intervention, it seems prudent to anticipate these complications and institute a mode of dialysis before morbid complications develop and a crisis supervenes [13, 35, 36]. For example, if the clinician notes that fluid balance is persistently positive in an oliguric patient, is unable to control serum potassium or acid-base balance with conservative measures, or notes early uremic signs such as nausea, anorexia, pruritis or lethargy, then dialysis should be commenced. On some occasions, the tempo of rise of the BUN or serum creatinine may be used as an indication for dialysis, the intention being to preempt uremic or metabolic problems in a patient who from experience will likely evolve metabolic or uremic problems without early dialytic intervention. Prospective controlled

Table 16.5. Indications for dialysis

Fluid overload
Hyperkalemia
Acidosis
Profound hyponatremia
Overt uremic complications, e.g.
   Pericarditis
   Encephalopathy
   Convulsions
   Bleeding
To provide for hyperalimentation
To remove toxins

---

studies have indicated that patients with acute renal failure who receive early and regular dialysis so as to keep pre-dialytic BUN levels below 80 to 100 mg/dl (29 to 36 mmol/L) have lower mortality and fewer episodes of bleeding or sepsis than those who receive only periodic dialysis that allows pre-dialytic BUN to climb above 120 mg/dl (43 mmol/L) [35, 36]. However, more aggressive dialysis with conventional techniques does not appear to render any additional benefit [37].

The goals of dialysis in the setting of acute renal failure are comprehensive. Some goals are immediate, such as lowering an elevated serum potassium concentration or removing excess fluid, while others have a larger perspective, such as controlling fluid to permit effective hyperalimentation, or controlling uremia to preclude pericarditis or improve platelet dysfunction. No single goal is less important than another, although control of some problems such as severe catabolism, recurrent hyperkalemia, ongoing acidosis, pericarditis, volume overload from vigorous hyperalimentation, and seizures may require daily dialysis [38]. In fact, data show that current dialytic techniques are quite effective in controlling electrolyte and fluid imbalances and preventing overt uremic complications such as convulsions and pericarditis, yet morbidity and mortality remain high from problems such as sepsis, bleeding, malnutrition, and other concurrent organ failures [30, 39]. While age, cause of the renal failure, and co-morbid conditions account for some of these complications, the uremic state contributes substantially and truly effective dialysis is central to their management. Commencing dialysis early, assuring that clearance goals are being met, restoring and maintaining fluid and electrolyte balances, and exercising care that dialysis is not causing harm or physiologic compromise are cardinal principles for dialytic intervention [13, 38].

Advances in dialytic techniques and introduction of new modalities for dialysis allow individualization of therapy toward specific needs or constraints of a given patient. Conventional hemodialysis and peritoneal dialysis remain the mainstays of dialytic intervention for most patients, but passive continuous arteriovenous hemofiltration/diafiltration (CAVH/CAVHD) or pump-driven continuous venovenous hemofiltration/diafiltration (CVVH/CVVHD) have certain advantages and applications that may be particularly suitable for a given patient [40, 41]. One particular advantage to CAVHD or CVVHD is the usual avoidance of hypotensive episodes, which complicate up to 50% of hemodialysis sessions in the intensive care setting [40, 42]. There is a suggestion that hypotensive episodes associated with conventional hemodialysis may initiate fresh ischemic injury to already injured kidneys and hence delay their recovery [37, 42]. Hypotensive episodes also predispose to cardiac problems and other organ ischemia.

There is evidence to suggest that CAVHD and CVVHD may be associated with reduced morbidity and mortality over conventional therapies in acute renal failure [40]. One explanation for these observations may be their continuous nature with less cardiovascular and renal stress from ischemia or blood pressure fluctuations. Another may relate to the observation that the dialyzers employed with CVVH and CAVH purify the blood more broadly, removing for example circulating mediators of ongoing inflammation, such as tumor necrosis factor, interleukins, thromboxanes, leukotrienes, and prostaglandins [40]. Removing such factors appears to impact favorably on the toxic problems engendered by sepsis and endotoxemia. Continuous diafiltration may manage the patient with pulmonary capillary leak syndrome more effectively as well [43].

On the other hand, conventional hemodialysis and peritoneal dialysis techniques have evolved since their initial application. Biocompatible dialyzer membranes with greater tensile strength and porosity, sodium modeling during hemodialysis, bicarbonate-based dialysate, and precise ultrafiltration controls on the dialysis machines offer greater efficiency and less stress or hazard to the patient. Accordingly, a dialytic strategy should incorporate not only the specific urgency and immediate indications for dialysis, but address other factors as well, such as hemodynamic stability and cardiac performance, bleeding tendencies, presence of sepsis, respiratory issues, nutritional needs, cost, personnel requirements, and local expertise [13, 38].

Conventional hemodialysis
Hemodialysis remains the most frequently-employed modality for dialytic treatment of patients with acute uremia. Hemodialysis requires secure vascular access, a safe dialysis machine, a commercial dialysis cartridge (dialyzer), a filtered water source, a water treatment apparatus such as a reverse osmosis unit which guarantees chemical and bacteria-free source-water, commercial dialysis concentrate which is mixed with the water emerging from the reverse osmosis unit, and a nurse experienced with the operation of dialysis and with problems that may arise during a given dialysis treatment. Vascular access is typically provided through a central venous catheter specially designed to withdraw blood from the patient and return just-dialyzed blood through a separate but juxtaposed lumen. Most often blood is heparinized to prevent clotting during its extracorporeal circulation through the dialyzer, a trip which takes about 1 minute. At any one time, approximately 160–200 ml of whole blood are circulating outside the body through the blood lines and dialyzer cartridge.

With hemodialysis, preferential solute and water removal from the blood occurs as blood courses through the dialyzer and comes in "contact" with dialysate across a closed network of semipermeable membranes housed in the dialyzer, which allows diffusive movement of nonprotein-bound solutes according to their molecular size and chemical gradients between the dialysate and blood. Diffusion down electrochemical gradients accounts for the removal of urea, creatinine, potassium, phosphate, uric acid, and other unmeasured substances that are accumulating because of renal failure. Water and sodium removal depends upon a hydrostatic transmembrane pressure gradient between the dialysate and blood that is set up by the head of pressure of blood moving into the dialyzer, resistance to blood return to the patient, and negative pressure in the dialysate compartment created by placing the dialysate pump on the outflow side of the dialyzer. Rate and extent of fluid removal is totally controllable with modern dialysis equipment that allows the nurse to precisely determine the amount of fluid removed during the treatment.

Despite the remarkable efficiency and control which modern hemodialysis affords, there are potential problems with its application. First of all, while vascular access is relatively easy to secure, the commonly-employed central venous catheters represent a source of sepsis, bleeding, and thrombus formation, and create a likelihood of scarring and stenosis of the vein in which the catheter resides if left in place for more than one or two weeks [44]. Secondly, the need for heparin compounds the bleeding risk which already exists from uremia itself. Hemodialysis without heparin is possible, but risk of dialyzer clotting is high [13]. Hemodialysis following very low-dose heparin protocols reduces incidence of clotting without increasing risk of bleeding in high-risk patients, provided clotting times are monitored closely during the hemodialysis procedure. Hypotension is probably the most serious concern with hemodialysis in the already-sick patient, for blood pressure reductions, whether abrupt or indolent, reduce cerebral, myocardial, splanchnic, and renal blood flows, sometimes with serious consequences. Reductions in renal blood flows with hemodialysis is speculated to retard or limit renal recovery from acute renal failure [42]. Hemodialysis also may lower arterial oxygen saturation, precipitate dysequilibrium syndromes, induce a transient leukopenia and cause degranulation of leukocytes, and increase tissue oxygen consumption in some patients [13, 40]. Use of bicarbonate-based dialysate and biocompatible dialyzes membranes obviates some of these problems. Although hemodialysis is efficient and generally well-tolerated, these issues may prompt clinicians to choose other modalities for renal replacement therapy in the acute setting.

Conventional hemodialysis equipment can also be used to perform *isolated hemofiltration*. This process removes an isotonic filtrate of plasma and accomplishes no diffusive dialysis. Accordingly, osmolality of the extracellular fluid does not decline during the procedure, which is one of the mechanisms for hypotension during conventional hemodialysis. Isolated hemofiltration therefore allows rapid removal of relatively large volumes of fluid from the patient with greater hemodynamic stability than with conventional hemodialysis. It may be employed sequential to a conventional hemodialysis treatment or as an isolated procedure.

Peritoneal dialysis

Peritoneal dialysis accomplishes removal of waste and fluid and correction of electrolyte disturbances at approximately one-fifth the efficiency of hemodialysis [45]. Yet, it is precisely for these reasons that peritoneal dialysis may be preferable for certain patients.

Peritoneal dialysis requires only the placement of a peritoneal dialysis catheter, air-tight connecting tubing, and peritoneal dialysate, which can either be commercially purchased or created from common intravenous fluid solutions. Peritoneal dialysis is performed either by a staff nurse or technician, and requires less technical knowledge than other modalities for dialysis.

The principle behind peritoneal dialysis is simple diffusion. Through the indwelling dialysis catheter, dialysate is instilled into the abdominal peritoneal cavity, allowed to dwell, and then drained out into a closed bag. While dialysate is dwelling, molecules and water diffuse down chemical and osmotic gradients, such that waste and excess solute is eliminated from the blood, chemical balance restored to the plasma, and bulk fluid removed. Rate and extent of solute and water removal can be adjusted by altering the chemical or osmotic content of the dialysate, volume of the dialysate, and dwell time of each instillation. By creating a larger osmotic gradient between the dialysate and blood, higher glucose concentrations in the dialysate remove more fluid and solute per unit time. Efficiency of dialysis is also proportional to volume of the dialysate and its dwell time in the abdomen: a larger volume and a shorter dwell time increase the efficiency of the dialysis. An average prescription for acute peritoneal dialysis would commence with 1.5–2 liter volumes dwelling for 30 to 90 minutes. Dialysate with 2.5% glucose content would ultrafiltrate approximately 200 ml per exchange.

The chief advantage of peritoneal dialysis is its relative ease and low-cost. As well, it does not invade the vascular system, does not require systemic heparin, is less stressful on the heart, reduces the likelihood of dialysis dysequilibrium syndrome, and lessens the risk of dialysis-associated hypotension or organ hypoperfusion injury [45]. Peritoneal dialysis remains the preferred modality for the uremic patient in whom heparin is contraindicated.

However, potential and real shortcomings exist. Catheter-associated peritonitis is frequent, particularly with temporary peritoneal catheters that have no fibrous cuff and are inserted without subcutaneous tunneling. Fresh dialysate, which is hypertonic owing to large amounts of glucose and relatively acidic, impairs leukocytic and macrophage function in the peritoneum [46]. Cells appear to recover their functions as dialysate dwells for 90–120 minutes, however, which allows dissipation of the hypertonicity and an increase in fluid pH. Fresh abdominal wounds and ostomies usually prohibit peritoneal dialysis, and existing internal adhesions from prior surgeries may preclude effective fluid exchanges. Respiratory compromise may occur with large volumes of intraperitoneal fluid due to limitations on diaphragm mobility and creation of atelectasis, and frank hydrothorax may appear from pleural-peritoneal leaks. Hyperglycemia owing to absorption of glucose from the dialysate is another potential concern, as is loss of amino acids and proteins through the dialysate. These latter problems tend to occur more often in the patient requiring frequent exchanges per day but can usually be managed through provision of insulin and adjustments of nutritional inputs. Perhaps most important for the critically ill hypercatabolic patient is the fact that peritoneal dialysis may not provide molecule clearances sufficient to ensure adequate control of uremia and its attendant problems [45]. In these patients, conventional hemodialysis or a continuous diafiltration modality is necessary.

Hemofiltration and hemodiafiltration
The hemodynamic instability that may accompany conventional hemodialysis and the inefficiency or anatomic constraints that sometimes prohibit use of peritoneal dialysis have led to the development of alternative forms of "hemodialysis." First to be introduced was a technique called "slow continuous ultrafiltration," which employed a small but highly permeable dialyzer that did not connect to a dialysis machine nor receive pump-driven blood flow [47]. Rather, a free-standing cartridge dialyzer would receive slow input of arterial blood driven by that patient's own blood pressure, and no dialysate would circulate against the semipermeable membranes. As heparinized blood flows through the dialyzer, large volumes of plasma water are simply sieved away into a collection container. Removed along with plasma water by solvent drag are any nonprotein-bound solutes that are dissolved therein, including electrolytes, wastes, and drugs. Since dialysate does not flow through this system, there are no solute or osmotic concentration gradients, so diffusive removal of solutes does not occur.

The principal advantage of this modality is that effective plasma osmolality does not rapidly fall as treatment is commenced. Accordingly, hemodynamic stability is greater because maintenance of effective plasma osmolality precludes movement of extracellular water to the intracellular compartment. Fluid removal can thus be accomplished steadily with a fairly brisk rate, often 500 ml per hour. Some solutes are lost from extracellular fluid with this technique, but only in proportion to their free concentration in plasma. Yet, if filtration rates are high enough (500–800 ml per hour), sufficient solute may be removed to attenuate a mild uremic condition and to prevent electrolyte accumulations [41].

Continuous ultrafiltration can be accomplished two different ways: (1) with arterial and venous cannulations, such that arterial blood flows under its own pressure through the hemofiltration cartridge and then back to the patient through a venous catheter – so-called "continuous arteriovenous hemofiltration" (CAVH), or (2) with two separate venous cannulations, such that blood from one vein passes through the hemofiltration cartridge and then returns through a separate vein – so-called "continuous venovenous hemofiltration" (CVVH) [41]. CVVH requires a blood pump, whereas CAVH does not. Yet, CVVH avoids arterial cannulation, which for CAVH must be accomplished with a large-bore catheter. For this reason, CVVH appears to have less morbidity than CAVH [48]. With either modality, heparin must be infused.

Either modality may be undertaken with or without a "replacement solution." If a replacement solution is not supplied, then the process simply achieves slow continuous ultrafiltration of plasma and volume control. However, if ultrafiltration rates exceed 200 or 300 ml per hour for several hours in a row, then sufficient solute removal occurs by convection to create a need for specific solute replacement. Most important is bicarbonate, calcium, potassium, and magnesium [41]. Replacement solutions are therefore constituted as isotonic crystalloids with ionic concentrations of sodium, chloride, potassium, bicarbonate, magnesium, and calcium close to that of normal plasma. This solution is typically administered at a rate selected to be less than the rate of ultrafiltration loss so that net fluid removal is achieved. Rate of net fluid loss can be modulated by providing less or more of the replacement solution per hour.

Enteral and parenteral nutrition solutions should be incorporated into the fluid and electrolyte management regime, and to the extent that these are provided per hour, the crystalloid replacement infusion should be decreased. In fact, one of the chief advantages of CAVH or CVVH is continuous fluid removal of sufficient volume to permit high-volume feeding without concern for cyclic fluid overloads which often occur with intermittent conventional hemodialysis [40, 41].

Finally, these hemofilter cartridges can possess dialysate ports so that a countercurrent flow of dialysate against the semipermeable membranes may be accomplished. This is referred to as "hemodiafiltration." [41] This addition to the modality provides diffusive removal of solutes (dialysis) which enhances individual solute clearance. Bulk fluid removal by ultrafiltration may also decline with the presence of dialysate in the cartridge, as dialysate will create an opposing force to fluid ultrafiltration.

The advantages of hemodiafiltration by CAVHD or CVVHD are multiple [40, 41, 49]. Fluid removal is gentle, continuous, and able to be modulated. Urea removal is usually sufficient to control uremia in even the very catabolic patient, yet the presence of dialysate in the cartridge allows control of potassium, bicarbonate, magnesium, and calcium removal so as to preclude untoward surfeits or deficits in their balance. Protein-rich nutrition can be continuously administered with-

out inducing fluid overload or interdialytic urea buildup, and because fluid control is continuous, volume stress on the heart and lungs is minimized. In essence, high clearance dialysis is continuously achieved with a remarkable degree of hemodynamic stability and little stress to the heart or kidneys.

Intriguing are the suggestions that continuous hemodiafiltration may improve outcomes in critically ill patients with multi-organ failure by offering better blood purification than conventional modalities [40, 49]. Indeed, to the extent that continuous hemodiafiltration avoids hypotensive episodes, precludes pulmonary edema, offloads volume and pressure burdens on the heart, and allows aggressive nutritional support with continuous control of uremia, these modalities would appear to offer unique advantage to the unstable, critically-ill patient with acute renal failure. Additionally, the filtration characteristics of these cartridges allow removal of prostaglandins, leukotrienes, thromboxanes, complement components, interleukins, and tumor necrosis factor [40]. Removal of these substances may have a favorable impact on the clinical course of sepsis and pulmonary capillary leak syndromes which often accompany acute renal failure in an intensive care unit [50, 51].

Adequacy of dialysis in the setting of acute renal failure should be judged with daily or pre-dialysis measurement of urea and electrolyte concentrations coupled to a bedside assessment of fluid volume status and signs or symptoms of uremia. A single quantitative parameter with which to judge adequacy of dialysis does not exist for the acutely uremic patient. However, in general, physicians will prescribe dialysis to maintain the urea nitrogen level below 80 to 100 mg/dl (29 to 36 mmol/L), upper limits generally accepted as precluding uremic complications in the setting of acute renal failure. The dialytic technique should also control acidosis, hyperphosphatemia, hyperkalemia, fluid overload and hypertension, minimize anticoagulation, hypotension, and cardiac stress, yet allow early and sufficient provision of nutrition. Which modality will serve which patient the best can only partially be predicted at outset, so the physician must remain critically observant and willing to switch modalities if one proves harmful or inadequate.

REFERENCES

1. Berl T and Schrier RW. Disorders of water metabolism. In: Schrier RW, editor. Renal and electrolyte disorders. Little, Brown and Co., Boston 1986: 1–77.

2. Sterns RH. The management of symptomatic hyponatremia. Seminars in Nephrology 1990; 10:503–14.

3. Sterns RH. The treatment of hyponatremia: first, do no harm. Am J Med 1990; 88:557–60.

4. Arieff AI and Guisdado R. Effects on the central nervous system of hypernatremic and hyponatremic states. Kidney Int 1976; 10:104–16.

5. Arieff AI. Hyponatremia, convulsions, respiratory arrest, and permanent brain damage after elective surgery in healthy women. N Engl J Med 1986; 314:1529–35.

6. Spital A and Sterns RD. The paradox of sodium's volume of distribution: why an extracellular solute appears to distribute over total body water. Arch Intern Med 1989; 149:1255–8.

7. Russo D, Memoli B and Andreucci VE. The place of loop diuretics in the treatment of acute and chronic renal failure. Clin Nephrol 1992; 38:S69–S73.

8. Ettinger PO, Regan TJ and Oldewurtel HA. Hyperkalemia, cardiac conduction, and the electrocardiogram. A review. Am Heart J 1974; 88:360–71

9. Adrogue HJ and Madias NE. Changes in plasma potassium concentration during acute acid-base disturbances. Am J Med 1981; 71:456–67.

10. Knochel JP. Biochemical, electrolyte, and acid-base disturbances in acute renal failure. In: Brenner BM and Lazarus JM, editors. Acute renal failure. WB Saunders Co., Philadelphia, 1983: 568–85.

11. Bennett WM, Aronoff G, Golper TA et al. Drug prescribing in renal failure: dosing guidelines for adults. Philadelphia, American College of Physicians, 1991: 1–143.

12. Bennett WM and Blythe WB. Use of drugs in patients with renal failure. In: Schrier RW and Gottschalk CW, editors. Disease of the kidney. Little, Brown and Co, Boston, 1988: 3437–506.

13. Brezis M, Rosen S and Epstein FH. Acute renal failure. In: Brenner BM and Rector FC Jr., editors. The kidney. W.B.Saunders Co., Philadelphia, 1991: 993–1061.

14. Wesson DE, Mitch WE and Wilmore DW. Nutritional considerations in the treatment of acute renal failure. In: Brenner BM and Lazarus JM, editors. Acute renal failure. W.B. Saunders Co., Philadelphia, 1983: 618–42.

15. Kudsk KA, Croce MA, Fabian TC et al. Enteral versus parenteral feeding: effects on septic morbidity after blunt and penetrating abdominal trauma. Ann Surg 1992; 215:503–11.

16. Moore F, Feliciano DV, Andrassy RJ et al. Early enteral feeding, compared with parenteral, reduces post-operative septic complications. Ann Surg 1992; 216:172–83.

17. Rutsky EA and Rostand SG. Treatment of uremic pericarditis and pericardial effusion: Am J Kidney Dis 1987; 1:2–8.

18. Ventura SC and Garella S. The management of pericardial disease in renal failure. Seminars in Dialysis 1990; 3:21–5.

19. De Pace N, Nestico P, Schwartz AB et al. Predicting success of intensive dialysis in the treatment of uremic pericarditis,

Am J Med 1984; 76:38–46.

20. Spector D, Alfred H, Siedlecki M et al. A controlled study of the effect of indomethacin in uremic pericarditis. Kidney Int 1983; 24:663.

21. Alcan KE, Zabetakis PM, Marino ND et al. Management of acute cardiac tamponade by subxiphoid pericardiotomy. JAMA 1982; 247:1143–8.

22. Kwasnik EM, Koster K, Lazarus JM et al. Conservative management of uremic pericardial effusions. J Cardiovasc Surg 1978; 76:629–32.

23. Buselmeier TJ, Davin TD, Simmons RL et al. Treatment of intractable uremic pericardial effusion. Avoidance of pericardiectomy with local steroid instillation. JAMA 1978; 240:1358–9.

24. Fuller TJ, Knochel JP, Brennan JP et al. Reversal of intractable uremic pericarditis by triamcinolone hexacetamide. Arch Intern Med 1976; 136:979–82.

25. Quigg RJ Jr, Idelson BA, Yoburn DC et al. Local steroids in dialysis-associated pericardial effusion. A single intrapericardial administration of triamcinolone. Arch Intern Med 1985; 145:2249–50.

26. Ghosh SC, Larrieu AJ, Ablaza SGG et al. Clinical experience with subxiphoid pericardial decompression. Int Surg 1985; 70:5–7.

27. Luft FC, Kleit SA, Smith RN et al. Management of uremic pericarditis with tamponade. Arch Intern Med 1974: 134:488–90.

28. Prager RL, Wilson Ch and Bender HW. The subxiphoid approach to pericardial disease. Annals Thoracic Surg 1982; 34:6–9.

29. DiMinno G, Martinez J, McLean ML et al. Platelet dysfunction in uremia. Am J Med 1985; 5:219.

30. Finn WF. Recovery from acute renal failure. In: Brenner BM and Lazarus JM, editors. Acute renal failure. WB Saunders Co., Philadelphia, 1983: 753–74.

31. Mannucci PM, Remuzzi G, Dusineri F et al. Deamino-8-arginine vasopressin shortens the bleeding time in uremia. N Engl J Med 1983; 308:8.

32. Eberst ME and Berkowitz LR. Hemostasis in renal disease: Pathophysiology and management. Am J Med 1994; 96:168–79.

33. Nissenson AR, Nimer SD and Wolcott DL. Recombinant human erythropoietin and renal anemia: molecular biology, clinical efficacy and nervous system effects. Ann Intern Med 1991; 114:402–16.

34. Parker S, Carlon GC, Isaacs M et al. Dopamine administration in oliguria and oliguric renal failure. Crit Care Med. 1981; 9:630–2.

35. Conger JD. A controlled evaluation of prophylactic dialysis in post-traumatic acute renal failure. J Trauma 1975; 15:1056–63.

36. Kleinknecht D, Jungers P, Chanard J et al. Uremic and non-uremic complications in acute renal failure: evaluation of early and frequent dialysis on prognosis. Kidney Int 1972; 1:190–6.

37. Gillum DM and Conger JD. The role of intensive dialysis in acute renal failure. Clin Nephrol 1986;25:249–55.

38. Hakim RM and Lazarus JM. Hemodialysis in acute renal failure. In: Brenner BM and Lazarus JM, editors. Acute

renal failure. WB Saunders Co., Philadelphia, 1983: 643–88.

39. Cameron JS. Acute renal failure – the continuing challenge. Q J Med 1986; 59:337–43.

40. Bellomo R and Boyce N. Does continuous hemodiafiltration improve survival in acute renal failure? Seminars in Dialysis 1993; 6:16–9.

41. Ronco C. Continuous renal replacement therapies for the treatment of acute renal failure in intensive care patients. Clin Nephrol 1983; 40:187–98.

42. Conger JD. Does hemodialysis delay recovery from acute renal failure? Seminars in Dialysis 1990; 3:146–8.

43. Coglutino F, Paganini E, Lockremm J et al. Continuous arteriovenous hemofiltration in the adult respiratory distress syndrome. Contrib Nephrol 1991; 93:94–7.

44. Bander SJ and Schwab SJ. Central venous angioaccess for hemodialysis and its complications. Seminars in Dialysis 1992; 5:121–8.

45. Nolph KD and Sorkin M. Peritoneal dialysis in acute renal failure. In Brenner BM and Lazarus JM, editors. Acute renal failure. WB Saunders Co., Philadelphia, 1983: 689–710.

46. Nolph KD. Peritoneal dialysis. In Brenner BM and Rector FC Jr., editors. The kidney. WB Saunders Co, Philadelphia, 1991: Ch. 50, 2299–335.

47. Kramer P, Wigger W, Rieger J et al. Arteriovenous hemofiltration: a new and simple method for treatment of over-hydrated patients resistant to diuretics. Klin Wochenschr 1977; 55:1121–2.

48. Bellomo R, Parkin G, Love J et al. A prospective comparative study of continuous arteriovenous hemodiafiltration and continuous venovenous hemodiafiltration in critically ill patients. Am J Kidney Dis 1993; 21:400–4.

49. Geronemus RP, Schneider NS and Epstein M. Survival in patients treated with continuous arteriovenous hemodialysis for acute renal failure and chronic renal failure. Contrib Nephrol 1991; 93:29–31.

50. Barzilay E, Kessler D, Lesmer C et al. Sequential plasmafilter-dialysis with slow continuous hemofiltration: Additional treatment for sepsis-induced MOSF patients. J Crit Care 1988; 3:163–6.

51. Barzilay E, Kessler D, Berlot G et al. Use of extracorporeal supportive techniques as additional treatment for septic induced multiple organ failure patients. Crit Care Med 1989; 17:634–7.

17. General management of the patient with chronic renal failure

REX L. MAHNENSMITH and DOUGLAS SHEMIN

Chronic renal failure denotes an irreversible reduction in GFR characterized by persistent elevations in BUN and Scr. While there are a number of disease processes which can result in chronic renal injury, two common features eventually emerge histologically: glomerulosclerosis and tubulointerstitial fibrosis. The physiologic consequences of these two processes are impairment in glomerular filtration and tubular functions. The former is characterized by azotemia, while the latter confers difficulty with sodium and water balance, potassium and acid excretion, and erythropoietin and 1,25 dihydroxycholecalciferol (activated vitamin D) synthesis.

CONSEQUENCES OF CHRONIC RENAL FAILURE

Adaptation to loss of nephrons

A common feature of progressive renal insufficiency is hypertrophy of undamaged nephrons [1]. Single nephron GFR (SNGFR) increases above normal and tubular transport processes augment. The increase in SNGFR evolves from sustained vasodilation of preglomerular arterioles and hypertrophy of remnant glomeruli. Augmentation of tubular transport processes derives from an increase in transporter number per cell and alteration of kinetic performance of existing transporters. Accordingly, solute and water transport by individual nephrons is adjusted proportionately to the GFR of that nephron, becoming either increased in hypertrophied nephrons or reduced in atrophied nephrons. Adaptive hypertrophy is minimal when renal insufficiency is mild: solute balance is easily maintained unless tubular injury is prominent, and waste excretion per nephron is only mildly augmented. But, as renal insufficiency progresses and the number of functional nephron units declines, remnant nephron functions hypertrophy more or less in proportion to the degree of renal insufficiency. Filtered load of waste and solute per nephron rises substantially. Total solute reabsorption per nephron also increases, but as a percentage of filtered load, solute reabsorption actually declines so that individual electrolyte homeostasis is remarkably maintained. For potassium which is excreted by secretion in the distal nephron, quantity secreted per nephron is augmented in proportion to degree of renal insufficiency. When renal insufficiency becomes advanced, however, filtration and tubular hypertrophy becomes inadequate and electrolyte imbalances emerge.

Mild renal insufficiency

Renal insufficiency causes few clinical problems while the GFR remains above 50 ml/min. Mild hypertension may develop and medication clearances will be altered, but the reduction in waste clearance which accompanies such a mild decline in GFR bears little consequence to the patient. Electrolyte balances are generally maintained by hypertrophy of remnant nephron functions.

The principal consequence of mild renal insufficiency is the *loss of renal clearance reserve* (i.e. the ability to increase GFR in response to dietary protein loads and other stimuli), which leaves the patient with increased vulnerability to clinically important renal failure from relatively minor pre-renal, intra-renal, or post-renal insults [2]. A decline in efficiency of autoregulation also occurs with mild renal insufficiency. This is the ability to maintain a stable renal blood flow and GFR in the face of moderate rises or falls in blood pressure [1, 2].

169

J.G. Abuelo (ed.), Renal Failure, 169–186.
© 1995 *Kluwer Academic Publishers.*

Moderate renal insufficiency

When GFR declines below 50 ml/min, clinically important consequences of renal insufficiency begin to emerge. *Hypertension* is more prevalent and derives from sodium and water retention and angiotensin-mediated vasoconstriction. Systemic blood pressures tend to be "salt sensitive" in this context, and rise abruptly or are relatively refractory to therapy if salt intake is high. A physiologic paradox of chronic renal insufficiency, however, is an *impairment in sodium conservation* when fluid depletion threatens, such as with vomiting or diarrhea. This paradox is due to the fact that tubular sodium reabsorption per nephron is already near-maximum in the steady state. When intravascular fluid depletion supervenes, further increase in tubular sodium reabsorption from the filtrate is either inadequate or not possible. An associated *loss of urinary concentrating ability* magnifies the vulnerability to fluid depletion. Annoying nocturia and polyuria may be the only manifestation of this, but substantial fluid depletion may emerge if oral intake declines in the face of non-renal fluid losses.

Measurable *phosphate retention* appears as GFR declines below 30 ml/min. Associated increases in parathyroid hormone secretion mitigate hyperphosphatemia by reducing tubular reabsorption of filtered phosphate as the GFR declines, but extract a biologic price by increasing bone turnover and inducing early osteodystrophy. *Hypocalcemia* typically accompanies hyperphosphatemia and is due to a reduction in renal synthesis of 1,25 dihydrocholecalciferol, which is essential for the absorption of calcium from the small intestine. *Acid* and *potassium* homeostasis are generally adequately maintained by hypertrophied remnant tubules unless tubulointerstitial involvement is a prominent feature of the renal disease. Then, *hyperkalemia* and a *hyperchloremic metabolic acidosis* appear even when GFR remains above 20 to 30 ml/min. *Anemia* is another expected accompaniment of progressive renal insufficiency due to declining erythropoietin production, but its appearance is variable. Some patients such as those with polycystic kidney disease retain erythropoietic capacity even as GFR declines below 10 ml/min, while others such as those with diabetic nephropathy evolve anemia much earlier in the course of their renal insufficiency.

Severe renal insufficiency

When glomerular filtration rates decline below 20 ml/min, electrolyte disturbances are more common and *uremia* is imminent. Nephron adaptations may still effectively mitigate imbalances such as hyperkalemia and hyponatremia, but a water load may result in severe hyponatremia or a potassium load may result in abrupt hyperkalemia. Uremia seems to impact nearly every tissue and organ system (Table 17.1).

Inexorable loss of renal function

A final aspect of renal insufficiency is its *progressive nature* [1, 3–5]. Progression may occur through activity of the primary disease process, as with diabetes mellitus, poorly controlled hypertension, polycystic kidney disease, or systemic lupus erythematosis, for example. If this is the case, accurate etiologic diagnosis and therapeutic intervention to interrupt the active pathogenetic mechanisms are cornerstones of management. However, even when the primary etiologic process is rendered inactive, eventual progression towards end stage renal failure seems inevitable in most patients. Several factors affect this progression and its rate: (1) extent of the original parenchymal injury; (2) presence and degree of systemic arterial hypertension; (3) nephron hypertrophy and associated intraglomerular hypertension; (4) intercurrent appearance of secondary problems such as obstruction, urinary tract infection, or injury from nephrotoxic medications or radiocontrast agents; and (5) co-existence of metabolic problems such as hyperlipidemia, diabetes mellitus, or hyperphosphatemia [4, 5].

Systemic and intraglomerular hypertension may be the dominant factors determining progression of renal insufficiency. Owing to the preglomerular vasodilation which adaptively evolves to augment single nephron GFR, remaining glomeruli of an already-diseased kidney become particularly vulnerable to the hemodynamic stresses of systemic hypertension and tend to undergo progressive sclerosis [1, 5, 6]. This has been conclusively demonstrated in diabetic nephropathy, where tempo of deterioration of renal function is clearly related to degree of systemic arterial pressure elevation, but animal and human data also suggest that systemic hypertension accelerates deterioration of renal function in nondiabetic contexts,

Table 17.1. Features of the uremic syndrome

Neurologic abnormalities
  Central
    Cognitive change
    Lethargy
    Stupor
    Coma
  Peripheral
    Motor neuropathy
    Sensory neuropathy
    Myoclonus
    Fasciculations

Cardiovascular abnormalities
  Hypertension
  Pericarditis
  Accelerated atherosclerosis
  Vascular calcifications

Hematologic abnormalities
  Anemia
  Leukocyte & lymphocyte dysfunction
  Platelet defect

Gastrointestinal abnormalities
  Anorexia, nausea, vomiting
  Gastroparesis
  Hypomotility of bowel
  Mucosal bleeding

Bone abnormalities
  Osteomalacia (impaired mineralization)
  Osteitis fibrosa (bone resorption)
  Osteosclerosis
  Aluminum associated osteomalacia

Rheumatologic abnormalities
  Myopathy
  Calcific bursitis
  Avascular necrosis
  Carpal tunnel syndrome (amyloid deposition)
  Articular amyloid deposition

Metabolic abnormalities
  Glucose intolerance
  Impaired protein synthesis
  Hyperlipidemia

Dermatologic abnormalities
  Pruritis
  Calcium-phosphate deposition

Pleural-pulmonary abnormalities
  Pleuritis and effusion
  Parenchymal calcification
  Edema

as well [5–10]. In experimental models of chronic renal failure induced by renal ablation or uncontrolled diabetes, intraglomerular hypertension exists even when systemic blood pressures are normal or just mildly elevated. Reduction of systemic hypertension with diuretic-adrenergic-blocker-vasodilator combinations in these models is not as effective in preserving renal function and lowering intraglomerular pressures as angiotensin converting enzyme (ACE) inhibitors, which uniquely lower glomerular capillary pressures by vasorelaxing postglomerular arterioles [5–10]. This latter finding strongly suggests that intraglomerular hypertension is an expected eventuality of chronic renal insufficiency, regardless of systemic blood pressure, and mitigation of intraglomerular hypertension attenuates progression of renal insufficiency.

GAUGING THE PROGRESSION OF RENAL INSUFFICIENCY

Sequential measurement of GFR through endogenous creatinine clearance is probably the most accurate and available way to assess changes in renal function over time. However, the clinician should realize that creatinine clearance overestimates true GFR because a small amount of creatinine can enter the urine via tubular secretion. The proportion of urinary creatinine deriving from tubular secretion and consequently the degree of overestimation of GFR rises as true GFR falls [11]. Alternative methods of assessing GFR include infusion inulin clearance, which is impractical and cumbersome, and radioactive iothalamate clearance, which is expensive and generally reserved for use in experimental protocols. Thus, sequential measurement of creatinine clearance remains the preferable clinical gauge for estimating changes in GFR in individual patients over time.

Longitudinal assessment of the Scr may be a suitable alternative for following progressive loss of renal function. The relationship between Scr and creatinine clearance is hyperbolic, such that the Scr changes little as the GFR falls from 100 ml/min to 50 ml/min, then rises in a brisk curvilinear fashion as GFR falls from 50 ml/min toward 0, so one cannot assume that a given change in Scr reflects a *proportional* change in GFR (Figure 17.1A). However,

A

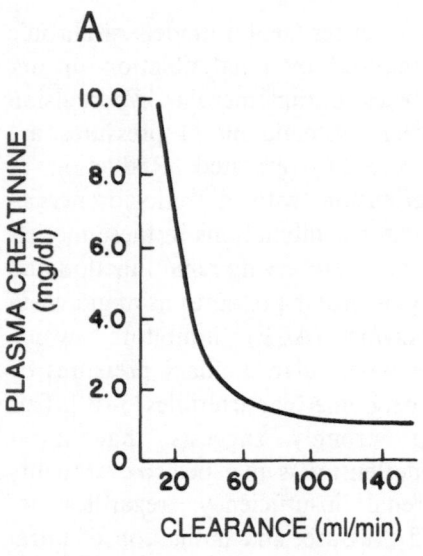

B

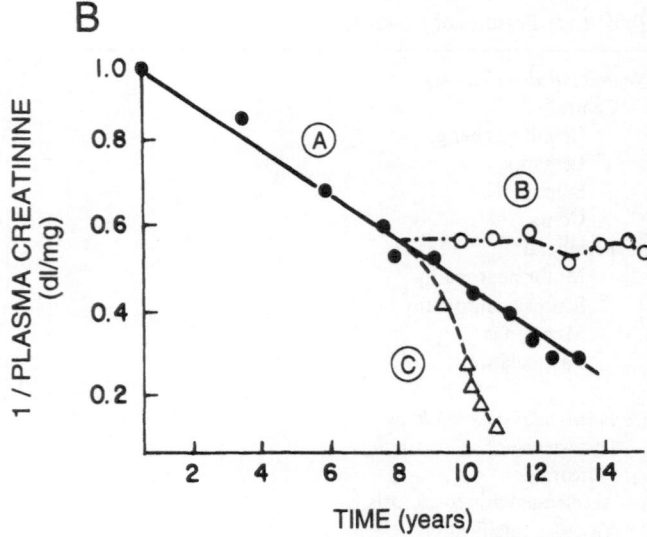

Fig. 17.1. (A) Graph depicting relationship between creatinine clearance and plasma creatinine concentration. This relationship is hyperbolic, such that creatinine clearance may decline from 100 ml/min to 50 ml/min with little change in the plasma creatinine concentration. However, when creatinine clearance is low, small changes in creatinine clearance will cause substantial increments in plasma creatinine concentrations. (B) Graphical plot of the reciprocal of plasma creatinine concentration (1/Scr) versus time in years. This relationship is typically linear (line A) unless forces intervene which either slow (line B) or accelerate (line C) the deterioration in renal function.

a plot of the reciprocal of serum creatinine (1/Scr) against time in an individual patient usually yields a linear relationship, which permits meaningful tracking of a given patient's clinical course and allows one to extrapolate clearance [12]. Thus, it has become a customary practice for physicians to follow individual patients with sequential Scr measurements and plot 1/Scr against time (in months or years) as a reliable gauge to their disease progression. A departure from the declining linearity in this relationship suggests either successful intervention on the part of the physician (if the relationship becomes more horizontal) or superimposition of aggressive factors accelerating loss of GFR (if the plot becomes more vertical). (Figure 17.1B)

PREVENTING LOSS OF RENAL FUNCTION

Limiting acute-on-chronic renal failure

Acute deterioration in GFR is a particular vulnerability in a person with established renal insufficiency, because of limitations of reserve function and impaired autoregulation of GFR. As discussed, sclerotic kidneys possess a reduced nephron population that is already maximally

adapted with preglomerular vasodilation and single nephron hyperfiltration. Thus, a hypotensive event or emergence of hypovolemia cannot be compensated by any further preglomerular vasodilation, such as would occur in a normal kidney, and GFR will fall.

The reduced nephron population is also relatively more vulnerable to toxic insults. For example, the leading risk factor for radiocontrast nephrotoxicity is chronic renal insufficiency [13]. This is due to the loss of renal reserve which accompanies chronic renal insufficiency and to the fact that the administered toxin is handled by fewer nephrons, implying that the toxic burden per nephron is greater than in a patient with normal kidney function.

It bears emphasis that a given toxic insult can precipitate a decline in renal function that is critical for a patient with renal insufficiency, whereas the same damage in a patient with normal renal function may be clinically unimportant. For example, radiocontrast and gentamicin administration to a patient with GFR 100 ml/min may precipitously cause a decline in GFR from 100 ml/min to 65 ml/min. This would not be clinically important. Yet, if that patient had a pre-existing GFR of 55 ml/min and experienced a loss of GFR to 20 ml/min, clinically significant complications would likely evolve.

A rise in Scr in a patient with otherwise stable renal insufficiency should provoke a comprehensive search for pre-renal, post-renal, and intrarenal factors that may be responsible. The approach should be identical to that followed in any patient with de novo acute renal failure. In patients with pre-existing renal insufficiency, hemodynamic or drug-related insults are the most common reasons for an acute loss of GFR. Hypovolemia from diarrhea, vomiting, or overdiuresis are common occurrences and easily discernible. A reduction in renal blood flow from evolving congestive heart failure is more subtle and will result in a decline in GFR if autoregulation of GFR is significantly impaired, as so often it is. Excessive decline in intravascular volume due to diuretics may compound the problem. This occurrence is diagnosed by careful history and physical examination and review of the patient's medication record. Nephrotoxic injury can be diagnosed from the history and by excluding other factors.

The most cogent management principle is to prevent such problems from arising. This translates into maintaining optimal cardiac output in any patient with impaired cardiac function, using diuretics judiciously to guard against hypovolemia, maintaining mean arterial pressure within the mid to high-normal range which will not subtend renal autoregulation, avoiding or minimizing potentially nephrotoxic medications and those which may further impair autoregulation, such as NSAIDs, and adjusting doses of drugs for the degree of their renal clearance.

Urinary tract obstruction is another mechanism for acute deterioration in function of chronically diseased kidneys. Obstruction of the urinary drainage system anywhere from the calyces to the urethral meatus can cause renal insufficiency. In a normal person, obstruction above the bladder must be bilateral to produce elevations in Scr and BUN, since GFR can decline nearly 50% without much effect on BUN and Scr concentrations. However, when a patient with stable renal insufficiency from bilateral parenchymal disease acutely obstructs one ureter, Scr and BUN will abruptly double their concentrations.

Urinary obstruction may be partial or complete. In either circumstance, intratubular hydrostatic pressures increase and oppose filtration, and renal blood flows decline, decreasing glomerular capillary pressures and forward filtration forces. Both result in worsening of renal insufficiency. Only the tempo of functional decline differs. Prolonged obstruction, whether partial or complete, can result in indolent tubular necrosis eventuating in additional permanent damage. If the urine is infected, then damage may be worsened by inflammatory mediators. These facts lend urgency to accurate diagnosis and treatment of obstructive processes and infection in any person with chronic renal insufficiency.

Slowing the progression of renal insufficiency
The progression of renal insufficiency and its prevention have been major focuses of nephrologic investigation [3, 4]. As discussed earlier, systemic and intraglomerular hypertension are acknowledged as leading factors in the progressive glomerulosclerosis and inevitable deterioration of GFR that occurs in most patients who have lost more than 75% of kidney function from processes as diverse as polycystic kidney disease, diabetes mellitus, chronic glomerulonephritis, and nephrosclerosis associated with poorly-controlled hypertension [1, 3, 4, 11, 13, 14].

Sustained reduction in systemic arterial blood pressure can limit this secondary glomerulosclerosis [5, 6, 15, 16]. Yet, even with normalization of systemic arterial pressures, intraglomerular hypertension can persist owing to preglomerular vasodilation and some degree of postglomerular vasoconstriction in chronically-scarred kidneys [4–6]. Further reduction in glomerular hypertension can be achieved with either *low protein diets* or *angiotensin converting enzyme (ACE) inhibitors* [4, 5, 10, 15]. Low protein diets constrict dilated preglomerular arterioles; ACE inhibitors relax postglomerular arterioles. Both actions reduce intraglomerular pressure and capillary wall tension, and both interventions appear to be effective towards retarding progression of renal insufficiency [4, 10, 15].

Whether the benefits of dietary protein restriction are additive to those of ACE inhibitors over a long period of time is unclear. Additive benefit in reducing proteinuria was documented in a three week crossover trial involving just 17 patients with nondiabetic nephrotic syndrome, but these findings require confirmation and extension to a longer term of trial observation [17]. Also, whether reduced proteinuria reflects reduced chronic injury or just some functional change needs more study.

Evidence exists that a protein-restricted diet probably confers renal-sparing benefit beyond systemic blood pressure control [18–21]. Yet, controlled human data suggest that this benefit may be small or countervailed by other forces, particularly when renal insufficiency is advanced [19–22]. For example, protein restriction will have little or no benefit if blood pressure is not controlled or if hyperglycemia persists in a diabetic patient.

Nevertheless, towards the goal of retarding progression of renal insufficiency, sufficient data now exist to support the following approach for patients with renal insufficiency: (1) reduce the systemic arterial blood pressures to values ≤ 140/85 mmHg with medications that are well-tolerated and do not aggravate existing clinical problems (e.g. avoid overdiuresis, and avoid beta blockers in patients with glucose intolerance or a congestive cardiomyopathy) [16]; (2) restrict protein in the diet to 0.6 to 0.8 gm/kg/day, but make certain calories remain approximately 30 to 35 kcal/kg/day; dietary protein restriction mandates isocaloric substitution with complex carbohydrates and polyunsaturated fats [18]; more restrictive diets with less than 0.6 gm/kg/day entail the risk of negative nitrogen balance and important nutritional compromise; dietary protein restriction may be of greatest benefit when renal insufficiency is mild and may lead to protein malnutrition when renal insufficiency is advanced; (3) for hypertensive individuals employ ACE inhibitors to the fullest dose tolerated, e.g. 75 mg captopril per day unless hyperkalemia, acute renal failure, or hypotension supervene (see below under Hypertension for further recommendations). Although short-term data suggest that normotensive diabetic individuals with albuminuria will experience a reduction in albuminuria excretion rates and stabilization of GFR over time with ACE inhibitor therapy, there is no proof that this correlates with histologic benefit [10]; longer-term and more comprehensive study is needed before such intervention can be recommended in this patient population.

Diabetic Nephropathy. Diabetic nephropathy is not only the most common chronic renal disease

that progresses to end-stage renal failure, it is the most studied with regards to factors that determine its progression and the value of specific therapeutic interventions. As already discussed, uncontrolled hypertension accelerates and blood pressure control slows its progression to end-stage failure, no matter what medication program one chooses [8, 9]. Additionally, several prospective controlled studies have concluded that diabetic patients in particular can expect benefit beyond systemic blood pressure control from *ACE inhibitor therapy*, benefit attributed to the unique action of ACE inhibitors to lower intraglomerular pressures [10, 23, 24]. It appears that relatively high doses of ACE inhibitors are required to achieve slowing of renal deterioration in diabetic patients. Where benefit has been shown, captopril dosage has been 75 or 100 mg per day and enalapril dosage has been 20 mg per day. Care must be taken that hyperkalemia or acute renal insufficiency not evolve from the ACE inhibitor. Low protein diets may provide additional benefit although human data are scanty in this regard [8, 15, 18, 19]. On the other hand, the renal benefits of *tight glycemic control* are now beyond refute. Three studies demonstrate conclusively that consistent glycemic control judged by glycosylated hemoglobin levels less than 8% results in at least retarded progression of diabetic nephropathy and perhaps its regression [25–27]. Superior glycemic control is achieved either by continuous infusion of insulin by portable pump or by three or more injections of insulin per day with multiple capillary blood glucose assessments by finger stick per day. It is important to point out that benefit was seen only after years of tight control and was most demonstrable in those who had little end-organ disease at the start of the study. Imposition of tight glycemic control with multiple doses of insulin when renal disease is advanced probably imputes little benefit to the kidney and may be harmful to the patient, since insulin is cleared by the kidneys and the danger of hypoglycemia is therefore high when GFR is low.

Pregnancy. A common practical question is whether pregnancy impacts negatively on the natural history of antecedent renal insufficiency. First of all, term pregnancies are unusual in the context of renal insufficiency, particularly if the BUN and Scr concentrations exceed 30 and 3 mg/dl respectively (urea: 10.7 mmol/L and Scr: 265 μmol/L) [28]. Conception is difficult due to irregular ovulation. Fertilized ova have difficulty establishing growth in the endometrium, and miscarriage is frequent. However, erythropoietin usage and near-normalization of hematocrits have altered this grim picture, improving both male and female fertility, intrauterine survival, and outcome of term pregnancies. If renal function is near-normal at conception, it is likely that the pregnancy will reach term.

Pregnancy has variable effects on function of already-diseased kidneys. The nature of the underlying kidney disease, the extent of renal insufficiency, and the blood pressure at conception appear to determine the impact of pregnancy on native kidney function [28]. For example, pregnancy appears to have little adverse effect on chronic latent glomerulonephritis and non-infectious tubulointerstitial disease unless hypertension and renal insufficiency (with GFR <80 ml/min) co-exist. Hypertension in association with renal insufficiency presents an increased risk of *accelerated hypertension, preeclampsia, and worsening of the renal insufficiency* that is permanent in up to one-third of cases. If proteinuria is a major component of a patient's renal disease, then pregnancy is likely to worsen it. This of itself is usually of no consequence unless nephrotic syndrome supervenes with its own set of complications, such as a hypercoagulable state, progressive edema, and intravascular fluid depletion. Fetal loss is high when there is heavy proteinuria associated with primary renal disease.

Pregnancy creates definite but limited risks in women with *diabetic nephropathy*. Preeclampsia and upper tract urinary infections occur more often than in nondiabetics, but renal insufficiency does not progress in the vast majority of gravid diabetics. Exacerbation of proteinuria in an already-proteinuric diabetic is common with pregnancy, as is a rise in systemic blood pressure, but these problems usually abate postpartum.

The impact of pregnancy on the kidney in patients with *lupus nephritis* is controversial. Aggravation of renal disease, no change in renal disease, and even transient improvement have been described in various series [28]. If lupus activity is in remission at the time of conception, gestation is usually uncomplicated. Hypertension and preeclampsia may be more frequent if some degree of chronic renal insufficiency exists, regardless of activity of lupus in the kidney. In all cases, close monitoring of renal function is warranted, since exacerbations of lupus can occur with pregnancy, especially in the puerperium [28].

Some general recommendations regarding pregnancy and renal disease are in order: (1) given the good maternal and fetal outcome with Scr <1.5 mg/dL, women with mild chronic renal disease should be advised to complete childbearing earlier rather than later; (2) women with Scr > 1.5 mg/dL should be informed of risks of pregnancy (preeclampsia, progression of chronic renal failure, and hypertension), and should be supported in their decision to avoid or proceed with conception; (3) pregnant women with underlying chronic renal failure who exhibit accelerated renal failure during pregnancy should be evaluated for reversible causes, such as infection or obstruction. If none is found, elective delivery should be performed if the fetus is viable, or hospitalization with intensive monitoring offered until the fetus is viable; however, many physicians recommend termination of pregnancy before this eventuality, since the loss of renal function may be recoverable with this action. Even if renal failure goes to endstage and the fetus is ultimately lost, renal transplantation may offer another chance for childbearing. On the other hand, the current pregnancy may be the last and many couples will choose to carry the baby to term or near-term in the hopes of a successful delivery. Women and their spouses should be thoughtfully and fully counseled regarding the risks and alternatives in this context.

In all cases, management of the pregnant azotemic woman requires a team of physicians that includes a high-risk pregnancy specialist and a neonatologist, frequent monitoring of blood pressure, blood chemistries, urine protein and urine cultures, and regular assessments of fetal well-being with nonstress monitoring and ultrasonographic measurements of growth and fetal activity [29].

NONDIALYTIC TREATMENT OF UREMIC COMPLICATIONS

Although renal replacement therapy with hemodialysis, peritoneal dialysis, or renal transplantation is the definitive treatment for patients with advanced renal disease, a number of adjunctive treatments may be used by the physician to treat uremic symptoms and complications and even to delay the necessity for dialysis.

Hypertension

Most patients with chronic renal insufficiency have systemic arterial hypertension either as a consequence of their renal disease or as a primary disorder responsible for their renal insufficiency. Persistent hypertension in the context of renal insufficiency promotes progression of the renal insufficiency, regardless of its etiology, and contributes to evolution of left ventricular hypertrophy, systolic and diastolic ventricular dysfunction, atherosclerosis, coronary insufficiency, and stroke [30]. Control of hypertension is central to cardiovascular well-being and longevity of the patient with renal insufficiency.

Hypertension in chronic renal insufficiency arises from sodium retention and two processes that heighten peripheral vascular resistance. First, renal parenchymal disease may be associated with inappropriate renin output in the face of intravascular volume overload and, second, hypertension persisting over months and years will lead to structural vascular narrowing. Hence, it is common that control of hypertension in patients with chronic renal insufficiency requires more than one pharmacological agent.

All antihypertensive regimens in the setting of chronic renal failure should contain *dietary sodium restriction and a loop diuretic*. Care must be taken to avoid overdiuresis, but relatively low doses of furosemide often are sufficient to sustain natriuresis and lower blood pressure. Once the retention of sodium has been managed, *ACE inhibitors* are the logical next choice antihypertensive agent. ACE inhibitors will lower intraglomerular pressures, reduce peripheral vascular resistance, and ameliorate left ventricular hypertrophy and congestive heart failure. ACE inhibitors may reduce GFR and promote hyperkalemia, however, so Scr and potassium concentrations must be monitored. Additionally, the combination of loop diuretics and an ACE inhibitor are particularly prone to precipitate ARF. *Calcium antagonists, beta adrenergic antagonists, and alpha adrenergic antagonists* are logical next choices. The peripheral

vasodilating effects of calcium antagonists are particularly effective toward lowering blood pressure in the context of renal insufficiency and have few side-effects. Calcium antagonists also ameliorate left ventricular hypertrophy. Beta adrenergic antagonists may aid blood pressure control in combination with other drugs, but may cause hyperkalemia, particularly in patients with diabetes mellitus and advanced renal insufficiency [30].

Hyperlipidemia

Lipid abnormalities often coexist or arise with chronic renal insufficiency [31]. Lipid surveillance should be part of one's semiannual assessment of patients with chronic renal disease. Hyperlipidemia probably exacerbates vascular disease and may contribute to the progression of renal insufficiency through a direct glomerular effect. Conventional parameters and means for intervention should be employed by the physician, starting with dietary restrictions and then pharmacological agents.

Renal osteodystrophy

Pathogenesis. Bone disease is a universal consequence of renal insufficiency but has a complex pathogenesis (Figure 17.2). Two central factors are responsible: 1,25 dihydroxycholecalciferol deficiency and hyperparathyroidism [32-35]. Phosphorus retention may be central to both. Phosphorus retention is apparent as GFR declines below 40 ml/min. Concomitant with phosphorus retention is a decline in 1,25 dihydroxycholecalciferol production by decreased or diseased renal tissue, which is exacerbated by a phosphate-induced reduction in the renal enzyme activity responsible for the production of 1,25 dihydroxycholecalciferol from 25 hydroxycholecalciferol. Deficiency of 1,25 dihydroxycholecalciferol leads to reduced intestinal absorption of dietary calcium and an impaired calcemic response of bone to parathyroid hormone (PTH). Hypocalcemia results from this as well as from hyperphosphatemia-induced calcium-phosphate precipitation. Reduced serum ionized calcium stimulates higher output of PTH. 1,25 dihydroxycholecalciferol deficiency also augments PTH output [32, 34]. PTH promotes resorption of formed bone.

Two kinds of bone lesions are seen in chronic

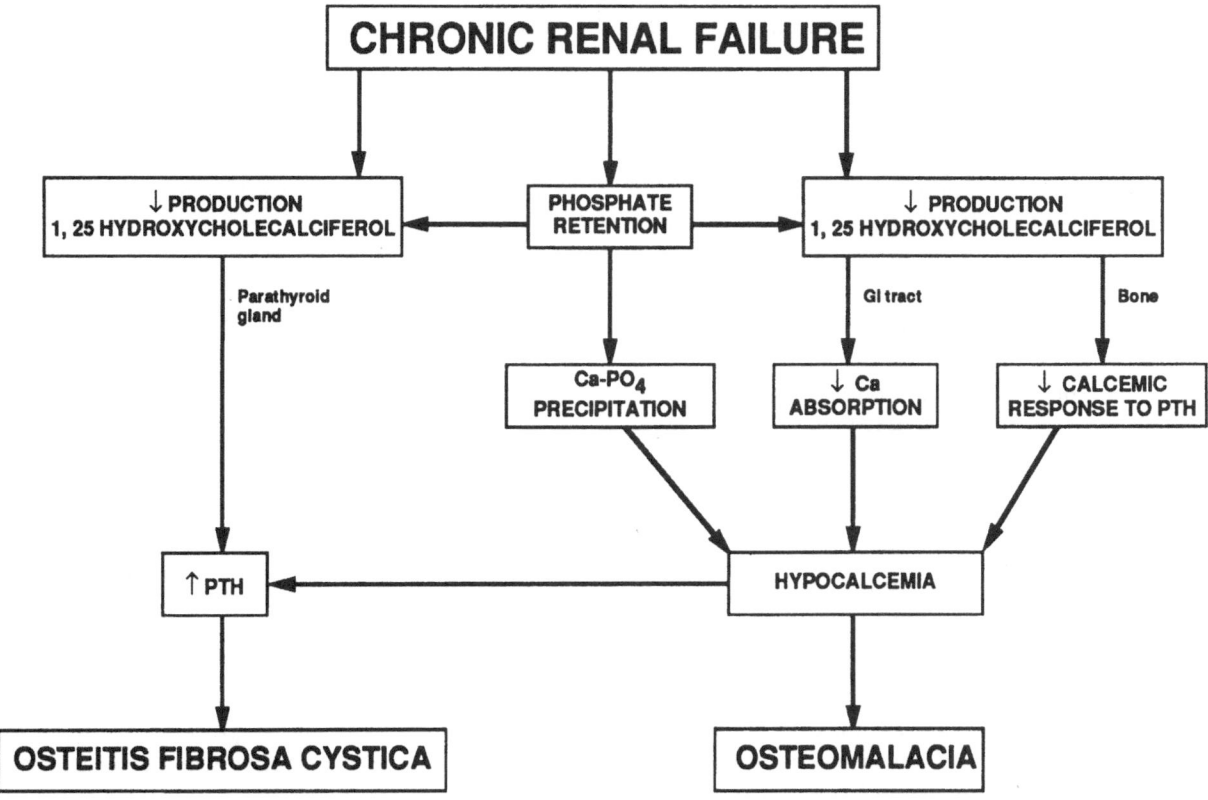

Fig. 17.2. Pathophysiology of renal osteodystrophy. Hyperphosphatemia, deficiency of 1,25 dihydroxycholecalciferol, and hyperparathyroidism are principal pathogenetic factors.

renal insufficiency: *osteitis fibrosa cystica*, which derives from excess cortical bone resorption owing to excess PTH, and *osteomalacia*, which results from prolonged deficiency of 1,25 dihydroxycholecalciferol [31]. Other features of osteitis fibrosa cystica include progressive fibrosis of marrow space and appearance of disorganized osteoid, which does not display normal mineralization. Osteomalacia evolves principally as a mineralization defect, which is manifested by unmineralized collagen seams and a reduction in calcified cortical bone. Bone from a given patient may exhibit a preponderance of either osteitis fibrosa cystica or osteomalacia or may exhibit both processes.

Metabolic acidosis results in loss of calcium carbonate from bone, which probably contributes to the skeletal demineralization of renal insufficiency. Chronic interstitial diseases associated with renal tubular acidosis predispose to this mechanism more than others [32].

Therapy. Treatment of renal osteodystrophy must be commenced early [32–34]. Prevention is the primary goal. Interventions should aim at pathogenetic forces. *Dietary phosphorus restriction* to less than 800 mg per day is central. Phosphorus binders are also essential and should be taken during meals to maintain serum phosphate levels below 5.5 mg/dl (1.8 mmol/L) [33, 35]. *Calcium acetate and calcium carbonate* are preferred over aluminum carbonate or aluminum hydroxide for this purpose because aluminum absorption can contribute to osteomalacia and absorption of calcium may aid in maintaining serum calcium levels in the normal range. Calcium acetate 667–1334 mg or calcium carbonate 500–1000 mg per meal are usual starting doses. One titrates the dose to serum calcium and phosphate levels, aiming to achieve serum calcium between 9.1 and 10.0 mg/dl (2.3 and 2.5 mmol/L) and the calcium × phosphate product less than 55 (4.4 in SI units).

Therapy with 1,25 dihydroxycholecalciferol should commence early, also [33, 34]. The usual starting dose is 0.25 to 0.5 μg per day. It is marketed by prescription as *calcitriol*. This agent is titrated principally against the serum PTH level. The therapeutic goal is to lower serum PTH levels to approximately 1.5 to 2 times normal. Further lowering may lead to an adynamic bone lesion. Use of calcitriol must be monitored closely. It can raise serum calcium levels above the normal range, causing lethargy, constipation, and mental status changes. It can also raise serum phosphate levels by promoting phosphate absorption from the diet. Hence, calcitriol must be administered in harmony with calcium salts, dietary phosphate restriction, and if need be, small amounts of aluminum hydroxide or aluminum carbonate. Since chronic acidosis slowly demineralizes bone, metabolic acidosis should be ameliorated as well [32, 34]. This is best done with sodium citrate or bicarbonate compounds. (See section on Metabolic Acidosis later in this chapter.)

If bone disease is advanced, then bone pain and pathologic fractures may occur and more aggressive intervention will be necessary. Accurate diagnosis of the type of bone disease is essential [32, 33]. This can be diagnosed indirectly by assessment of bone X-rays, serum PTH, calcium, and phosphorus levels, and concentration of serum alkaline phosphatase. Osteitis fibrosa cystica will usually be associated with very high PTH levels, bony erosions on X-ray, and high alkaline phosphatase. Osteomalacia exhibits a less erosive change on bone X-rays and lower PTH levels, yet hypercalcemia easily emerges with calcium and calcitriol therapy in the context of osteomalacia because the bone cannot utilize available calcium. However, clinical features or clues such as these do not accurately predict type of bone lesion, and a bone biopsy is really necessary to discriminate between the two types. Bone biopsy is also critical when aluminum-associated bone disease is entertained. Aluminum will deposit along the mineralization front of cortical bone and prevent effective mineralization, and a form of osteomalacia is the result. This must be treated with chelation therapy and can be particularly problematic if left undiagnosed.

Treatment options for advanced bone disease include *high-dose daily calcitriol, intermittent pulse calcitriol therapy* (e.g. every other day with hemodialysis, or twice a week with peritoneal dialysis), *parathyroidectomy*, and *deferoxamine*

chelation therapy, if aluminum-associated bone disease is diagnosed [32–35]. Indications for high-dose calcitriol include refractory hyperparathyroidism and advancing osteodystrophy. *Parathyroidectomy* should be undertaken only when conservative measures fail and bone disease is advancing or there is a large burden of soft-tissue calcification [32–35].

Volume overload

Most patients with advancing renal insufficiency will develop an expansion of their intravascular volume as a result of decreased urinary excretion of sodium and water. Symptoms and signs of volume overload may include weight gain, pulmonary congestion, an S3 gallop, and peripheral edema, or may be limited to systolic and diastolic hypertension. This problem should be initially managed with *dietary sodium restriction*; an 88 mEq/day sodium diet (corresponding to a 2 gram/day sodium diet) is much lower than the average American intake of 200 mEq/day and is palatable enough to satisfy most patients and ensure an adequate caloric intake.

In those patients who do not respond to dietary intervention alone, *diuretics* are necessary for natriuresis and normalization of intravascular volume. *Loop diuretics*, such as furosemide and bumetanide, are generally the agents of choice; thiazides lose efficacy when the GFR drops below 30 ml/minute. Furosemide is usually begun at a dose of 40 mg daily, in two divided doses. The duration of action of furosemide is about six hours and once-daily dosing is commonly inadequate, as tubular reabsorption of sodium may rebound following a furosemide-induced diuresis. Although some authorities advocate up to four grams daily, the general consensus is that doses above 400 mg do not yield added benefit [36]. Because furosemide is protein-bound and exerts its effect from inside the nephron lumen, proteinuria interferes with its efficacy, and a higher initial dose is usually necessary in azotemic patients with nephrotic syndrome [37]. *Metolazone*, a thiazide-like agent with a primary effect in the distal tubule, may be added to furosemide for synergistic effect; the dose ranges from 2.5 to 10 mg daily.

Since loop diuretics and metolazone enhance urinary potassium excretion, hypokalemia is a potential risk of therapy. This development is less common in patients with renal failure and decreased renal potassium excretion, so that treatment with potassium chloride should be reserved for patients with potassium levels consistently below 3.0 mEq/L, on digoxin, or with cardiac arrhythmias. Excessive diuresis is a potential hazard of diuretic therapy, and may lead to volume depletion, prerenal azotemia, and worsening of renal insufficiency. Body weight, BUN and Scr levels should be followed regularly to screen for this complication.

Hyperkalemia

Many patients with chronic renal failure have hyperkalemia, as defined by a serum potassium level above 5.0 mEq/L. Azotemic patients with primary tubulointerstitial disease, such as obstructive or reflux nephropathy, analgesic nephropathy, or sickle cell nephropathy with papillary injury, are at particularly high risk, as they will tend to have decreased tubular secretion of potassium as well as decreased GFR. Hyperkalemia is also more common in patients with diabetic nephropathy and hyporeninemic hypoaldosteronism; a hyperchloremic metabolic acidosis is also often present. In addition, many patients with renal failure are treated with pharmacologic agents that tend to increase the potassium level, including ACE inhibitors, beta blockers, and NSAIDs.

If the potassium level is consistently above 6.0 mEq/L, dietary restriction of potassium to less than 50 mEq/day is indicated, and medications which can induce hyperkalemia should be discontinued or decreased in dose. *Volume depletion, metabolic acidosis*, and *hyperglycemia* all potentially contribute to hyperkalemia, and should be investigated and corrected. In patients with hypertension or volume expansion who remain hyperkalemic despite dietary potassium restriction, *diuretics* may be employed to augment renal potassium excretion. The mineralocorticoid agonist *fludrocortisone acetate* also increases renal tubular secretion of potassium at doses of 0.1 to 0.2 mg daily, but it promotes sodium retention and is relatively contraindicated in renal insufficiency associated with volume expansion. It may be combined with diuretics to control hyperkalemia and maintain a neutral sodium balance. As a final measure, the cation exchange resin *sodium polystyrene sulfonate* may be used chronically to increase gastrointestinal potassium excretion; it is generally given as a 15 to 60

gram/day dose in a solution of sorbitol for a cathartic effect. It can also be given intrarectally as a dose of 30 to 60 grams if a patient is unable to tolerate oral feedings; sorbitol should not be used intrarectally because of the risk of colonic necrosis [38]. Cation exchange resins have variable and unpredictable effects on the serum potassium level, and chronic daily use requires frequent checks of potassium levels. Their effect depends on intestinal absorption of sodium in exchange for potassium, and their use is therefore problematic in patients with volume overload. The cost may be prohibitive for most patients.

Chronic renal failure increases the risk of acute rises in the serum potassium concentrations to critical or life-threatening levels (above 6.5 mEq/L). Management of such emergencies is discussed in Chapter 16.

Metabolic acidosis

Metabolic acidosis with an elevated anion gap is a feature of progressive renal failure because of decreased glomerular filtration of dietary and endogenous acids. This is generally mild with serum bicarbonate levels ranging from 18 to 20 mEq/L. Patients with renal failure due to primary tubulointerstitial or obstructive disease tend to have even lower bicarbonate values because of decreased tubular secretion of hydrogen ion and decreased renal tubular bicarbonate production.

The catastrophic consequences of acidemia, such as decreased myocardial contractility and cardiac arrhythmias, are rare at these levels of acidosis. However, in chronic metabolic acidosis the bony skeleton acts as a buffer, resulting in increased bone resorption and impaired bone growth. *Sodium bicarbonate or sodium citrate therapy* improves acidosis and decreases bone turnover. A reasonable approach would be to treat all acidemic patients who have bicarbonate levels below 15 mEq/L with sodium citrate or bicarbonate, starting with a dose of 0.5 mEq/kg/day in two or three divided doses and aiming for a bicarbonate level above 18 mEq/L. The target level should ideally be higher (above 21 mEq/L) in children and adolescents in order to maximize growth. Since sodium bicarbonate and sodium citrate increase intravascular volume and blood pressure, some patients may require initiation of or an increased dose of a diuretic.

Anemia

A normochromic, normocytic anemia is present in most patients with chronic renal failure. This is due to a number of factors, including decreased renal synthesis of erythropoietin, which normally stimulates the production of erythrocytes in the bone marrow, inhibition of the erythropoietin effect on erythrocyte precursors by uremia, a shortened erythrocyte life span, and occult bleeding due to uremic platelet defects [39].

In the 1980s, the human erythropoietin gene was identified and then introduced into mammalian cells, allowing erythropoietin to be produced commercially in large quantities. Erythropoietin has proven effective in patients with end-stage renal disease treated with dialysis as well as in patients with azotemia not yet on dialysis [40]; this suggests that higher levels of erythropoietin can overwhelm any uremic inhibitors of erythropoietic action. Concomitant with or because of a rise in the hematocrit, erythropoietin administration leads to a host of other beneficial effects, including improvement in appetite, sexual function, and exercise tolerance [41].

Erythropoietin must be given parenterally. When administered subcutaneously, the peak level is lower than with intravenous administration, but the duration of action and efficacy is greater. The subcutaneous route is the most practical one in patients not treated with hemodialysis. There are many approaches to dosing; most authorities suggest an initial dose of 100 to 200 units/kg/week in one or two divided doses, with initiation of treatment when the hematocrit is below 30%. It typically takes two to six weeks for erythropoietin to have a measurable effect on the hematocrit; an increase in the reticulocyte count precedes a rise in the hematocrit and should be noted within the first two weeks of therapy. The goal should be a hematocrit of about 35%; the dose of erythropoietin should be gradually increased after the initial six week period if that goal is not achieved.

Iron deficiency is the principal cause of failure to respond to erythropoietin; it will also develop in most patients during therapy. *Plasma ferritin* and *percent transferrin saturation* should be measured prior to initiation of therapy and periodically thereafter; iron deficiency, characterized by a plasma ferritin of less than 100 ng/mL and a transferrin saturation less than 20%, mandates

treatment with iron [42]. A reasonable starting dose is 50 to 100 mg of elemental iron by mouth two to three times daily. Gastrointestinal side effects may occur with this dose, and it may be necessary to try several different iron preparations. If patients are unable to tolerate oral iron, it may be given intravenously as iron dextran in 100 mg doses for a total dose of 500 to 1000 mg. Administration of parenteral *iron dextran* involves some risk of anaphylaxis, and patients should be pretreated with a test dose of 25 mg with emergency equipment available in the event of a reaction.

The major side effect of erythropoietin therapy is *hypertension*, which is probably due to an increase in peripheral vascular resistance. This has been reported in up to a third of hemodialysis patients treated with erythropoietin, but may be less common in pre-dialysis patients [40]. *Seizures* were initially reported in patients receiving 500 to 1000 units/kg/week in association with rising blood pressure; seizures are probably less common at lower doses and with controlled blood pressures.

Bleeding

Patients with progressive azotemia typically exhibit a bleeding tendency characterized by easy bruisability, ecchymoses, and bleeding from mucous membranes, especially in the gastrointestinal tract. This is probably due to a number of uremic-induced abnormalities of platelet aggregation and platelet adhesion to vessel walls. Patients have normal prothrombin and partial thromboplastin times and normal platelet counts, but the *bleeding time* is abnormally prolonged [43].

Severe bleeding due to platelet dysfunction in an azotemic patient is an indication for dialysis, but there are a number of therapies that may be employed in nondialyzed individuals to control minor bleeding or prevent hemorrhage. Improvement of anemia with either red blood cell transfusions or erythropoietin (see above) to a hematocrit above 30% will improve the bleeding time. Intravenous *desmopressin acetate*, a derivative of vasopressin, at a dose of 0.3 µg/kg also improves the bleeding time and decreases clinical bleeding; the mechanism relates to release of von Willebrand factor multimers from storage pools [44]. Desmopressin acetate loses therapeutic efficacy eight hours after administration and with multiple doses and is thus unsuitable for long-term administration. *Estrogens* are also effective in improving uremic bleeding, although the mechanism is unclear; the onset of action is two to five days. Estrogen may be given intravenously, as a dose of 0.6 mg/kg/day for five days [45] or orally, as a dose of 50 mg conjugated estrogens daily for five to ten days [46]. Low doses of estrogen in the form of oral contraceptives have been shown to control chronic gastrointestinal bleeding in patients with renal failure and angiodysplastic lesions [47].

Pruritus
Pruritus is a frequent symptom in patients with chronic renal failure. Potential causes are deposition of uremic solutes in the skin, an elevated calcium-phosphorus product with intradermal microcalcifications, and secondary hyperparathyroidism [48]. As an approach to this problem, potentially reversible causes of pruritus, including xerosis, fungal skin infections, scabies, and allergic reactions, should be addressed first. Hyperphosphatemia should be vigorously treated with dietary phosphorus restriction, (less than 800 mg of phosphorus daily), and *oral phosphate binders*. Calcitriol should be prescribed if the parathyroid hormone level is elevated, but as calcitriol increases gastrointestinal absorption of calcium and phosphorus, it should be withheld until the serum phosphorus level is below 6 mg/dl (1.9 mmol/L) and the dose decreased once the calcium level is above 11 mg/dl (2.75 mmol/L). Oral *antihistamines*, including diphenhydramine, hydroxyzine, or trimeprazine, may provide short term relief. Unfortunately, these measures do not always improve uremic itching, which if severe enough is an indication for dialysis. Ultraviolet phototherapy, topical capsaicin, and erythropoietin have been reported to be effective antipruritic modalities in patients treated with hemodialysis.

Nausea and vomiting
Gastrointestinal side effects become more common as renal failure progresses and may be quite disabling. Dysgeusia, nausea, anorexia, and vomiting lead to volume depletion and malnutrition. Potentially reversible etiologies, including peptic ulcer disease, gastric outlet obstruction, diabetic gastroparesis, and constipation, should be investigated and treated. If symptoms are severe or

accompanied by other manifestations of uremia, dialysis should be initiated. However, *dietary protein restriction*, to less than 0.6 g/kg/day, may eliminate gastrointestinal uremic symptoms for a short term, a two to three week period pending the maturation of an arteriovenous fistula, for example. *Antiemetics*, such as prochlorperazine, promethazine, or metoclopramide, may be beneficial for short periods.

Restless legs and leg cramps
A variety of symptoms involving the musculoskeletal and neurologic systems accompany progressive azotemia. Spontaneous muscle cramps, involuntary myoclonic jerks, and "restless legs" are most common. "Restless legs" is a neurologic symptom described as an aching, jittery sensation felt deep within the muscles of the legs; patients describe an irresistible urge to move their legs, and symptoms are relieved by movement and massage. The mechanisms for all of these symptoms are poorly defined and probably relate to uremic toxic effects on muscle and peripheral nerve. They improve with dialysis. Prior to initiation of dialysis, muscle cramps may be treated with restoration of any volume deficit and *quinine sulfate*, at a dose of 325 mg every eight hours. Myoclonic jerks may respond to low doses of *benzodiazepines*; narcotic analgesics have an exacerbating effect and should be discontinued.

DIALYSIS AND RENAL TRANSPLANTATION

When irreversible manifestations of uremia and volume overload complicate renal failure, either *chronic dialysis therapy* or *renal transplantation* is necessary to improve symptoms and maintain life. The two forms of chronic dialysis therapy employed in end stage renal disease care are *hemodialysis* and *peritoneal dialysis*.

Chronic hemodialysis
The hemodialysis process was described in Chapter 16. Three hemodialysis treatments weekly, each lasting three to four hours, control most manifestations of uremia and volume overload in outpatients with chronic renal failure.

Vascular Access. Since subcutaneous blood vessels are insufficiently capacious to provide the high blood flows required for effective treatment, a fistula between a superficial artery and vein in an extremity or a synthetic graft between an artery and vein must be surgically created as a *permanent vascular access.* Fistulae constructed from endogenous blood vessels are superior to synthetic grafts, but may require eight weeks or longer to mature for hemodialysis use; they should be created far in advance of their anticipated use. Arteriovenous grafts usually may be used two to three weeks after their construction. *Temporary vascular access* with a dual lumen catheter inserted into a femoral, internal jugular, or subclavian vein may be necessary if dialysis must be started prior to maturation of the vascular access. Vascular access may be difficult to create in patients with arterial or venous insufficiency. Access thrombosis, infection, aneurysm, and ischemia of the extremity distal to the arteriovenous anastamosis are other potential complications; the incidence of infection may be decreased with meticulous attention to aseptic technique during needle placement [49].

Complications. Besides access problems, a wide variety of complications may be associated with hemodialysis treatments; these range from minor problems such as headaches or itching to rare fatal events such as anaphylaxis. *Hypotension,* from rapid ultrafiltration of fluid and rapid decreases in serum osmolality, is the most common [50].

Prognosis. Morbidity and mortality in patients treated with maintenance hemodialysis is high; there is an annual mortality rate of over 20% among patients in the United States. Clinical outcomes on dialysis are influenced by a host of factors, including age, comorbid medical conditions, the presence or absence of diabetes mellitus, nutritional status, psychosocial issues, and the adequacy of the dialysis prescription. The relationship between the amount of dialysis prescribed and patient outcome has, to date, been incompletely explored. Three weekly treatments of more than three and a half hours each, with a drop in the BUN level of at least 65% over the course of each treatment, may correlate with a decreased mortality and morbidity [51, 52].

Chronic peritoneal dialysis

Peritoneal dialysis is performed with a silicone rubber or polyurethane catheter permanently implanted in the peritoneal cavity through the anterior abdominal wall. The distal end of the catheter has multiple side holes and rests in the intraperitoneal space, allowing instilled fluid to enter and then drain from the peritoneal cavity. In *chronic ambulatory peritoneal dialysis (CAPD),* patients instill one to three liters of peritoneal dialysate through the catheter into the intraperitoneal space. The fluid is allowed to dwell intraperitoneally for three to eight hours, and then drain out (see Figure 17.3). This cycle is serially repeated, for a total of three to six cycles daily. Uremic toxins diffuse across peritoneal capillary basement membranes and gradually accumulate in the peritoneal cavity, reaching equilibration over a two or four hour period before they are drained out. The dialysate contains high concentrations of dextrose, from 1.5 to 4.25 g/dl (83 to 264 mmol/L). This acts as an osmotic agent and promotes the movement of water and sodium into the peritoneal space, ultrafiltering excess fluid from the patient. Peritoneal dialysate solution typically contains concentrations of sodium and chloride that are similar to those in plasma, low concentrations of potassium and magnesium, and high concentrations of calcium and lactate, which is converted to bicarbonate by the liver.

There are a number of variations on this method. In *chronic cycled peritoneal dialysis (CCPD),* a machine delivers a set volume of dialysate and regulates the inflow, dwell, and drain phases; this process is usually performed at night during sleep, and a variable amount of fluid is left dwelling during the day. In *intermittent peritoneal dialysis (IPD),* the peritoneal exchanges are done rapidly, over a 20 to 40 hour period twice weekly; during the remainder of the week, no dialysis occurs.

Although prescribed in fewer patients than hemodialysis, peritoneal dialysis has a number of attractive features. There is no need for a vascular access in patients with severe arterial or venous insufficiency. Since dialysis and ultrafiltration are gradual and continuous during the course of the day, compartmental fluid shifts, fluid removal, and changes in osmolality occur more slowly than in hemodialysis. Thus, hypotension, or dise-

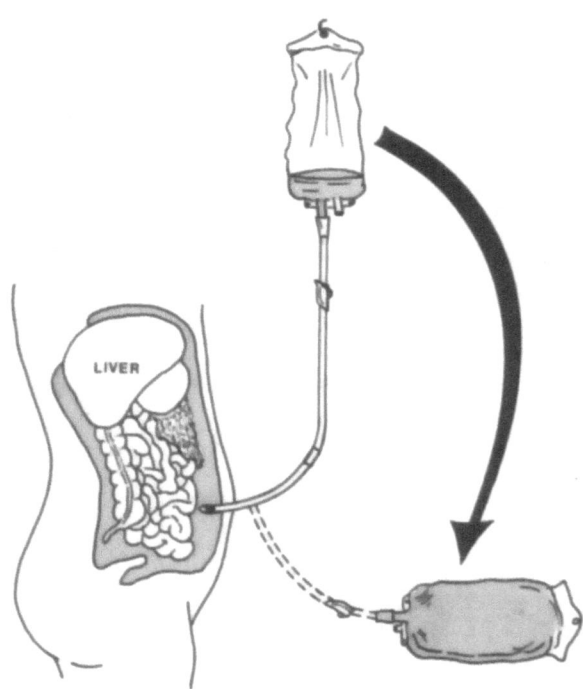

Fig. 17.3. Peritoneal dialysis. Dialysate is instilled into the peritoneal cavity, dwells for a defined period of time, and then drains out by gravity.

quilibrium from a sudden decrease in extracellular osmolality occurs much less often than in hemodialysis. Patients on CAPD may have less uremic symptoms than patients treated with hemodialysis. This may be explained by the notion that larger molecular weight solutes are responsible for the uremic syndrome and peritoneal membranes allow more diffusion of those solutes than hemodialysis membranes. This is controversial, but it seems clear that there is less anemia, probably due to decreased blood loss, and greater maintenance of residual renal function in patients treated with CAPD [53].

The principal risk of CAPD is *peritonitis*, which occurs about once every one to two years in treated patients. The cause is *Staphylococcus aureus* or *Staphylococcus epidermitis* in about 75% of patients, and gram negative bacilli in most of the remainder. Fungi and mycobacteria have been reported in immunosuppressed patients. Most infections can be treated in an outpatient setting with intraperitoneal antibiotics, but some gram negative infections and virtually all fungal infections require removal of the peritoneal catheter and temporary

discontinuation of peritoneal dialysis. CAPD may also be complicated by *hypoalbuminemia* because of albumin loss in dialysate and *hypertriglyceridemia* because of excessive glucose absorption; these abnormalities can usually be handled with dietary therapy [54].

Mode of dialysis therapy
There is no evidence to date that one form of dialysis is significantly superior to another in improving morbidity from renal failure or long term survival in adults [55]. The choice of hemodialysis or peritoneal dialysis in a patient with chronic renal failure is one the physician and the patient should make in concert after analysis of the drawbacks and benefits of each form of treatment in the context of the patient's clinical status. Lifestyle and personality issues are also relevant; hemodialysis is completely performed by nursing and technical staff and peritoneal dialysis requires extensive involvement in the procedure by the patient. Peritoneal dialysis seems to permit a greater degree of growth in children and allows for a less restricted dietary intake; most sources believe it is the best dialysis modality for children and adolescents [56].

Renal transplantation
Renal transplantation is the treatment of choice over hemodialysis and peritoneal dialysis for the majority of patients with end-stage renal failure. The mortality rate is much lower in transplant recipients than in patients treated with chronic dialysis. Patients with chronic renal failure who are less than 70 years of age and free of infection and active malignancy should be considered possible renal transplant recipients. Renal allografts are either donated to a patient with renal failure from a living, healthy family member with normal renal function, or are harvested from brain dead individuals with a compatible blood type and previously normal renal function. Living related kidney transplants have a higher chance of success than cadaveric transplants, but the one year graft survival is greater than 80% in both groups [57]. More than three quarters of the renal transplants performed in the United States involve cadaver donors; because of the shortage of available cadaver kidneys, most patients with renal failure wait two or more years on dialysis before receiving a cadaveric transplant.

Immunosuppression. Donors, whether living related or cadaveric, must be matched with recipients to decrease the risk of transplant rejection. Donors and recipients must have *compatible ABO blood types.* Additionally, the *major histocompatibility antigens* on donor and recipient leukocytes are identified; these are three loci on the sixth chromosome coding for six cell surface antigens which govern immunologic rejection. With greater similarity of donor and recipient major histocompatibility antigens, there is a decreasing risk of transplant rejection. To prevent rejection, all transplant recipients are routinely treated with lifetime immunosuppressive therapy. The specifics of this therapy vary, but generally involve *azathioprine,* *prednisone,* and *cyclosporine.* Azathioprine inhibits purine nucleotide synthesis and has a general myelosuppressive effect. Prednisone has a variety of immunosuppressive and anti-inflammatory effects, including inhibition of both lymphocyte and monocyte migration. Cyclosporine interferes with production of interleukin by T-cells and, thereby, blocks the proliferation of activated T-cells. In addition, many transplant centers prescribe *polyclonal* or *monoclonal antibodies against T-cells,* either at the time of transplantation, or during episodes of acute rejection [58].

Complications. Besides acute or chronic progressive rejection, complications of renal transplantation are generally due to the effects of immunosuppressive therapy. The side effects of long term prednisone therapy are well known to most physicians and include predisposition to infection, osteopenia, glucose intolerance, impaired wound healing, cataracts, and cosmetic effects. The adverse effects of azathioprine are primarily due to bone marrow depression. The most important complication of cyclosporine use is *renal arteriolar disease,* which may acutely or chronically decrease renal perfusion and the GFR and cause hypertension. Cyclosporine may also cause hepatotoxicity, hirsutism, gingival hyperplasia, and peripheral neuropathy. The dose should be titrated according to blood levels; nephrotoxicity and hypertension are linked to high levels [59].

Renal transplant recipients are at higher risk for *infection,* particularly with opportunistic organisms, cytomegalovirus, and hepatitis C. There is also a higher incidence of *malignancies,* especially skin cancers; patients who have received monoclonal antibodies are at particularly high risk for lymphoma [60].

Long-Term Results. Nevertheless, with careful and compulsive medical attention and faithful compliance with immunosuppression, many transplant recipients have a good prognosis and maintain excellent allograft function over years of therapy. Five year graft survival rate is about 70% with cadaveric allografts, and is over 80% with living related donors.

REFERENCES

1. Brenner BM. Nephron adaptation to renal injury or ablation. Am J. Physiology 1985; 249:F324–F37.
2. Toto RD, Mitchell HC, Lee HC et al. Reversible renal insufficiency due to angiotensin converting enzyme inhibitors in hypertensive nephrosclerosis. Ann Intern Med 1991; 115:513–9.
3. Klahr S, Schreiner G and Ichikawa I. The progression of renal disease. N Engl J Med 1988; 318:1657–66.
4. Narins RG and Cortes P. The role of dietary protein restriction in progressive azotemia. N Engl J Med 1994; 330:929–30.
5. Anderson S, Meyer TW, Renneke HG and Brenner BM. Control of glomerular hypertension limits glomerular injury in rats with reduced renal mass. J Clin Invest 1985; 76:612–9.
6. Anderson S, Rennke HG, Garcia DL et al. Short and long term effects of antihypertensive therapy in the diabetic rat. Kidney Int 1989; 36:526–36.
7. Tierney WM, McDonald CJ and Luft FC. Renal disease in hypertensive adults: effect of race and type II diabetes mellitus. Am J Kidney Dis 1989; 13:485–93.
8. Noth RH, Krolewski AS, Kaysen GA et al. Diabetic nephropathy: hemodynamic basis and implications for disease management. Ann Intern Med 1989; 110:795–813.
9. Kasiske BL et al. Effect of antihypertensive therapy on the kidney in patients with diabetes: a meta-regression analysis. Ann Intern Med 1993; 118:129–38.
10. Mogensen CE. Angiotensin converting enzyme inhibitors and diabetic nephropathy. Lancet 1992; 304:327–8.
11. Carrie BJ, Golbetz HV, Michaels AS and Myers BD. Creatinine: an inadequate filtration marker in glomerular diseases. Am J Med 1980; 69:177–82.
12. Mitch WE, Walser GA, Buffington GA and Lemann J Jr. A simple method of estimating progression of chronic renal failure. Lancet 1976; 2:1326–8.
13. Bennett WM, Elzinga LW and Porter GA. Tubulointerstitial disease and toxic nephropathy. In: Brenner BM and Rector FC Jr., editors. The kidney. WB Saunders Co, Philadelphia, 1991:4th ed., 1430–96.
14. Gabow P. Autosomal dominant polycystic kidney disease. N Engl J Med 1993; 329:332–42.

15. Hunsicker LG. Studies of therapy of progressive renal failure in humans. Semin Nephrol 1989; 321:1773–7.

16. Bergstrom J, Alvestrand A, Bucht H and Gutierrez A. Progression of chronic renal failure in man is retarded with more frequent clinical follow-ups and better blood pressure control. Clin Nephrol 1986; 25:1–6.

17. Ruilope LM, Casal MC, Praga M, Alcazar JM et al. Additive antiproteinuric effect of converting enzyme inhibition and a low protein intake. J Am Soc Nephrol. 1992; 3:1307–11.

18. Zeller K, Whittaker E, Sullivan L et al. Effect of restricting dietary protein on the progression of renal failure in patients with insulin-dependent diabetes mellitus. N Engl J Med 1991; 324:78–84.

19. Zeller KR. Low-protein diets in renal disease. Diabetes Care 1991; 14:856–66.

20. Klahr S, Levey AS, Becvk GJ et al. The effects of dietary protein restriction and blood-pressure control on the progression of chronic renal disease. N Engl J. Med 1994; 330:877–84.

21. Locatelli F, Alberti D, Graziani G et al. Prospective, randomised, multicentre trial of effect of protein restriction on progression of chronic renal insufficiency. Lancet 1991; 337:1299–1304.

22. Oldrizzi L, Rugiu C, Valvo et al. Progression of renal failure in patients with renal disease of diverse etiology on a protein-restricted diet. Kidney Int 1985; 27:553–7.

23. Lewis EJ, Hunsicker LG, Bain RP et al. The effect of angiotensin-converting enzyme inhibition of diabetic nephropathy. N Engl J Med. 1993; 329:1456–62.

24. Ravid M, Savin H, Jutrin I et al. Long-term stabilizing effect of angiotensin-converting enzyme inhibition on plasma creatinine and on proteinuria in normotensive type II diabetic patients. Ann Intern Med 1993; 118:577–81.

25. Reichard P, Nilsson BY and Rosenqvist U. The effect of long-term intensified insulin treatment on the development of microvascular complications of diabetes mellitus. N Engl J Med 1993; 329:304–9.

26. Feldt-Rassmussen B, Mathiesen ER, Jensen T et al. Effect of improved metabolic control on loss of kidney function in type I diabetic patients: an update of the Steno studies. Diabetologia 1991; 34:164–70.

27. Diabetes Control and Complications Trial Research Group. The effect of intensive treatment of diabetes on the development and progresion of long-term complications in insulin-dependent diabetes mellitus. N Engl J Med 1993; 329:977–86.

28. Katz AI and Lindheimer MD. Kidney disease and hypertension in pregnancy. In: Massry SG and Glassock RJ, editors. Textbook of nephrology. Williams and Wilkins, Baltimore, 1989: 1003–19.

29. Sibai BM and Fairlie FM. Renal disease in pregnancy. In: Depp R, Eschenbach DA and Sciarra JJ, editors. Gynecology and obstetrics revised edition – 1993. J.B. Lippincott Co. Philadelphia, 1993; 1–16.

30. Joint National Committee on Detection, Evaluation, and Treatment of High Blood Pressure. The fifth report of the Joint National Committee on Detection, Evaluation, and Treatment of High Blood Pressure. Arch Intern Med 1993; 153:154–83.

31. Anderson S, Garcia DL and Brenner BM. Renal and systemic manifestations of glomerular disease. In: Brenner BM and Rector FC Jr, editors. The kidney. WB Saunders Co, Philadelphia, 1991: 1831–70.

32. Massry SG. Divalent ion metabolism and renal osteodystrophy. In: Massry SG and Glassock RJ, editors. Textbook of nephrology. Williams and Wilkins, Baltimore, 1989: 1278–1311.

33. Ott SM, Kaye M, Delmez JA et al. What are the most common errors in the management of renal osteodystrophy? Semin Dialysis. 1989; 2:145–57.

34. Cunningham J. The prevention of secondary hyperparathyroidism. Current Opinion in Nephrology and Hypertension. 1993; 2:552–7.

35. Ghazali A, Hamida FB, Bouzernidj M et al. Management of hyperphosphatemia in patients with renal failure. Current Opinion in Nephrology and Hypertension. 1993; 2:566–79.

36. Rose BD. Diuretics. Kidney Int 1991; 39:336–52.

37. Rane A, Villeneuve JP, Stone WJ et al. Plasma binding and disposition of furosemide in the nephrotic syndrome and in uremia. Clin Pharm Ther 1978; 2:199–207.

38. Wootton FT, Rhodes DF, Lee WM et al., Colonic necrosis with kayexalate-sorbitol enemas after renal transplantation. Ann Intern Med 1990; 111:947–9.

39. Eschbach J. The anemia of chronic renal failure: pathophysiology and the effects of recombinant erythropoietin. Kidney Int 1989; 35:134–48.

40. Lim VS, DeGowin RL, Zavala D et al. Recombinant human erythropoietin in pre-dialysis patients: a double-blind placebo-controlled trial. Ann Intern Med 1989; 110:108–14.

41. Evans R W, Rader B, Manninen DL et al. The quality of life of hemodialysis patients treated with recombinant human erythropoietin. JAMA 1990; 263:825–30.

42. Van Wyck DB. Iron management during recombinant human erythropoietin therapy. Am J Kidney Dis 1989; 14:9–13.

43. Remuzzi G. Bleeding in renal failure. Lancet 1988; i:1205–8.

44. Mannucci PM, Remuzzi G, Pusineri F et al. Deamino-8-D-arginine vasopressin shortens the bleeding time in uremia. N Engl J Med 1983; 308:8–12.

45. Livio M, Mannuci PM, Vigano G et al. Conjugated estrogens for the management of bleeding associated with renal failure. N Engl J Med 1986; 315:731–5.

46. Shemin D, Elnour M, Amarantes B et al. Oral estrogens decrease bleeding time and improve clinical bleeding in patients with renal failure. Am J Med 1990; 89:436–40.

47. Bronner MH, Pate M, Cunningham JT et al. Estrogen-progesterone therapy for bleeding gastrointestinal telangiectasias in chronic renal failure. Ann Intern Med 1986; 105:371–4.

48. Francos G. Uremic pruritis. Semin Dialysis 1988; 1:209–12.

49. Fan P-Y and Schwab SJ. Vascular access: concepts for the 1990s. J Am Soc Nephrol 1992; 3:1–11.

50. Abuelo JG, Shemin D and Chazan JC. Acute symptoms produced by hemodialysis: a review of their causes and associations. Semin Dialysis 1993; 6:59–69.

51. Held PJ, Levin NW, Bovbjerg RR et al. Mortality and duration of hemodialysis treatment. JAMA 1991; 265:871–5.

52. Owen WF, Lew NL, Liu Y et al. The urea reduction ratio and serum albumin concentration as predictors of mortality in patients undergoing hemodialysis. N Engl J Med 1993; 329:1001–6.

53. Nolph KD. Is residual renal function preserved better with CAPD than with hemodialysis? AKF Nephrology Letter 1990; 7:1–4.

54. Nolph KD, Lindblad AS and Novak JW. Continuous ambulatory peritoneal dialysis. N Engl J Med 1988; 318:1595–600.

55. Nelson CB, Port FK, Wolfe RA et al. Comparison of continuous ambulatory peritoneal dialysis and hemodialysis survival with evaluation of trends during the 1980s. J Am Soc Nephrol 1992; 3:1147–55.

56. Stewart CL and Fine RN. Growth in children with renal insufficiency. Semin Dialysis 1993; 6:37–45.

57. Excerpts from the United States Renal Data System: 1993 Annual Report. Am J Kidney Dis 1993: 22: Suppl 2 58–69.

58. Lu CY, Sicher SC and Vazquez MA. Prevention and treatment of renal allograft rejection: new therapeutic approaches and new insights into established therapies. J Am Soc Nephrol 1993; 4:1239–56.

59. Kahan BD. Cyclosporine. N Engl J Med 1989; 321:1725–38.

60. First MR. Long-term complications after transplantation. Am J Kidney Dis 1993; 22:477–86.

18. Treatment of specific causes of renal failure

J. GARY ABUELO, AUGUST ZABBO, DOUGLAS SHEMIN and AARON SPITAL

The general management of patients with renal failure was addressed in the last two chapters. The therapy of the individual conditions that produce renal failure will now be discussed.

PRERENAL CAUSES

J. GARY ABUELO

A certain number of cases of prerenal azotemia are iatrogenic, and can be prevented by *increased awareness of the risk factors* for this condition. One set of risk factors are obviously those that reduce blood pressure and renal perfusion – hypovolemia, fall in systemic vascular resistance and fall in cardiac output due to heart disease. The other set of risk factors are those that impair the kidneys' ability to autoregulate GFR in the face of moderate reductions in perfusion – chronic renal failure, renal artery stenosis, NSAID's and converting enzyme inhibitors (see Chapter 8). Thus, physicians should avoid therapies that increase the risk of prerenal azotemia in susceptible patients. For example, NSAID's ought not be given to hypovolemic patients. Alternatively, if benefits of such therapies outweigh their risk, they may be employed, but Scr should be monitored during their use. Converting enzyme inhibitors are often used in this way in the management of congestive heart failure. In such cases a limited rise in Scr may be acceptable. In the above example, the Scr might rise from 1.0 mg/dL to 1.7 mg/dL (88 μmol/L to 150 μmol/L) as the patient's heart failure comes under control. The benefit from improvement of cardiac function outweighs the detriment of a slight loss of renal function.

One avoidable cause of prerenal azotemia is seen in individuals taking long-term diuretics, usually for hypertension or congestive heart failure. If such patients abruptly reduce their salt intake, the continued use of diuretics can lead to hypovolemia and prerenal azotemia. Common examples of this might be individuals who begin a low sodium diet after seeing a public health announcement or individuals who develop anorexia during intercurrent illnesses. On prescribing diuretics, physicians need to educate their patients about the need to maintain a constant daily salt intake. Patients unable to eat normally should contact their physician for instructions about their diuretic dose.

The treatment of prerenal renal failure centers on correcting the patient's hemodynamic status. This is usually straightforward, and typically involves *intravenous volume repletion*. Four situations require comment.

In sicker patients with multiple problems, the true cause of hypotension may be obscure. For example, the physician may initiate fluid resuscitation in a hypotensive patient with minor fluid loss, when the fall in blood pressure is really due to a painless myocardial infarction or early sepsis. It is necessary in such cases to recognize the possibility of alternative causes for the hypotension, and to insert a central vein catheter. One then may determine cardiac output, systemic vascular resistance and pulmonary capillary wedge pressure, and *make an accurate hemodynamic diagnosis*.

In patients without frank hypotension, volume repletion may take place over several days and use the *oral rather than intravenous route*. An example might be a patient with acute-on-chronic renal failure associated with a fall in blood pressure from 140/85 to 115/60 mmHg due to transient gastrointestinal fluid loss. The methods to raise intravascular volume are discontinuation or dose reduction of diuretics, discontinuation of salt-

J.G. Abuelo (ed.), Renal Failure, 187–229.
© 1995 *Kluwer Academic Publishers.*

restricted diets, and addition of foods with high salt content. These include commercial soups, salted snack foods, and ham, anchovies and other salted meats and fish. One gram salt tablets (17 mEq) may also be used to replete volume. Three tablets three times a day provide the equivalent of a liter of normal saline, the water portion coming from fluids consumed in response to salt-induced thirst. The rate of volume replenishment is best monitored with daily weights. A weight gain of two pounds per day is a reasonable goal in most patients.

In patients who do not recover renal function with repletion of volume, the continued administration of fluid may produce pulmonary edema. The diagnosis of prerenal azotemia is usually wrong in such patients who actually have acute tubular necrosis or another process unresponsive to fluids. Individuals with congestive heart failure are similarly at risk of pulmonary edema, if fluid replacement exceeds the volume deficit. Unfortunately, some physicians address the risk of volume overload by administering fluids too slowly or by using hypotonic solutions such as 0.45% saline. Often the result is inadequate fluid replenishment or hyponatremia, or both. Instead, volume repletion should employ normal saline given at maximum intravenous flow rates until the patient no longer has hypotension or orthostatic changes in pulse and blood pressure. To avoid excessive fluid administration, the patient should be checked frequently for signs of volume overload – orthopnea, edema, distended neck veins, third heart sound and basilar rales. It is helpful to know the patient's usual blood pressure range since 110/60 mmHg might be normal for one individual and 140/85 mmHg for another. When fluid administration produces hypervolemia in a patient with continued oliguria, it usually indicates a cause of renal failure other than prerenal azotemia. The physician should stop fluid administration immediately, and should institute diuretics and fluid restriction in order to restore euvolemia.

In patients with *prerenal azotemia due to severe congestive heart failure*, a trial of *angiotensin converting enzyme inhibitors* may be considered. While the drug's renal vasomotor action may compromise GFR in some cases, in others the converting enzyme inhibitor produces such an increase in cardiac function and renal perfusion that GFR rises despite the adverse vasomotor effect [1, 2].

REFERENCES

1. Packer M, Lee WH, Medina N, Yushak M and Kessler PD. Functional renal insufficiency during long-term therapy with captopril and enalapril in severe chronic heart failure. Ann Intern Med 1987; 106:346–54.
2. Oster JR and Materson BJ. Renal and electrolyte complications of congestive heart failure and effects of therapy with angiotensin-converting enzyme inhibitors. Arch Intern Med 1992; 152:704–10.

POSTRENAL CAUSES

AUGUST ZABBO

Postrenal azotemia results from disruption of the normal egress of urine from the kidneys out of the body. This can occur at any point along the urinary collecting and delivery system and therapy is dictated by the level at which the disruption of urinary flow occurs. Initial treatment always involves drainage of urine proximal to the point of disruption, allowing for stabilization of renal function, and then definitive treatment of the etiology of the obstruction to urinary flow. The causes of postrenal renal failure are listed in Table 9.1.

Postobstructive Diuresis

Upon relief of urinary obstruction, there is normally a brisk diuresis as the kidneys mobilize retained fluid and solutes. Ordinarily when these solutes have reached normal levels, the urine output returns to normal. This is a normal physiologic diuresis.

However in some patients there is a pathologic postobstructive diuresis [1]. The proposed mechanisms for this are:
(1) Impaired urinary concentrating ability.
(2) Impaired tubular sodium reabsorption.
(3) Osmotic diuresis due to retained urea.

In these situations, urine output may be extreme with rates reported up to 69 ml per minute [2]. Untreated the patient could develop major fluid and electrolyte depletion and vascular collapse due to hypovolemia. These patients should be managed with careful monitoring of the daily weight and blood pressure, and orthostatic signs should be taken. If the urine volume exceeds 200 ml per hour and signs of hypovolemia develop, the physician should be notified and *intravenous replacement therapy* instituted usually with 0.45% sodium chloride. In the awake and alert patient, the thirst mechanism will allow for much of the fluid replacement. Monitoring of the urine electrolytes will guide replacement therapy. This pathologic postobstructive diuresis generally resolves over a few days but can last for several weeks.

Bladder Outlet Obstruction

Bladder outlet obstruction is diagnosed when the bladder is distended with urine in the face of some obstructive process involving the urethra anywhere along its course from the prostate to the urethral meatus.

Initial treatment
Initial therapy is to drain the bladder usually by placement of a *urethral Foley catheter*, but if the process obstructing the urethra is impassable, the bladder can be drained by placing a *suprapubic tube* percutaneously. This is safe only when there has not been previous lower abdominal surgery. In the face of previous lower abdominal surgery, there is potential entry into adherent bowel so open surgical suprapubic tube placement may be necessary.

Palliative treatment
In the palliative situation where the patient is unable to undergo corrective surgery for whatever process is causing the urethral obstruction, a chronic indwelling tube may be necessary. In males a *suprapubic tube* is preferable for this purpose, as a chronic indwelling urethral catheter can result in epididymoorchitis and urethral erosion. In females urethral catheters may produce urethral erosion with a vesicovaginal fistula. Since this is more likely to occur when the patient has lost sensation in the perineum, such cases should also be considered for a suprapubic tube. It should be noted that with any chronic indwelling urinary tract tube sterility of the urine cannot be maintained. There will always be colonizing bacteriuria and likely candiduria; generally treatment of urinary tract infections in this setting is only undertaken when there are signs of systemic infection.

When the bladder outlet obstruction is easily passable by a catheter, another option for treatment is *chronic intermittent catheterization* [3].

Either the patient or an attendant catheterizes the patient and drains the bladder four to five times a day, or more often depending on the patient's urinary volume and bladder capacity.

Definitive treatment

Benign Prostatic Hypertrophy. Definitive treatment of bladder outlet obstruction is directed at the underlying etiology. For benign prostatic hypertrophy, transurethral or suprapubic *prostatectomy* is usually successful in relieving the obstruction. However, if the obstruction has been very longstanding and the bladder has been chronically dilated, it may have lost much of its normal capacity to contract and therefore may still be unable to expel urine and thus require intermittent catheterization or a chronic indwelling tube. *Newer methods* of treating benign prostatic hypertrophy such as prostatic hyperthermia, laser therapy to the prostate and indwelling prostatic urethral stents may offer additional options for treatment of this condition. Recently finasteride, a five alpha-reductase inhibitor, has become available for the treatment of benign prostatic hypertrophy [4]. Administration of the drug results in reduction of the size of the prostatic adenoma. Since this may take several months, it is not appropriate for the treatment of acute urinary retention with postrenal renal failure where more immediate relief of the obstruction is desirable.

Prostatic Carcinoma. Prostatic carcinoma can also cause bladder outlet obstruction generally when the disease has advanced to a stage beyond surgical cure. In these patients a so called *"channel" transurethral prostatectomy* can be undertaken, but as the prostatic carcinoma can also infiltrate under the bladder neck and obstruct the distal ureters, this may not be entirely successful in relieving the obstruction to urinary flow. This usually would be noted by failure of the Scr to return to normal with urethral Foley catheter drainage. In these cases treatment for ureteral obstruction (see below) could be employed until therapy of the prostatic carcinoma has become effective. Generally, *hormonal therapy* to lower the patient's serum testosterone level is undertaken in the hopes of causing regression of the tumor.

Other causes of urethral obstruction such as stricture and urethral valves and urethral carcinoma are rare causes of postrenal renal failure, but would be treated in a similar manner of draining the bladder first and then doing surgical repair on an elective basis.

Neurogenic Bladder

The discussion of the treatment of neurogenic bladder is an extensive subject but can be briefly summarized by dividing patients into two types [5]. The first includes patients with chronic retention of urine secondary to the loss of motor or sensory function of the bladder. The bladder is "flaccid" or chronically dilated and the dilation and elevated pressure is transmitted back to the ureters and kidneys resulting in hydronephrosis. The second type of patient has a "spastic" neurogenic bladder, in which there has been disruption of the normal inhibitory nerves that allow the normal bladder to accommodate the filling of urine. Thus, despite small volumes of urine the bladder spastically contracts and causes high pressure within the bladder. This high pressure is transmitted back to the ureters and kidneys.

Flaccid neurogenic bladder
The "flaccid" neurogenic bladder is often seen with lower spinal cord lesions, but chronic urinary retention on this basis can also be caused by anticholinergic drugs or multiple sclerosis. Some patients with diabetes mellitus and tabes dorsalis lose sensation of bladder filling and this results in chronic overfilling of the bladder and a picture similar to the flaccid bladder.

Treatment of these patients is with *initial bladder drainage* and then most patients are best managed with *chronic intermittent catheterization*.

Spastic neurogenic bladder
The "spastic" neurogenic bladder results mostly from upper spinal cord trauma. It may be associated with autonomic dysfunction, in which distention of the bladder and a lack of normal inhibitory reflexes lead to a sympathetic neuron discharge. This results in extreme hypertension, sweating, and nausea, and is relieved by drainage of the bladder. In these patients, the bladder capacity is very limited because of the spasticity of the bladder.

Treatment of this condition can be by *chronic indwelling bladder drainage*. More often in males the urethral sphincter is purposefully cut and then the patient is placed on *condom catheter drainage*. In those patients that have the capacity to do it, *chronic intermittent catheterization* coupled with reduction of spasm of the bladder with anticholinergic medications may be an effective approach. Some patients require expansion of their bladder capacity by augmentation with a segment of small bowel. In the past, urinary diversion to an ileal conduit or other cutaneous diversion was common and still may be done in selected patients.

Ureteral Obstruction

Ureteral obstruction causes postrenal renal failure only if it blocks both ureters or the ureter of a solitary kidney.

Initial treatment
The initial therapy of ureteral obstruction is to drain the kidney; this is most often done with a *percutaneous nephrostomy* [6]. The alternative is an indwelling *ureteral stent which is passed retrograde* from the bladder to the kidney. The former procedure is better tolerated by the critically ill individual; the latter procedure is more convenient for patients, since the stent drains urine into the bladder and a urine collection bag is not needed. The decision between the two therapies is situational and is up to the urologist or other treating physician.

Definitive treatment
The renal function is allowed to stabilize and then definitive treatment of the cause of ureteral obstruction is carried out. Thus, one must define the etiology and prognosis of the obstructing disease process. In those patients who have a retroperitoneal malignancy, it is important to consider the overall outlook before embarking on "palliative" treatment. One should discuss with the patient and the family the prognosis and whether or not they desire continued invasive attempts at palliative treatment. It may also be important in these cases to salvage as much renal function as possible before potentially nephrotoxic chemotherapy. For example, in those patients who will receive cisplatin, bilateral nephrostomy tubes may be placed to preserve maximal renal paren-

chyma. Conversely, in a patient who will not undergo any nephrotoxic chemotherapy, there is probably no need to do percutaneous nephrostomy of both sides as relief of obstruction on one side will relieve the azotemia.

Specific treatment is based on the etiology of the obstruction. In patients with inoperable malignancies, one may try to bypass the ureteral obstruction in an antegrade fashion passing a tube from the kidney to the bladder. A chronic indwelling stent, the so-called *nephroureteral tube*, can be used. This allows the patient to clamp the nephroureteral tube and void through the bladder normally. Chronic indwelling tubes of any sort would need to be changed every four to twelve weeks depending on the nature of the tube, the patient's condition, and his urinary output. Failure to change the tubes periodically results in encrustation and obstruction of the tubes.

If the ureter is obstructed by a benign process, such as retroperitoneal fibrosis, then releasing the ureter from its entrapment is often successful in a procedure known as *ureterolysis*. In this procedure, the ureter is moved into the intraperitoneal space or laterally into the retroperitoneal fat away from the area of obstruction. In those patients with a distal ureteral obstruction, generally the ureter is transected above the level of obstruction and reanastomosed into the bladder.

In patients with obstruction due to stones, management is directed at *removal of the stones*. Some stones such as uric acid are amenable to chemodissolution [7], whereas others will require urologic procedures such as shock wave lithotripsy, percutaneous or ureteroscopic extraction, or possibly open stone surgery.

Recovery of Renal Function after Relief of Obstruction

Recovery of kidney function after relief of obstruction varies with the time and degree of obstruction as well as with other factors such as infection within the kidney, and anatomic configuration of the kidney (intrarenal or extrarenal pelvis). In the dog, studies have shown approximately 50% recovery of function after relief of two weeks of total obstruction. After six weeks of total obstruction in the dog, function is not recoverable [8].

No reliable data are available for recoverablility of renal function in humans after relief of obstruc-

tion. Predicting recovery then is problematic and in doubtful cases the obstruction should be relieved with a maneuver such as a percutaneous nephrostomy and the clinical effect monitored to see if kidney function returns. If there is not significant return of renal function within two to three months, it can be assumed that the kidney will not recover. Renal scans using various agents together with mathematical analysis of cortical zones of interest have been proposed to predict recoverability of function [9]. Certainly if a renal scan shows no cortical perfusion, then there is not likely to be any recoverable renal function.

REFERENCES

1. Vaughan ED, Jr. and Gillenwater JY. Diagnosis, characterization and management of postobstructive diuresis. J Urol 1973; 109:286–92.
2. Eiseman B, Vivion C and Vivian J. Fluid and electrolyte changes following relief of urinary obstruction. J Urol 1955; 74:222–6.
3. Frankel HL. Intermittent catheterization. Urol Clin North Am 1974; 1:115–24.
4. Stoner E and the Finasteride Study Group. The clinical effects of a 5α reductase inhibitor, finasteride, on benign prostatic hyperplasia. J Urol 1992; 147:1298–302.
5. Barrett D and Wein AJ. Voiding dysfunction: diagnosis, classification and management. In: Gillenwater JY, Grayhack JT, Howards ST and Duckett JW, editors. Adult and pediatric urology. Year Book Medical Publishers, 1987; 863–952.
6. Stables DP. Percutaneous nephrostomy: techniques, indications and results. Urol Cl North Am 1982; 9:15–29.
7. Sheldon CA and Smith AD. Chemolysis of calculi. Urol Clin North Am 1982; 9:121–30.
8. Vaughan ED Jr., Shenasky JH II and Gillanwater JY. Mechanism of acute hemodynamic response to ureteral occlusion. Invest Urol 1971; 9:109–12.
9. Kalika V, Bard RH, Iloreta A et al. Prediction of renal functional recovery after relief of upper urinary tract obstruction. J Urol 1981; 126:301–5.

VASCULAR CAUSES

J. GARY ABUELO

Vasomotor Disturbances

Hepatorenal syndrome

Prevention of hepatorenal syndrome would be desirable, but is probably not possible in most patients, in whom the cause is advanced and irreversibly worsening liver disease. In contrast, in cases with stable hepatic failure avoidance of situations that reduce renal perfusion may protect against kidney insufficiency. Thus, NSAIDs should be avoided, infections should be evaluated and treated early, and any gastrointestinal blood and fluid losses should be replaced promptly. Also, treatment of ascites with diuretics and paracentesis is more likely to produce renal failure in the absence of edema [1], and should be approached with caution.

Hepatorenal syndrome is theoretically curable if liver failure resolves. Thus, those patients with hepatorenal syndrome fortunate enough to receive a *liver transplant* experience improvement in renal function [2, 3]. Other specific measures to reverse hepatorenal syndrome are limited. As discussed in Chapter 10 under Vasomotor Disturbances, the clinical picture may suggest prerenal azotemia; this should be excluded by a trial of volume expansion or by hemodynamic measurements through a Swan-Ganz catheter (Figure 10.3). The physician is cautioned against "overinterpretation" of the response to intravenous fluid. Patients with hepatorenal syndrome frequently have a transient and limited increase in urine output and GFR after a trial of volume expansion, but continued fluid administration worsens ascites and peripheral edema and may cause variceal bleeding without significantly improving azotemia [1, 4–6].

> Peritoneovenous shunts, such as the LeVeen shunt, have been used to relieve ascites and improve renal function in the hepatorenal syndrome. While a fall in Scr may follow shunt placement in some cases, the procedure often causes consumption coagulopathy, sepsis or other serious complications and does not prolong average survival [7]. Thus, while they are possibly effective in mobilizing ascites and improving GFR, peritoneovenous shunts are not recommended in the management of hepatorenal syndrome. A variety of vasoactive agents that induce peripheral vasoconstriction or renal vasodilation have been used without success to treat hepatorenal syndrome [5, 8].

Individuals with hepatorenal syndrome often die of another complication of liver disease, before their renal failure reaches the point of requiring dialysis [8, 9]. Occasionally, however, loss of GFR leads to uremic symptoms or other indications for dialysis. In the typical case of end stage alcoholic cirrhosis

with no reversible exacerbating factors dialysis does not reduce morbidity or significantly prolong survival, and in general should not be performed. On the other hand, if reason exists to believe that the liver failure may be reversible, *dialysis* should be used to tide the patient over. Thus with dialytic support, hepatorenal syndrome can improve in patients who recover from acute fulminant liver disease [10] or who receive a liver transplant [1, 2]. Hemodialysis is usually tolerated, but hypotension during the treatment may be a contraindication in some cases. Peritoneal dialysis or continuous arteriovenous hemofiltration may be used in such patients [10].

Prognosis in hepatorenal syndrome has been grim with death due to complications of liver disease occurring in most patients within several weeks [8, 9, 11]. Even with dialytic support, patients with fulminant hepatic failure who survive are unusual [10, 11]. The rare patients with cirrhosis who recover with conservative treatment tend to have milder degrees of liver disease and presumably have healing of alcoholic hepatitis or another reversible component [8, 9, 12]. The situation is more favorable for individuals with liver disease who undergo liver transplantation. Some 70% of patients survive and experience recovery of renal failure [2, 3]. However, alcoholics with cirrhosis are not considered candidates for transplantation at most centers for moralistic and socioeconomic reasons.

Hypercalcemia

Renal failure may have several mechanisms. Initially, the most important factor is a reversible fall in glomerular capillary pressure caused by arteriolar vasoconstriction and hypovolemia secondary to renal salt wasting. After weeks or months, nephrocalcinosis and interstitial fibrosis add irreversible structural elements to the picture.

Reduction of serum calcium levels involves specific treatment of the etiology of hypercalcemia (e.g. surgery for hyperparathyroidism) and nonspecific treatment [13–15]. *Intravenous saline administration* is the most important nonspecific measure, since it will repair the hypovolemia that occurs with renal salt wasting. In addition, volume repletion increases urinary calcium excretion and improves hypercalcemia. Normal saline should be administered intravenously at 3 to 4 liters per day.

Patients need to be observed for fluid overload, which should be treated with a loop diuretic and not a thiazide.

Once hypovolemia has been corrected, *furosemide* may be given 80 to 100 mg every 1 to 2 hours to further increase urinary calcium excretion. However, one must measure serum electrolyte and magnesium concentrations every six hours and sodium, potassium, and magnesium concentrations in four-hour urines so that urine losses may be replaced with intravenous fluids [16]. The additional efficacy of furosemide compared with that of volume expansion alone is modest, and fluid and electrolyte management is so complicated that few patients should receive this therapy.

Another means of removing calcium from the body is *peritoneal or hemodialysis* using a low-calcium dialysate. It is used in patients with severe renal failure and is very effective.

One may also reduce bone resorption of calcium. *Calcitonin* given intramuscularly, 4 to 8 units per kg every 6 to 12 hours, is safe and may lower calcium concentrations within a few hours. However, its effect may be weak and tachyphylaxis is common. Therefore, it is mainly useful in the first day or so of treatment until slower acting measures become effective. Bisphosphonates reduce high serum calcium levels by inhibiting osteoclastic bone resorption. *Pamidronate* is preferred over etidronate and clodronate, which may be nephrotoxic [14]. The excretion and dosage of pamidronate in renal failure has not been well studied. Amounts of 15 to 90 mg given intravenously over 24 hours have been used safely in a few patients with renal failure. The hypocalcemic effect begins within two days, is maximal at four to seven days, and may last from one to several weeks [14, 17–19]. Correction of hypophosphatemia, if it is present, may reduce bone resorption of calcium. Initially 500 mg of *phosphorus* 3 or 4 times a day may be given orally. Hyperphosphatemia may occur rapidly in patients with renal failure, so that serum phosphate levels must be followed daily. Intravenous phosphate replacement may produce metastatic calcification and should be reserved for severe hypophosphatemia. *Plicamycin* (mithramycin) may also be used intravenously to inhibit bone resorption at a dose of 16 µg/kg when GFR is 10 to 50 ml/minute and 12.5 µg/kg when GFR is less than 10 ml/minute. The dose may be repeated the following day if the response is inadequate. The

hypocalcemic effect lasts several days. Renal failure and thrombocytopenia are rare complications, and one must obtain daily platelet counts [13]. Gallium nitrate is an effective drug, but is contraindicated by renal failure [20].

Glucocorticoids reduce excess vitamin D-mediated calcium absorption from the gut, which is the mechanism of hypercalcemia in patients with vitamin D overdose, sarcoid and other granulomatous diseases. These patients may be given intravenous hydrocortisone, 200 to 300 mg per day, or oral prednisone, 60 mg per day, in divided doses. Oral nonabsorbable *cellulose sodium phosphate* can reduce calcium absorption from the gut by binding calcium [21]. *Hydroxychloroquine* or *ketoconazole* may be employed in sarcoidosis to inhibit activation of vitamin D [21].

Sepsis

The most important measure in treating sepsis-induced vasomotor renal failure is the proper diagnosis and treatment of the infection with antibiotics, surgical drainage or both. In addition, the hypotension commonly seen in septic individuals must be evaluated and aggressively treated. For many cases this is best carried out in an intensive care unit, where measurements of pulmonary capillary wedge pressure, cardiac output, and peripheral vascular resistance may be made with a Swan-Ganz catheter, and monitoring may be continued as treatment progresses. A common error in septic patients is to assume that the hypotension is just due to volume depletion. Sepsis may produce hypovolemia through capillary leakage and venous dilatation and some septic patients may have undetected fluid loss. However, more often the main mechanism for low blood pressure is reduced vascular resistance complicated in some cases by an abnormal ventricular function [22]. Thus, in many cases volume expansion does not raise the blood pressure and may be harmful. Instead, the therapy of hypotension should include *vasopressors* to increase vascular resistance, and *inotropic drugs* to increase ventricular performance [23]. The sorting out of the various mechanisms of hypotension usually requires central line measurements.

Research into the cause of the hypotension and renal failure observed with bacterial sepsis suggests a pathogenic role of bacterial endotoxins and the cascade of inflammatory mediators that endotoxins trigger [24, 25]. Intravenous administration of anti-endotoxin antibodies [26] or human immunoglobulin G [27] may block some of these mechanisms. Preliminary evaluations of these agents in septic patients suggest a beneficial effect on survival, but further studies are needed.

The prognosis for patients with vasomotor renal failure due to sepsis is not good. In many patients renal ischemia goes on to produce acute tubular necrosis. Moreover, septic patients are critically ill, often with multiple organ failure, and even with availability of dialysis mortality is about 50% [28–30].

Drugs and contrast media
Prevention of renal failure with these agents involves recognizing the predisposing factors (Table 18.1), and either avoiding the agent in question or using it with frequent monitoring of Scr. *Sulindac* may have a somewhat less adverse renal vasomotor action than other NSAID's [32].

Contrast Media. Various methods have been proposed to prevent contrast-mediated nephrotoxicity in patients at risk. These include avoidance of volume depletion, intravenous administration of normal saline during the procedure [33], mannitol [34, 35], furosemide [35], or nitrendipine [36]. Unfortunately, nephrotoxicity can occur despite these measures, and the studies that support the various recommendations either did not have adequate controls or did not study an adequate number of patients at risk. In fact, one group found that mannitol or furosemide increased contrast nephrotoxicity [37]! However, this adverse effect may be limited to diabetics [38]. Given the mild and self-limited nature of most episodes of contrast media-induced renal failure, it is probably best to await future definitive studies before accepting any of these prophylactic protocols. It is prudent, however, to replete the fluid deficit in hypovolemic patients before carrying out the procedure. Also, nonionic low-osmolarity contrast media have less nephrotoxicity than conventional media, and, despite their high cost, should be used in patients at particularly high risk (Scr > 4.0 mg/dL or 354 μmol/L) [39–41].

Table 18.1. (See Chapter 10) Factors predisposing to production of vasomotor renal failure by drugs and contrast media

NSAID	Cyclosporine A
↓ Effective volume	NSAID
Hepatorenal	
syndrome	ACE inhibitor
Cyclosporine A	*Contrast media* [31]
Chronic renal failure	Chronic renal failure
ACE inhibitor	Diabetes mellitus
↓ Effective volume	Less certain
Renal artery stenosis	Dehydration
Cyclosporine A	Large contrast loads
Chronic renal failure	Low cardiac output
Nifedipine (rare)	Repeated contrast exposure
Chronic renal failure	Old age
	Prior contrast nephrotoxicity

Discontinuation of the responsible medication is the usual treatment of vasomotor-type renal failure. However, patients with severe heart failure may have a worsening of cardiac function after stopping an ACE inhibitor. Therefore, it may be preferable in such cases to try to improve GFR through measures which increase ventricular filling: oral or intravenous administration of sodium chloride and dosage reduction or temporary discontinuation of diuretics [41a].

The prognosis for recovery of renal function in patients with vasomotor renal failure caused by drugs or contrast media is good. A fall in Scr begins within a day or two of stopping the drug and is usually complete in a week or two. With contrast media-induced nephrotoxicity, the Scr usually peaks 2 to 5 days after the procedure, and recovery is complete by two weeks (see Chapter 10). Contrast media-induced renal impairment severe enough to require dialysis is uncommon, and is seen mainly in patients with advanced underlying chronic renal failure. While recovery is the rule, chronic dialysis may be necessary in some individuals with low GFR to begin with [31].

Small Vessel Involvement

Atheroembolic disease
Prevention of renal failure caused by cholesterol emboli is theoretically possible by avoiding arterial manipulation in susceptible patients. Unfortunately, the individuals most at risk for atheroemboli are usually those most in need of cardiac

catheterization, arteriography or vascular surgery. Therefore, the benefits of the procedure being considered usually outweigh the risk of precipitating this form of renal failure.

There is little specific therapy available for patients with atheroembolic disease. Any anticoagulation should be stopped, if possible, and one should discourage efforts of other physicians to use anticoagulation to prevent further embolization [42]. The embolized cholesterol crystals may stimulate an inflammatory cascade. Therefore, one group has used colchicine to reduce pain in the ischemic feet and toes, and other workers have given corticosteroids to patients, a few of whom had a beneficial response of extrarenal manifestations [43–46]. However, it is premature to recommend using these anti-inflammatory agents, given the paucity of published information. One group mentions axillobifemoral bypass with iliac ligation in order to stop recurrent painful atheroemboli to the feet [46]. Other authors discourage unnecessary vascular surgical procedures in these patients [44].

The prognosis in atheroembolic disease is poor. The mortality over the ensuing months is 70 to 80% with death resulting from a variety of causes, including myocardial infarction, other atherosclerotic complications and infections [44, 47]. Renal failure usually progresses in stepwise progression and patients often become dialysis dependent, if they live long enough [44, 48, 49]. Nevertheless, some patients may experience substantial recovery of renal function even after months on dialysis [48–50].

Scleroderma

The treatment of scleroderma renal crisis is *ACE inhibitors*. Captopril has been used most commonly, but enalapril has also been effective [51]. Daily doses of captopril as high as 150 mg may be used to control hypertension. Other antihypertensive agents, such as nifedipine or minoxidil, may be added, if needed, for control of blood pressure.

A further rise in Scr following a dose increase of the ACE inhibitor would suggest an adverse effect on renal hemodynamics. If this happens, one should go back to the lower dose and add another blood pressure medication.

ACE inhibitors improved renal function in 56% of cases with scleroderma renal crisis in one recent study; even among those patients needing dialysis, after treatment with ACE inhibitors 35% of individuals were able to come off dialysis [51]. On the other hand, 22% of patients died and 16% developed end stage renal disease. Hemodialysis, chronic peritoneal dialysis and renal transplantation all have been used in this situation, but morbidity and mortality are generally high because of complications of scleroderma [52].

Malignant hypertension [53, 54]

Hospitalization and prompt reduction of blood pressure is the treatment of malignant hypertension. However, abrupt lowering of blood pressure into the normal range with antihypertensive drugs may produce a stroke, myocardial ischemia or a marked fall in GFR. Therefore, blood pressure should only be lowered to about 150/100–110 mmHg, and mean blood pressure should not fall by more than 25%.

Cases with acute target organ damage limited to the kidneys and retina are *hypertensive urgencies*. They can usually be managed with oral administration of drugs, such as *nifedipine*, *clonidine* or *minoxidil* (Table 18.2). *Captopril* is indicated in hypertensive crises associated with scleroderma, but because of possible adverse renal vasomotor actions should probably be avoided in other patients with malignant hypertension and azotemia. A β-blocker may be needed to prevent the tachycardia often seen with minoxidil. Addition of a *loop diuretic* may help optimize blood pressure control.

Also, renal failure and certain antihypertensive drugs, especially minoxidil, both tend to cause accumulation of salt and water. Since this may impede blood pressure control, daily weights should be obtained and any fluid retention should be treated with diuretics.

Cases with malignant hypertension complicated by hypertensive encephalopathy, pulmonary edema, acute aortic dissection, unstable angina, eclampsia or severe adrenergic crises are *hypertensive emergencies*. They should be managed with parenteral administration of drugs. Although other agents have some advantages in special circumstances, *sodium nitroprusside* is the drug of choice in most cases (Table 18.3). Because of its short time of onset and duration, it must be given with an infusion pump, and blood pressure must be followed

Table 18.2. Drugs for oral treatment of hypertensive urgencies

Drug	Initial		Usual daily		Maximum
	Dose (mg)	Frequency	Dose (mg)	Frequency	Dose (mg/day)
Nifedipine	10	Repeat in 1/2 h	30–60	3–4	160
Minoxidil*	2.5 to 10	Every 4 to 6 h	10–40	1–2	100
Clonidine hydrochloride	0.2	0.1 mg per hr (0.8 mg total)	0.2–0.8	2	2.4
Captopril	6.25–25	Repeat every 1/2 h	25–150	2–3	450

* Usually given with a loop diuretic and a β-blocker.

Table 18.3. Drugs for parenteral treatment of hypertensive emergencies

Drug	Indication	IV dose
Sodium nitroprusside	Hypertensive encephalopathy, pulmonary edema, cerebrovascular accident	0.3–10 μg/kg/min
Nitroglycerine	Unstable angina*, myocardial infarction*, post coronary bypass*	5–100 μg/min
Hydralazine hydrochloride	Eclampsia	5–20 mg (or 10–40 mg IM), give as needed every 20 min
Trimethaphan camsylate	Dissecting aneurysm*	0.5–5 mg/min[†]
Phentolamine mesylate	Pheochromocytoma*, clonidine withdrawal*, cocaine use*	0.5–5 mg/min

* Nitroprusside + beta blocker can also be used.
[†] Target systolic blood pressure is 100–120 mmHg.

with a continually reinflated sphygmomanometer or preferably, an intra-arterial line.

> Frank overdosage of nitroprusside may produce *cyanide toxicity*, manifested by hypotension, metabolic acidosis, changes in mental status, bright red venous blood and pink skin color. If this occurs, a cyanide level should be obtained. Without awaiting the results the nitroprusside should be discontinued, sodium nitrite 4 to 6 mg/kg should be injected over 2 to 4 minutes to be followed by sodium thiosulfate, 150–200 mg/kg (typically 12.5 Gm) over 15 to 20 minutes.
>
> High dosage of nitroprusside for over 48 hours in patients with renal failure may produce *thiocyanate toxicity*, which is manifested by nausea, vomiting, headache and changes in mental status. Plasma thiocyanate levels should be obtained periodically in patients receiving high doses of nitroprusside, especially if GFR is reduced. If toxicity develops, the nitroprusside infusion should be stopped; thiocyanate may be removed with dialysis.

If pulmonary edema is present, a loop diuretic should be used. To reduce the duration of parenteral antihypertensives, oral therapy should be started as soon as practicable. As the blood pressure responds to increasing doses of oral medications, the parenteral therapy may be tapered and stopped. The addition of oral minoxidil, may facilitate control of blood pressure in those rare patients refractory to parenteral drugs.

Most patients with malignant hypertension respond to antihypertensive treatment with a fall in blood pressure, healing of fibrinoid necrosis, and a resolution of neurologic and cardiac symptoms. Nevertheless, 10 to 20% of patients die during the first year of strokes, myocardial infarctions, hypertensive encephalopathy, and conditions unrelated to the hypertension such as infections or cancer [55–58]. After the blood pressure is controlled, a small number of patients ($\sim$10%) will experience a prompt improvement in renal failure. A greater number of patients ($\sim$30%) will have a progressive worsening in renal function; while a majority of patients ($\sim$60%) will experience a transient deterioration lasting a week or two and then an improvement in renal function (Figure 18.1) 55–57, 59]. However, with the passage of weeks

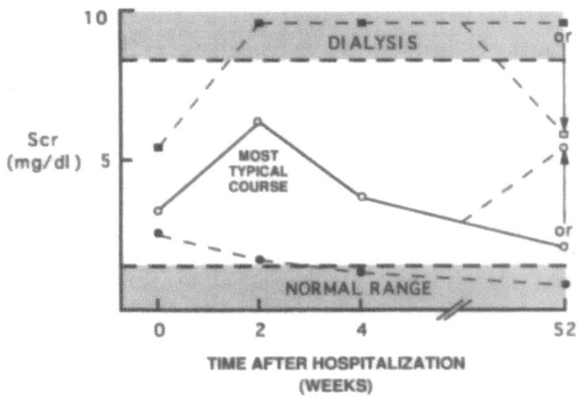

Fig. 18.1. Schematic representation of time course of renal function in different patients with malignant hypertension.

Table 18.4. Complications of hemolytic uremic syndrome and nonspecific treatment measures

Complication	Treatment
Bleeding due to thrombocytopenia	Platelet transfusion*
Anemia due to hemolysis & bleeding	Red cell transfusion
Seizures due to neurologic involvement	Anticonvulsants
Ischemic bowel lesions	Abdominal surgery
GI fluid losses	Fluid and electrolyte therapy
Malnutrition due to coma or GI disease	Enteral or parenteral nutrition
Hypertension	Antihypertensive drugs
Renal failure	Dietary restrictions & dialysis

* May exacerbate disease.

and months some patients whose GFR was improving will have permanent loss of renal function, and other patients on chronic hemodialysis will regain enough renal function to discontinue dialysis [55, 60, 61].

Hemolytic uremic syndrome
Classical childhood post-diarrheal hemolytic uremic syndrome is usually caused by toxin-producing enteric bacteria. It may occur in epidemics, spread either by consumption of contaminated undercooked ground beef or by person-to-person contact in institutions like day care centers and in families [62–64]. Many of these cases could be prevented by adequate cooking of beef products and by handwashing and other infection control measures. In contrast, the treatment of bacterial colitis with antibiotics or antidiarrheal medication may increase the risk of hemolytic-uremic syndrome without improving the colitis [62, 63].

The treatment of patients with hemolytic uremic syndrome often involves nonspecific measures to manage the various complications of the disease (Table 18.4).

Antiplatelet agents, plasma exchange, intravenous IgG and a number of other specific measures have been used to reverse the disease process in hemolytic uremic syndrome. However, in classical childhood post-diarrheal hemolytic uremic syndrome, these therapies are of no proven benefit and are not recommended [65]. On the other hand, *plasma exchange* is now the treatment of

choice for adult and non-classic childhood hemolytic uremic syndrome. While protocols vary, a typical plasma exchange involves the removal and replacement of 1 to 1.5 volumes of plasma (50 to 75 ml/kg of body weight) with fresh frozen plasma. Continuous-flow centrifuge machines are most commonly used, but intermittent-flow centrifuge machines and membrane plasma separation have also been used successfully. Initially, plasma exchanges are performed daily, but exchanges are performed less often and are discontinued as the disease process abates, as judged by correction of platelet counts and serum lactic dehydrogenase levels. If a relapse occurs after plasma exchanges are stopped, treatments should be reinstituted. The number of exchanges to treat a patient averages about 10, but may range from 2 to over 30 [66–69]. In addition to plasma exchange, most patients receive *dipyridamole* (~300 mg/day), *aspirin* (325 mg/day), and *prednisone* (60–200 mg/day) [66, 67, 69]. Some patients also receive *plasma infusions* (~15 ml/kg body weight) on days that they do not have plasma exchanges. Patients unresponsive to this treatment may become responsive to plasma exchange following vincristine (1–2 mg once or twice a week) or splenectomy [66, 69, 70]. *Protein A immunoadsorption* of plasma has been described as a treatment of mitomycin-C-associated disease [71].

Partial or complete recovery is the rule in children with typical hemolytic uremic syndrome; less than 10% develop end stage renal disease or die of complications [65, 71a, 72]. Most adult patients, including some that require dialysis, respond to plasma exchange with partial or complete recovery of renal function [66, 67, 69]. However, only about 30% of cases of mitomycin-C-associated disease appear to resolve with plasma exchange [73, 74]. In this mitomycin-C variant, 45% response rate was described with protein A immunoadsorption, but renal failure stabilized rather than improved [71]. Spontaneous recovery may be observed in adults with diarrhea-associated illness [75], but rarely with other types [75a–77]. A certain number of adults develop end stage renal disease, and a few succumb to complications of the disease (e.g. hemorrhage) or of the treatment (e.g. sepsis due to corticosteroids) [66]. Some patients (13–73%) with end stage renal disease caused by hemolytic uremic syndrome have been observed to experience recurrent hemolytic uremic syndrome in a renal transplant [78–80].

Thrombotic thrombocytopenic purpura

The standard treatment of thrombotic thrombocytopenic purpura is the same as that outlined above for hemolytic uremic syndrome. *Plasma exchange therapy* is almost always accompanied by adjunctive *corticosteroids* and/or *dipyridamole* and *aspirin*. Plasma infusions are sometimes given in between plasma exchanges. *Vincristine* or *splenectomy* should be considered in the occasional cases resistant to this combined therapy; they may produce remission or make patients responsive to plasma exchange [66, 69, 81, 82]. *Intravenous immunoglobulin G* (1 g/kg infused over 4 hours) has been reported to be effective in refractory patients [83, 84]. Favorable responses have also been seen with cyclosporine in one case [85], and high dose intravenous methylprednisolone in two cases [86]. These therapies are unproven and should only be tried in patients who fail standard treatment. Patients with thrombotic thrombocytopenic purpura are best managed in conjunction with a hematologist.

The prognosis with this regimen has improved mortality from the 95% rate before 1970 and the 50% rate between 1970 and 1980 [87, 88]. Currently, response rate and overall survival are about 80% [66, 81, 82, 87]. Anywhere from 2 to over 30 plasma exchanges (average about 12) may be required to obtain a remission [66, 81, 82, 89], and anywhere from one to thirteen days of treatment (average 5

days) may be needed to see an increase in platelet count. Neurological improvement often begins after two days, and a 50% decrease in lactic dehydrogenase after three days of treatment [66]. Recovery of renal function usually is obtained in one to five weeks after initiating treatment [66, 89, 90]. Permanent neurological deficits or seizure disorders may occur despite hematologic resolution [66]. Death usually is caused by cerebral involvement and is preceded by seizures and coma [91].

About 30% of patients have anywhere from one to six relapses, which can usually be managed successfully with plasma exchange; splenectomy may induce a long remission in frequently relapsing patients [81].

Acute cortical necrosis

Acute cortical necrosis has become an unusual cause of renal failure in the developed world and obstetric cases are now quite rare [92]. The major factors responsible for prevention of this condition are undoubtedly more prompt and effective repletion of blood and fluid losses, better management of infections, increased proportion of hospital births, better prenatal care and the marked decrease in illegal abortions [92, 93].

There is no specific treatment for acute cortical necrosis. Patients with acute cortical necrosis are often critically ill and many die early on of sepsis and other complications. Of those cases surviving, about 25% require chronic hemodialysis. Other patients experience partial improvement of renal function for up to a year; some patients requiring dialysis may be able to come off even after months of oliguria [93–95].

Large Vessel Involvement

Renal artery stenosis

The treatment of renal artery stenosis is correction by percutaneous transluminal angioplasty or surgery. However, before deciding that a given patient should undergo one of these procedures, one must consider the factors that increase the risk of complications and those that militate against a subsequent improvement in GFR.

The risk of angioplasty or surgery rises with the overall debility of the patient from a nutritional, cardiac or other standpoint. Cholesterol emboli and other complications are more common when angioplasty is carried out via aortas with widespread endophytic atheromatosis or with large aneurysms [96]. Surgical mortality is greater in operations on badly diseased aortas [97], in combined repairs of renal arteries and the aorta [98–100], and in patients with left ventricular hypertrophy and extrarenal atherosclerotic disease [101].

Certain circumstances reduce the chance that correction of the stenosis will improve renal function. An initial Scr of greater than 3 mg/dl (265 μmol/L) or the need for dialysis forecasts a lower success rate of both surgery and angioplasty; only 30% or less of such patients have a fall in Scr [96, 98, 102, 103]. An improvement of Scr is even less likely in such patients, if they have a stenotic renal artery on one side and a *normal renal artery* on the other [96, 101, 104]. In these cases the marked azotemia indicates that neither the ischemic kidney nor the well perfused kidney are functioning well, and that probably both sides have nephrosclerosis or some other irreversible intrinsic process. With angioplasty a higher technical failure rate is seen with total renal artery occlusions or with osteal lesions* [105], although some workers have had good success in these situations [96, 103]. Another drawback in the use of angioplasty is that restenosis occurs in up to 50% of patients within one year of the procedure [106, 107]. This compares to a less than 15% occurrence of restenosis or thrombosis following vascular surgery [97, 100].

The proportion of cases experiencing a fall in Scr is about 40% after angioplasty, and somewhat higher (37 to 77%) following surgery (Table 18.5). Presumably, favorable outcomes are precluded in many cases by nephrosclerosis, ischemic atrophy, cholesterol emboli, or other parenchymal disease. In addition, inability to dilate the stenosis and traumatic renal artery occlusions are responsible for some of the failures with angioplasty [96, 102, 103], while thrombosed grafts and anastomoses adversely affect the results with vascular surgery [98, 100, 109].

The lower success rate of angioplasty (compared to surgery) is probably balanced by a lower morbidity and mortality. Surprisingly, recent series show that serious complications after angioplasty (e.g. renal artery perforation, cholesterol emboli) occur almost as often as they do after surgery (Table 18.5). This is possibly due to the selection of lower risk cases for vascular surgery than for angioplasty.

With the modest rate of success in improving Scr and the significant level of risk, the decision to recommend angioplasty or vascular surgery for renal failure caused by renal artery stenosis is often not a simple one. Given the number of factors affecting outlook, each case must be considered individually.

Patients who are at the highest risk for complications are best not subjected to a corrective procedure, even if they will need dialysis. In cases with advanced azotemia (Scr greater than 3.5 mg/dl or 309 μmol/L), the frequent lack of success in improving Scr militates against doing angioplasty or surgical reconstruction in all but the lowest risk candidates. Individuals with mild and stable

Table 18.5. Correction of renal artery stenosis: benefits and risks of surgery and angioplasty in recent series

	Total patients	Percent of patients with			Reference
		Improved Scr	Major complications	Fatal outcome	
Surgery	46	58	15	0	108
	17	76	24	12	109
	43	37	12	7	98
	17	77	29	0	110
Combined results	*123*	*56*	*18*	*4*	
Angioplasty	19	16	25	8	108
	79	43	8	1	96
	17	41	12	6	103
	60	40	15	0	102
Combined results	*175*	*40*	*13*	*4*	

azotemia (Scr less than 2 to 2.5 mg/dl or 177 to 221 μmol/L) and controlled hypertension can be corrected right away or, alternatively, may be observed under medical management. Several of these individuals will die early on of extrarenal atherosclerotic disease, since the mortality rate is about 10% per year in this population [100, 107]. At the same time many, perhaps the majority, will not experience a rise in Scr for several years [111]. The best candidates for a corrective procedure are those with low risk and a Scr between 2.0 and 3.5 mg/dl (177 and 309 μmol/L). *Angioplasty* is the preferred procedure unless the patient has a severely diseased aorta, in which case *a surgical approach* that avoids the aorta might be considered. With an osteal lesion or a complete renal artery occlusion, surgery may be performed either initially or in the case that angioplasty fails. It has been recommended that surgical candidates have screening for and correction of coronary or cerebrovascular disease before undergoing renovascular repair [97]. In addition, aortorenal bypass should be avoided when the aortic wall is markedly irregular; other revascularization techniques such as splenorenal bypass may be used [97].

Renal infarction

The most important measure we have to prevent renal infarction is the prevention of emboli in patients with atrial fibrillation using prophylactic heparin or warfarin. In addition, even in the absence of atrial fibrillation, patients with renal or other emboli from the heart, occurring for example after a myocardial infarction, should also be anticoagulated to prevent further emboli.

> Surgical embolectomy, systemic or intra-arterial thrombolytic agents, and percutaneous transcatheter aspiration of the clot may reestablish blood flow after renal embolization. However, these modalities do not prevent renal infarction. Irreversible renal infarction occurs within a few hours of *complete* arterial obstruction and is a *fait accompli* when the patient first presents. Consequently, the affected kidney fails to function and atrophies despite return of renal blood flow [112, 113]. Moreover, surgical embolectomy increases mortality compared to more conservative approaches [112, 114].
>
> The few reports of successful prevention of infarction after complete arterial occlusion by procedures that promptly reestablish renal blood flow do not stand up to scrutiny. In some cases the "rescued" kidney recovered some function on intravenous pyelography or radionuclide scan, but a reduced GFR or renal size revealed serious permanent damage [115–117]. In other cases the embolus did not completely occlude the renal artery, which together with collateral vessels provided enough flow to prevent infarction and to keep the kidney tissue viable [112]. In contrast to renal artery emboli, preservation of critical blood flow often does occur with renal artery *thrombosis*, because there has been progressive renal artery stenosis with development of collateral blood supply over months or years before the actual thrombosis occurs [113, 118].

Arteriography should be performed in cases suspected of renal infarction, if not contraindicated by the patient's condition. Ideally, arteriography will confirm the renal artery occlusion, show any preservation of blood flow from partial obstruction or collaterals, and will indicate the etiology (embolism, thrombosis, dissection). Patients with complete arterial obstruction due to an embolus should be *anticoagulated*; tissue infarction in the affected kidney has already occurred and function will not recover. There appears to be no reason to use surgery, intraarterial thrombolytics or transluminal clot aspiration in this situation [113]. Patients with partially obstructing emboli should also be anticoagulated; the emboli will be reabsorbed [114] and renal function will probably be preserved [112]. Intraarterial thrombolytics have produced similar results in these cases. However, they cannot be recommended because of the absence of data on their risks and benefits compared with those of anticoagulation. Patients with an acute thrombosis complicating renal artery stenosis and with evidence for collateral blood supply should be managed as if they have renal artery stenosis as outlined in the previous section [118].

Renal Vein Thrombosis. Prophylactic oral anticoagulation can probably prevent renal vein thrombosis in nephrotic patients. However, it is not clear that the benefits of this therapy are greater than the risks from iatrogenic bleeding. A recent decision analysis concluded that the benefits do outweigh the risks [119], but, in the absence of a controlled study of such prophylactic anticoagulation, it is not generally recommended unless the patient has already had a vascular thrombosis or pulmonary embolism [120, 121].

In an adult, an acute renal vein thrombosis is more likely to cause renal failure by reducing blood flow rather than by frank infarction, and should be treated with *thrombolytic therapy*. If successful, a rapid fall in Scr will be seen, and anticoagulation should be maintained with heparin and then warfarin for six months. The warfarin may be stopped before this, if the proteinuria improves and the serum albumin concentration rises above 3 g/dl (30 g/L). Such an improvement in serum albumin will end the hypercoagulable state.

Thrombolysis may be achieved in different ways. Several of the cases described in the literature were treated systemically with *intravenous streptokinase* (250,000 IU bolus followed by 100,000 IU per hour for 72 hours) [122–124]. Another case responded successfully to *intravenous urokinase* (300,000 IU over 20 minutes. followed by 150,000 IU per hour for 12 hours) [125]. Still another patient who was anuric recovered a normal Scr with *intraarterial urokinase* at 120,000 IU per hour for 17 hours, reduced to 50,000 IU per hour for 24 hours when bleeding occurred [126]. Tissue plasminogen activator would probably also be effective, but has not been reported. Each of these techniques has theoretical advantages and disadvantages. A comparative study has not been done. These thrombolytic agents are contraindicated by active bleeding, recent surgery or trauma, intracranial lesions and history of a cerebrovascular accident. The risk of bleeding with thrombolytic therapy may also be increased in patients with renal vein thrombosis. In one study, three of seven such patients so treated died of bleeding complications [127].

NOTES

* These are caused *by aortic* plaques rather than by *renal artery* atherosclerosis.

REFERENCES

1. Rodes J, Bosch J and Arroyo V. Clinical types and drug therapy of renal impairment in cirrhosis. Postgraduate Med J 1975; 51:492–7.
2. Gonwa TA, Morris CA, Goldstein RM. Husberg BS and Klintmalm GB. Long-term survival and renal function following liver transplantation in patients with and without hepatorenal syndrome-experience in 300 patients. Transplantation 1991; 51:430.
3. Seu P, Wilkinson AH, Shaked A and Busuttil RW. The hepatorenal syndrome in liver transplant recipients. Am J Surg 1991; 57:806–9.
4. Vaamonde CA. Selected renal and electrolyte abnormalities in liver disease. AKF Nephrology Letter 1992; 9:13–28.
5. Gentilini P and Laffi G. Renal functional impairment and sodium retention in liver cirrhosis. Digestion 1989; 43:1–32.
6. Cade R, Wagemaker H, Vogen S, Mars D, Hood-Lewis D, Privette M et al. Hepatorenal syndrome. Am J Med 1987; 82:427–38.
7. Epstein M. Role of the peritoneovenous shunt in the management of ascites and the hepatorenal syndrome. In: Epstein M, editor. The kidney in liver disease. Williams and Wilkins, Baltimore, 1988:3rd ed., 593–612.
8. Levenson DJ, Skorecki KL, Newell GC and Narins RG. Acute renal failure associated with hepatobiliary disease. In: Brenner BM and Lazarus JM, editors. Acute renal failure. Churchill Livingstone, New York, 1988; 535–80.
9. Epstein RG. Hepatorenal syndrome. In: Epstein M, editor. The kidney in liver disease. Williams and Wilkins, Baltimore, 1988:3rd ed., 89–118.
10. Perez GO, Epstein M and Oster JR. Role of dialysis and ultrafiltration in the treatment of the renal complications of liver disease. In: Epstein M, editor. The kidney in liver disease. Williams and Wilkins, Baltimore, 1988:3rd ed., 613–24.
11. Ring-Larsen H and Palazzo U. Renal failure in fulminant hepatic failure and terminal cirrhosis: a comparison between incidence, types, and prognosis. Gut 1981; 22:585–91.
12. Baldus WP, Feichter RN and Summerskill WHJ. The kidney in cirrhosis. I. Clinical and biochemical features of azotemia in hepatic failure. Ann Intern Med 1964; 60:353–65.
13. Burns Schaiff RA, Hall TG and Bar RS. Medical treatment of hypercalcemia. Clin Pharm 1989; 8:108–21.
14. Bilezikian JP. Management of acute hypercalcemia. N Engl J Med 1992; 3261196–1203.
15. Attie MF. Treatment of hypercalcemia. Endocrinol and Metab Clin N Amer 1989; 18:807–28.
16. Suki WN, Yium JJ, Von Minden M, Saller-Hebert C, Eknoyan G and Martinez-Maldonado M. Acute treatment of hypercalcemia with furosemide. N Engl J Med 1970; 283; 836–40.
17. Yap AS, Hockings GI, Fleming SJ and Khafagi FA. Use of aminohydroxypropylidene bisphosphonate (AHPrBP, "APD") for the treatment of hypercalcemia in patients with renal impairment. Clin Nephrol 1990; 34:225–9.
18. Nussbaum SR, Younger J, VandePol CJ, Gagel RF, Zubler MA, Chapman R et al. Single-dose intravenous therapy with pamidronate for the treatment of hypercalcemia of malignancy: comparison of 30–60-, and 90-mg dosages. Am J Med 1992; 95:297–304.
19. Pamidronate. The Medical Letter 1992; 34:1.
20. Todd PA and Fitton A. Gallium nitrate: a review of its pharmacological properties and therapeutic potential in cancer related hypercalcaemia. Drugs 1991; 42:261–73.
21. Casella FJ and Allon M. The kidney in sarcoidosis. J Amer Soc Nephrol 1993; 3:1555–62.
22. Parrillo JE, Parker MM, Natanson C, Suffredini AF, Danner RL, Cunnion RE et al. Septic shock in humans. Ann Intern Med 1990; 113:227–42.

23. Parrillo JE. Pathogenetic mechanisms of septic shock. N Engl J Med 1993; 328; 1471–6.

24. Zager RA. Endotoxemia, renal hypoperfusion, and fever: interactive risk factors for aminoglycoside and sepsis-associated acute renal failure. Am J Kidney Dis 1992; 20:223–30.

25. Badr KF, Kelley VE, Rennke HG and Brenner BM. Roles for thromboxane A$_2$ and leukotrienes in endotoxin-induced acute renal failure. Kidney Int 1986; 30:474–80.

26. Wolff SM. Monoclonal antibodies and the treatment of gram-negative bacteremia and shock. NEJM 1991; 324:486–8.

27. Keane WF, Hirata-Dulas CAI, Bullock ML, Ney AL, Guay DRP, Kalil RSN et al. Adjunctive therapy with intravenous human immunoglobulin G improves survival of patients with acute renal failure. J Am Soc Nephrol 1991; 2:841–7.

28. Frost L, Pedersen RS and Hansen HE. Prognosis in septicemia complicated by acute renal failure requiring dialysis. Scand J Urol Nephrol 1991; 25:307–10.

29. Van der Merwe WM and Collins JF. Acute renal failure in a critical care unit. N Z Med J 1989; 102:96–8.

30. Rayner BL, Willcox PA and Pascoe MD. Acute renal failure in community-acquired bacteraemia. Nephron 1990; 54:32–5.

31. Berns AS. Nephrotoxicity of contrast media. Kidney Int 1989; 36:730–40.

32. Murray MD and Brater DC. Renal toxicity of the nonsteroidal anti-inflammatory drugs. Annu Rev Pharmacol Toxicol 1993; 32:435–65.

33. Eisenberg RL, Bank WO and Hedgock MW. Renal failure after major angiography can be avoided with hydration. AJR 1981; 136:859–61.

34. Old CW, Duarte CM, Lehrner LM, Henry AR and Sinnott RC. A prospective evaluation of mannitol in the prevention of radiocontrast acute renal failure. Clin Res 1981; 29:472.

35. Porush JG, Chou S-Y, Anto HR, Oguagha C, Shapiro WB and Faubert PF. Infusion intravenous pyelography and renal function: effects of hypertonic mannitol and furosemide in patients with chronic renal insufficiency. In: Eliahou HE editor. Acute renal failure. John Libbey & Co., London, 161–7.

36. Neumayer HH, Junge JW, Kufner A and Wenning A. Prevention of radiocontrast-media-induced nephrotoxicity by the calcium channel blocker nitrendipine: a prospective randomised clinical trial. Nephrol Dial Transplant 1989; 4:1030–6.

37. Solomon R, D'Elia J and Mann D. Prevention of contrast induced acute renal failure (CIARF) in a high risk group. J Am Soc Nephrol 1992; 3:730.

38. Weisberg LS, Kurnik PB and Kurnik BRC. Risk of radiocontrast nephropathy in patients with and without diabetes mellitus. Kidney Int 1994; 45:259–65.

39. Katholi RE, Taylor GJ, Woods WT, Womack KA, Katholi CR, McCann WP et al. Nephrotoxicity of nonionic low-osmolality versus ionic high-osmolality contrast media: a prospective double-blind randomized comparison in human beings. Radiology 1993; 186:183–7.

40. Lautin EM, Freeman NJ, Schoenfeld AH, Bakal CW, Haramiti N, Friedman AC et al. Radiocontrast-associated renal dysfunction: a comparison of lower-osmolality and conventional high-osmolality contrast media. AJR 1991; 157:59–65.

41. Barrett BJ and Carlisle EJ. Metaanalysis of the relative nephrotoxicity of high- and low-osmolality iodinated contrast media. Radiology 1993; 188:171–8.

41a. Oster JR and Materson BJ. Renal and electrolyte complications of congestive heart failure and effects of therapy with angiotensin-converting enzyme inhibitors. Arch Intern Med 1992; 152:704–10.

42. Hyman BT, Landas SK, Ashman RF, Schelper RL and Robinson RA. Warfarin-related purple toes syndrome and cholesterol microembolization. Am J Med 1987; 82:1233–7.

43. Cosserat J, Bletry O, Frances C, Wechsler B, Piette JC, Kieffer E et al. Embolies multiples de cholesterol simulant une periarterite noueuse. Presse Med 1992; 21:557–64.

44. Dahlberg PJ, Frecentese DF and Cogbill TH. Cholesterol embolism: experience with 22 histologically proven cases. Surgery 1989; 105:737–46.

45. Rosansky SJ. Multiple cholesterol emboli syndrome. South Med J 1982; 75:677–80.

46. Kaufman JL, Stark K and Brolin RE. Disseminated atheroembolism from extensive degenerative atherosclerosis of the aorta. Surgery 1987; 102:63–70.

47. Fine MJ, Kapoor W and Falanga V. Cholesterol crystal embolization: a review of 221 cases in the English literature. J Vasc Dis 1987; 38:769–84.

48. Mannesse CK, Blankestijn PJ, Man in 't Veld AJ and Schalekamp MADH. Renal failure and cholesterol crystal embolization: a report of 4 surviving cases and a review of the literature. Clin Nephrol 1991; 36:240–5.

49. Smith MC, Ghose MK and Henry AR. The clinical spectrum of renal cholesterol embolization. Am J Med 1981; 72:174–80.

50. Colt HG, Begg RJ, Saporito J, Cooper WM and Shapiro AP. Cholesterol emboli after cardiac catheterization. Medicine 1988; 67:389–400.

51. Steen VD Costantino, JP, Shapiro AP and Medsger TA Jr. Outcome of renal crisis in systemic sclerosis: relation to availability of angiotensin converting enzyme (ACE) inhibitors. Ann Intern Med 1990; 113:352–7.

52. Donohoe JF. Scleroderma and the kidney. Kidney Int 1992; 41:462–77.

53. Gifford RW Jr. Management of hypertensive crises. JAMA 1991; 266:829–35.

54. Prisant LM, Carr AA and Hawkins DW. Treating hypertensive emergencies. Postgrad Med 1993; 93:92–110.

55. Lawton WJ. The short-term course of renal function in malignant hypertensives with renal insufficiency. Clin Nephrol 1982; 17:277–83.

56. Yu S-H, Whitworth JA and Kincaid-Smith PS. Malignant hypertension: aetiology and outcome in 83 patients. Clin and Exper Theory and Practice 1986; A8:1211–30.

57. Patel R, Ansari A and Grim CE. Prognosis and predisposing factors for essential malignant hypertension in predominantly black patients. Am J Cardiol. 1990; 66:868–9.

58. Guelpa G, Lucsko M, Chaignon M and Guedon J. Hypertension arterielle maligne, aspect semiologique et

pronostique. Schweiz. med. Wschr. 1984; 114:1870–7.

59. Mroczek WJ, Davidov M, Gavrilovich L and Finnerty FA Jr. The value of aggressive therapy in the hypertensive patient with azotemia. Circulation 1969; 40:893–904.

60. Cordingley FT, Jones NF, Wing AJ and Hilton PJ. Reversible renal failure in malignant hypertension. Clin Nephrol 1980; 14:98–103.

61. Isles CG, McLay A and Boulton Jones JM. Recovery in malignant hypertension presenting as acute renal failure. Quart J Med 1984; 53:439–52.

62. Robson WLM and Leung AKC. Hemolytic-uremic syndrome in children. A serious hazard of undercooked beef. Postgraduate Med 1990; 88:135–140.

63. Pavia AT, Nichols CR, Green DP, Tauxe RV, Mottice S, Greene KD et al. Hemolytic-uremic syndrome during an outbreak of *Escherichia coli* 0157 : H7 infections in institutions for mentally retarded persons: clinical and epidemiologic observations. J Pediatr 1990; 116:544–51.

64. Griffin PM and Tauxe RV. The epidemiology of infections caused by *Escherichia coli* 0157 : H7, other enterohemorrhagic *E. coli*, and the associated hemolytic uremic syndrome. Epidemiologic Reviews 1991; 13:60–98.

65. Siegler RL. Management of hemolytic-uremic syndrome. J Pediatr 1988; 112:1014–20.

66. Thompson CE, Damon LE, Ries CA and Linker CA. Thrombotic microangiopathies in the 1980s: clinical features, response to treatment, and the impact of the human immunodeficiency virus epidemic. Blood 1992; 80:1890–5.

67. Hakim RM, Schulman G, Churchill WH Jr. and Lazarus JM. Successful management of thrombocytopenia, microangiopathic anemia, and acute renal failure by plasmapheresis. Am J Kidney Dis 1985; 5:170–6.

68. Cattran DC. Adult hemolytic-uremic syndrome: successful treatment with plasmapheresis. Am J Kidney Dis 1984; 3:275–9.

69. Bell WR, Braine HG, Ness PM and Kickler TS. Improved survival in thrombotic thrombocytopenic purpura-hemolytic uremic syndrome. N Engl J Med 1991; 325:398–403.

70. Gutterman LA, Levin DM, George BS and Sharma HM. The hemolytic-uremic syndrome: recovery after treatment with vincristine. Ann Intern Med 1983; 98:612–4.

71. Snyder HW Jr., Mittelman A, Oral A, Messerschmidt GL, Henry DH, Korec S et al. Treatment of cancer chemotherapy-associated thrombotic thrombocytopenic purpura/hemolytic uremic syndrome by protein A immunoadsorption of plasma. Cancer 1993; 71:1882–92.

71a Siegler RL, Milligan MK, Burningham TH, Christofferson RD, Chang S-Y and Jorde LB. Long-term outcome and prognostic indicators in the hemolytic-uremic syndrome. J Pediatr 1991; 118:195–200.

72. Rowe PC, Orrbine E, Wells GA, McLaine PN and members of the Canadian Pediatric Kidney Disease Reference Centre. Epidemiology of hemolytic-uremic syndrome in Canadian children from 1986 to 1988. J Pediatr 1991; 119:218–24.

73. Lesesne JB, Rothschild N, Erickson B, Korec S, Sisk R, Keller J et al. Cancer-associated hemolytic-uremic syndrome: Analysis of 85 cases from a national registry. J Clin Oncol 1989; 7:781–9.

74. Poch E, Almirall J, Nicolas JM, Torras A and Revert L. Treatment of mitomycin-C-associated hemolytic uremic syndrome with plasmapheresis. Nephron 1990; 55:89–90.

75. White DJ, Yong F and McKendrick MW. Haemolytic uraemic syndrome in adults. BMJ 1988; 296:899.

75a Ponticelli C, Rivolta E, Imbasciati E, Rossi E and Mannucci PM. Hemolytic uremic syndrome in adults. Arch Intern Med 1980; 140:353–7.

76. Clarkson AR, Lawrence JR, Meadows R and Seymour AE. The haemolytic uraemic syndrome in adults. Quart J Med 1970; 39:227–44.

77. Segonds A, Louradour N, Suc JM and Orfila C. Postpartum hemolytic uremic syndrome: a study of three cases with a review of the literature. Clin Nephrol 1979; 12:229–42.

78. Eijgenraam FJ, Donckerwolcke RA, Monnens LAH, Proesmans W, Wolff ED and Van Damme B. Renal transplantation in 20 children with hemolytic-uremic syndrome. Clin Nephrol 1990; 33:89–93.

79. Van Den Berg-Wolf MG, Kootte AMM, Weening JJ and Paul LC. Recurrent hemolytic uremic syndrome in a renal transplant recipient and review of the Leiden experience. Transplantation 1988; 45:248–51.

80. Hebert D, Sibley RK and Mauer SM. Recurrence of hemolytic uremic syndrome in renal transplant recipients. Kidney Int 1986; 30:S51–8.

81. Onundarson PT, Rowe JM, Heal JM and Francis CW. Response to plasma exchange and splenectomy in thrombotic thrombocytopenic purpura. Arch Intern Med 1992; 152:791–6.

82. Rock GA, Shumak KH, Buskard NA, Blanchette VS, Kelton JG, Nair RC, Spasoff RA and the Canadian Apheresis Study Group. Comparison of plasma exchange with plasma infusion in the treatment of thrombotic thrombocytopenic purpura. N Engl J Med 1991; 325:393–7.

83. Raniele DP, Opsahl JA and Kjellstrand CM. Should intravenous immunoglobulin G be first-line treatment for acute thrombotic thrombocytopenic purpura?: Case report and review of the literature. Am J Kidney Dis 1991; 18:264–8.

84. Kondo H. Effect of intravenous gammaglobulin infusion on recurrent episodes of thrombotic thrombocytopenic purpura (TTP). Eur J Hematol 1993; 50:55–6.

85. Kierdorf H, Maurin N and Heintz B. Cyclosporine for thrombotic thrombocytopenic purpura. Ann Intern Med 1993; 118:987–8.

86. Toyoshige M, Zaitsu Y, Okafuji K, Inoue Y, Hiroshige Y, Matsumoto N et al. Successful treatment of thrombotic thrombocytopenic purpura with high-dose corticosteroid. Am J Hematol 1992; 41:69.

87. Lichtin AE, AD Schreiber, S Hurwitz, TL Willoughby and LE Silberstein. Efficacy of intensive plasmapheresis in thrombotic thrombocytopenic purpura. Arch Intern Med 1987; 147:2122–6.

88. Kwaan HC. Clinicopathologic features of thrombotic thrombocytopenic purpura. Semin Hematol 1987; 24:71–81.

89. Rock G, Shumak K, Kelton J, Blanchette VS, Buskard N, Nair R, Spasoff R and The Canadian Apheresis Studyedit Group. Thrombotic thrombocytopenic purpura: outcome in 24 patients with renal impairment treated with plasma

exchange. Transfusion 1992; 32:710–4.

90. Eknoyan G and Riggs SA. Renal involvement in patients with thrombotic thrombocytopenic purpura. Am J Nephrol 1986; 6:117–31.

91. Amorosi EL and Ultmann JE. Thrombotic thrombocytopenic purpura: report of 16 cases and review of the literature. Medicine 1966; 45:139–59.

92. Turney JH, Ellis CM and Parsons FM. Obstetric acute renal failure 1956–1987. Brit J Obstet and Gynaecol 1989; 96:679–87.

93. Chugh KS, Singhal PC, Kher VK, Gupta VK, Malik GH, Narayan G et al. Spectrum of acute cortical necrosis in Indian patients. Am J Med Sci 1983; 286:10–20.

94. Matlin RA and Gary NE. Acute cortical necrosis. Am J Med 1974; 56:110–8.

95. Kleinknecht D, Grunfeld J-P, Gomez PC, Moreau J-F and Garcia-Torres R. Diagnostic procedures and long-term prognosis in bilateral renal cortical necrosis. Kidney Int 1973; 4:390–400.

96. Martin LG, Casarella WJ and Gaylord GM. Azotemia caused by renal artery stenosis: treatment by percutaneous angioplasty. AJR 1988; 10:839–44.

97. Novick AC, Ziegelbaum M, Vidt DG, Gifford RW Jr., Pohl MA and Goormastic M. Trends in surgical revascularization for renal artery disease. JAMA 1987; 257:498–501.

98. Mercier C, Piquet P, Alimi Y, Tournigand P and Albrand J-J. Occlusive disease of the renal arteries and chronic renal failure: The limits of reconstructive surgery. Ann Vasc Surg 1990; 4:166–70.

99. Torsello G, Sachs M, Kniemeyer H, Grabitz K, Godehardt E and Sandmann W. Results of surgical treatment for atherosclerotic renovascular occlusive disease. Eur J Vasc Surg 1990; 4:477–82.

100. Lawrie GM, Morris GC Jr., Glaeser DH and DeBakey ME. Renovascular reconstruction: factors affecting long-term prognosis in 919 patients followed up to 31 years. Am J Cardiol 1989; 63:1085–92.

101. Simon N, Franklin SS, Bleifer KH and Maxwell MH. Clinical characteristics of renovascular hypertension. JAMA 1972; 220:1209–18.

102. Pattison JM, Reidy JF, Rafferty MJ, Ogg CS, Cameron JS, Sacks SH et al. Percutaneous transluminal renal angioplasty in patients with renal failure. Quart J Med 1992; 85:883–8.

103. O'Donovan RM, Gutierrez OH and Izzo JL Jr. Preservation of renal function by percutaneous renal angioplasty in high-risk elderly patients: short-term outcome. Nephron 1992; 60:187–92.

104. Dean RH, Englund R, Dupont WD, Meacham PW, Plummer WD, Pierce R et al. Retrieval of renal function by revascularization. Ann Surg 1985; 202:367–75.

105. Jacobson HR. Ischemic renal disease: an overlooked clinical entity? Kidney Int 1988; 34:729–43.

106. Wise KL, McCann RL, Dunnick NR and Paulson DF. Renovascular hypertension. J Urol 1988; 140:911–24.

107. Weibull H, Bergqvist D, Jonsson K, Hulthen L, Mannhem P and Bergentz S-E. Long-term results after percutaneous transluminal angioplasty of atherosclerotic renal artery stenosis – the importance of intensive follow-up. Eur J Vasc Surg 1991; 5:291–301.

108. Ziegelbaum M, Novick AC, Hayes J, Vidt DG, Risius B and Gifford RW Jr. Management of renal arterial disease in the elderly patient. Surgery, Gynecol & Obstet 1987; 165:130–4.

109. Mestres CA, Campistol JM, Ninot S, Botey A, Abad C, Guerola M et al. Improvement of renal function in azotaemic hypertensive patients after surgical revascularization. Br J Surg 1988; 75:578–80.

110. Messina LM, Zelenock GB, Yao KA and Stanley JC. Renal revascularization for recurrent pulmonary edema in patients with poorly controlled hypertension and renal insufficiency: a distinct subgroup of patients with arteriosclerotic renal artery occlusive disease. J Vasc Surg 1992; 15:73–82.

111. Schreiber MJ, Pohl MA and Novick AC. The natural history of atherosclerotic and fibrous renal artery disease. Urol Clin N Amer 1984; 11:383–92.

112. Gasparini M, Hofmann R and Stoller M. Renal artery embolism: clinical features and therapeutic options. J Urol 1992; 147:567–72.

113. Ouriel K, Andrus CH, Ricotta JJ, DeWeese JA and Green RM. Acute renal artery occlusion: when is revascularization justified? J Vasc Surg 1987; 5:348–53.

114. Moyer JD, Rao CN, Widrich WC and Olsson CA. Conservative management of renal artery embolus. J Urol 1973; 109:138–43.

115. Lessman RK, Johnson SF, Coburn JW and Kaufman JJ. Renal artery embolism. Ann Intern Med 1978; 89:477–82.

116. Steckel A, Johnston J, Fraley DS, Bruns FJ, Segel DP and Adler S. The use of streptokinase to treat renal artery thromboembolism. Am J Kidney Dis 1984; 4:166–70.

117. Gagnon RF, Horosko F and Herba MJ. Local infusion of low-dose streptokinase for renal artery thromboembolism. Can Med Assoc J 1984; 131:1089–91.

118. Schneider JR, Wright A and Mitchell RS. Successful percutaneous balloon catheter treatment of renal artery occlusion and anuria. Ann Vasc Surg 1992; 6:533–6.

119. Sarasin FP and Schifferli JA. Prophylactic oral anticoagulation in nephrotic patients with idiopathic membranous nephropathy. Kidney Int 1994; 45:578–85.

120. Bernard DB. Extrarenal complications of the nephrotic syndrome. Kidney Int 1988; 33:1184–1202.

121. Cameron JS. The nephrotic syndrome and its complications. Am J Kidney Dis 1987; 10:157–71.

122. Rowe JM, Rasmussen RL, Mader SL, DiMarco PL, Cockett ATK and Marder VJ. Successful thrombolytic therapy in two patients with renal vein thrombosis. Am J Med 1984; 77:1111–4.

123. Burrow CR, Walker WG, Bell WR and Gatewood OB. Streptokinase salvage of renal function after renal vein thrombosis. Ann Intern Med 1984; 100:237–8.

124. Crowley JP, Matarese RA, Quevedo SF and Garella S. Fibrinolytic therapy for bilateral renal vein thrombosis. Arch Intern Med 1984; 144:159–60.

125. Cagnoli L, Viglietta G, Madia G, Gattiani A, Orsi C, Rigotti A et al. Acute bilateral renal vein thrombosis superimposed on calcified thrombus of the inferior vena

cava in a patient with membranous lupus nephritis. Nephrol Dial Transplant Suppl. 1990; S1:71–4.

126. Vogelzang RL, Moel DI, Cohn RA, Donaldson JS, Langman CB and Nemcek AA Jr. Acute renal vein thrombosis: successful treatment with intraarterial urokinase. Radiology 1988; 169:681–2.

127. Laville M, Aguilera D, Maillet PJ, Labeeuw M, Madonna O and Zech P. The prognosis of renal vein thrombosis: a re-evaluation of 27 cases. Nephrol Dial Transplant 1988; 3:247–56.

GLOMERULAR CAUSES

J. GARY ABUELO

Acute Nephritic Disease

Primary glomerular disease

Idiopathic (Necrotizing and) Crescentic GN. Treatment is most likely to improve GFR early in the course of crescentic GN when fewer glomeruli are affected, and glomerular healing is possible because crescents are still small and cellular. Within a few weeks of onset of rapidly progressive disease, crescents may become fibrotic and completely circumferential, glomeruli obsolescent and renal failure irreversible. Thus, the diagnosis by renal biopsy and the initiation of treatment should be carried out with some urgency. When crescentic GN is suspected, some physicians will start immunosuppressive treatment or even plasmapheresis before having a histologic diagnosis, especially if unavoidable circumstances, like high risk of bleeding, delay the renal biopsy. This practice of treatment before diagnosis should be used infrequently, since the biopsy might reveal a disease, for which the treatment is not helpful, such as chronic GN, or a lesion for which immunosuppressives might be harmful, such as ATN due to sepsis.

The treatment of crescentic GN varies with the immunofluorescent pattern (see Chapter 11). Management of patients with a linear pattern of IgG deposition due to anti-GBM antibodies is discussed below in the section on *Goodpasture's syndrome*.

Patients with pauci-immune or immune complex patterns are both treated with 1 g *methylprednisolone, given intravenously* over 30 minutes each day for three successive days. Such pulse therapy may cause slight rises in blood pressure, temporary glucose intolerance, facial flushing, headache and bitter taste [1]. The pulse is followed by *oral prednisone*, 60 mg per day, for a month, although some authorities recommend an alternate day dosing of 2 mg/kg as a way of reducing adverse effects [2]. The prednisone is then tapered and discontinued, gradually over three or more months if there has been a clinical response, and more rapidly if there has been no response. Initially, patients started on corticosteroids must be monitored at least weekly for hyperglycemia, hypertension, volume overload, hypokalemia, and change in Scr. Patients should be warned about changes in facial appearance, mood and appetite, and should be instructed to promptly report symptoms of infection or peptic ulcer. Dietary counseling may be necessary in order to avoid weight gain. Cataracts, acne vulgaris, aseptic necrosis and osteoporosis with fractures are other possible complications of long-term corticosteroids. In order to prevent osteoporosis due to long-term corticosteroids, weight bearing exercise should be encouraged, and estrogen replacement should be given in women with ovarian failure or menopause [3]. Calcium deficits can be prevented by ensuring adequate vitamin D intake, and giving calcium supplements to achieve an intake of 1200 to 1500 mg per day. If a diuretic is needed, thiazides are preferred over furosemide.

Plasmapheresis does not generally improve the results of treatment when added to a regimen of corticosteroids and cytotoxic drugs [4, 5]. Nevertheless, as an alternative to discontinuing treatment in patients without a response to corticosteroids, some authorities recommend adding cyclophosphamide and plasmapheresis [5, 6]. Typically, the cyclophosphamide is given orally, 1–2 mg per day, for three weeks or until the Scr falls, if sooner. Plasmapheresis consists of replacement of one plasma volume, about 5% of body weight, with the same volume of albumin and saline. It is performed three times per week for three weeks or until the Scr falls, if sooner. In support of adding plasmapheresis with a cytotoxic drug is a report that adding plasmapheresis improved renal function in three out of five cases who had not responded to the initial therapy of azathioprine, cyclophosphamide and corticosteroids [7]. However, the improvement in renal function seen in dialysis-dependent patients treated with plasmapheresis (77% of cases) [5] was about the same as in a similar group treated with pulse methylprednisolone and oral prednisone (70% of cases) [2]. Furthermore, plasmapheresis is only thought to be effective when used with cytotoxic drugs, and these drugs are associated with a 19% incidence of infection, almost half of cases being fatal [7–10]. In comparison, in one report pulse methylprednisolone and oral prednisone had only a 7% incidence of infection [2]. Thus, it would seem prudent to avoid plasmapheresis and cytotoxic drugs in idiopathic crescentic GN, given the questionable advantage and greater toxicity of this therapy.

The response of azotemia caused by crescentic GN to treatment is similar in the pauci-immune and immune complex types [2, 8–10]. A worse prognosis is observed with oliguria, high initial Scr, high percentage of crescents (>80%), particularly if they are fibrocellular, and a high percentage of obsolescent glomeruli (>33%) [2, 4, 9], but some studies found no predictive value of oliguria or a high percent of crescents, especially if patients received pulse methylprednisolone [2, 8, 10]. With pulse methylprednisolone 79% of cases of crescentic GN had an improvement in Scr, including 70% of those requiring hemodialysis [2]. A fall in Scr is usually noted within a week of the pulse. Following a response to treatment a variable number of patients lose renal function again, and progress to end stage renal disease [2, 8, 9] or have a relapse that responds once more to therapy [8]. There is a suggestion that the late deterioration of renal function may be prevented with long-term immunosuppression [8, 9], but it is not clear if the benefit of the prolonged medication outweighs the added risk. Thus, while relapses should be retreated, long-term immunosuppression is not recommended.

IgA Nephropathy. This condition produces an acute nephritic picture with azotemia in less than 12% of patients [11–14]. Most of these cases are males and are characterized by prodromal pharyngitis, gross hematuria and spontaneous recovery over 2 to 20 weeks. In addition to the underlying IgA nephropathy, the renal biopsy typically shows red cells in the tubules, acute tubular necrosis and few (0–30%) crescents [15, 16]. After identifying such a case, the physician should manage the renal failure with the usual measures (see Chapter 16) in anticipation of a spontaneous recovery of function. On the other hand, a smaller group of nephritic patients is characterized by a *crescentic IgA nephropathy* (30 to over 90% crescents) on renal biopsy and progressive renal failure. Many patients already have irreversible changes (25 to 50% sclerotic glomeruli) when they

are biopsied, and usually do not respond to corticosteroid or cytotoxic therapy [17, 18]. Nevertheless, since treatment sometimes produces partial recovery of renal function [19–21], if extensive irreversible lesions are not present on renal biopsy, the physician should consider *a trial of pulse methylprednisolone* followed by oral prednisone (see above – *Idiopathic Crescentic GN*).

Membranoproliferative GN. This entity sometimes causes an acute nephritic syndrome with azotemia. For the most part, there is no treatment available for these patients, who may either improve spontaneously or progress to end stage renal disease (see Chapter 11). Nevertheless, an occasional case will have a crescentic GN complicating the underlying membranoproliferative GN [22]. Such patients may respond to *pulse methylprednisolone* followed by oral prednisone (see above – *Idiopathic Crescentic GN*) [23]. For management of membranoproliferative GN associated with hepatitis C virus infection, see *Essential Mixed Cryoglobulinemia* below.

Secondary glomerular disease

Poststreptococcal and Other GN Associated with Infection. The treatment of these conditions primarily involves the prompt diagnosis and eradication of the causative infection. This may entail surgical interventions such as drainage of abscesses, replacement of a heart valve, or removal of a ventriculo-atrial shunt [24, 25], in addition to medical therapy with specific antibiotic regimens. Control of infection stops the production of microbial antigens and the glomerular deposition of antigen-antibody complexes, and permits glomerular healing to occur. Because of the immunologic and inflammatory nature of the glomerular lesions, it has been suggested that immunosuppressive or anticoagulant therapy may have an ancillary role, particularly, if there are crescents involving more than half the glomeruli [24, 26–29a]. No study has been done to evaluate such treatment in post-infectious GN, but it is more generally believed that the renal prognosis is so good with effective eradication of the infection that not enough additional benefit accrues from immunosuppressive or anticoagulant therapy to justify the added risk [30, 31]. Infections are also more difficult to control when immunosuppressives are used. However, if the renal biopsy shows cellular crescents and recovery of renal function does not occur after successful treatment of an infection, a *trial of pulse methylprednisolone* followed by oral prednisone might be considered (see above – *Idiopathic Crescentic GN*).

The prognosis of post streptococcal GN with azotemia is quite good with over 75% of patients having a normal Scr after two to three months [32–34]. Patients with diffuse crescent formation tend not to recover renal function and to progress to end stage renal failure [33–35], although many patients with predominantly small, cellular crescents are able to recover renal function [36]. With modern drug and dialytic therapy, deaths due to uremia, acute pulmonary edema and hypertensive crisis are now rare.

Bacterial endocarditis is thought to be prevented by giving *prophylactic antibiotics* to susceptible individuals during procedures known to cause bacteremia, such as dental extraction. Although the effectiveness of this is not known, it sems prudent to follow recommendations for prophylaxis as outlined in standard textbooks or recent articles [37, 38].

The prognosis of GN caused by bacterial endocarditis is marked by greater than 30% mortality rate due to unremitting infection and other complications [39]. In surviving patients, Scr usually peaks during the first two weeks, if not during the first few days of antibiotic treatment, and partial or complete recovery usually ensues [39]. However, some individuals develop significant chronic renal failure or require dialysis; they usually have an initial Scr greater than 3 mg/dL (265 μmol/L) and on renal biopsy have crescents involving more than half the glomeruli [39].

GN associated with visceral abscesses has a similar prognosis to that of GN in bacterial endocarditis. A certain number of patients succumb to persistent infection. Most other individuals show varying degrees of recovery, except those with delayed control of infection or marked crescent formation who go on to chronic renal failure [24].

Shunt nephritis is largely prevented nowadays by the use of ventriculoperitoneal shunts.

When shunt nephritis occurs in an individual with a ventriculoatrial shunt, therapy involves complete shunt replacement, systemic and intraventricular antibiotics [25].

Azotemia completely resolves in most cases when the infection is controlled. Less than 10 percent of patients are left with chronic renal failure, due in large part to a delay in diagnosis and the extensive scarring that has occurred by the time that treatment is instituted [40, 41].

Lupus Nephritis. Prevention of exacerbations of lupus may reduce the occurrence of lupus nephritis. This can be accomplished in some cases by reducing exposure to sunlight with sunscreen, appropriate dress and moderation of outdoor activity, and by avoiding or minimizing pharmacologic doses of estrogens, as in oral contraceptives.

Individuals with azotemia due to lupus nephritis present three therapeutic problems. The first is treatment of *extrarenal symptoms*. Fatigue is managed with increased rest. Skin involvement may respond to oral *hydroxychloroquine*, 200 to 600 mg per day. Arthritis, serositis and fever can often be controlled with *nonsteroidal anti-inflammatory drugs*, which, however, may cause a vasomotor type of renal insufficiency, and must be used with caution [42, 43]. If nonsteroidals do not improve the symptoms of lupus, oral *prednisone*, 20 to 30 mg per day, is usually effective. After extrarenal manifestations are controlled, the dose should be gradually tapered to an alternate-day schedule if symptoms permit. Consultation with a rheumatologist is often helpful in treating manifestations of lupus, and is essential in the management of major extrarenal organ involvement, such as lupus cerebritis.

The second therapeutic problem is induction of a *remission of the acute nephritic syndrome*. This picture is most often associated with the diffuse proliferative form of lupus nephritis, and less often with the focal proliferative and membranous forms [44, 45]. The goal of therapy is improvement in renal function through a decrease in cellular proliferation and other histologic activity. The classic treatment is *oral prednisone*, 60 mg per day [46]; large individuals may take 1 mg/kg per day. Scr may continue to rise for one to two weeks before responding to therapy, and take several weeks to return to baseline. At this point, the prednisone is slowly tapered over two to four months. A low dose (0.2 to 0.4 mg/kg/day) may be continued long-term to control extrarenal symptoms. During steroid withdrawal lupus flares are common, and should be managed by returning to the previous dose of prednisone for up to several weeks. These flares must be distinguished from manifestations of steroid withdrawal, which last one to three days, and may include fever, hypotension, malaise and joint symptoms. (For adverse effects of corticosteroids and recommended precautions see above – *Idiopathic Crescentic GN*).

If Scr is still rising after one to two weeks of oral prednisone therapy, *pulse methylprednisolone* treatment should be considered. This was described above in the section on *idiopathic crescentic GN*. Oral prednisone is stopped during the pulse and then continued at 60 mg per day afterwards. Pulse methylprednisolone is relatively safe, and is believed to return deteriorating renal function to baseline more quickly than oral prednisone alone [47]. Although a fall in Scr may be seen in a day or two, this may not occur for several weeks, and maximum improvement in GFR often takes months [48–50]. Chronic azotemia is usually due to irreversible glomerular scarring and tubular atrophy, and is unlikely to respond [48]. Proteinuria improves over months and eventually resolves in about half of cases [49].

One study that compared pulse methylprednisolone followed by oral prednisone to oral prednisone alone showed that the pulse treatment returned the GFR to baseline in 17 ± 11 weeks compared with 29 ± 17 weeks for oral prednisone alone; final GFR's were not different between the groups [50]. Another study showed better overall control of lupus activity two weeks after pulse treatment than two weeks after starting oral prednisone alone; however, four weeks after starting therapy, lupus activity was equally well controlled in the two groups [51].

Most patients will experience a fall in Scr with oral or intravenous steroids [48, 52]. The proper management of patients whose renal function does not improve after three or four weeks of corticosteroids is uncertain. Intravenous or oral cyclophosphamide is often used together with prednisone in such individuals, who may subsequently have a fall in Scr. It is not known, however, if the improvement is due to the cyclophosphamide or merely to a delayed effect and additional duration of oral prednisone. Remarkably, the only controlled study that looked at the remission of azotemia in lupus nephritis showed no advantage of adding oral cyclophosphamide to steroids [52]. Meanwhile the adverse effects of cyclophosphamide are well-known, and include nausea, vomiting, alopecia, infection, ovarian failure, malignancy and hemorrhagic cystitis [53–56]. Thus, the benefit, if any, of cyclophosphamide may not outweigh its risk. Until further information becomes available, the physician may with clear conscience choose any of the following regimens to attempt to improve refractory azotemia: continue oral prednisone alone in the hopes of a late response, give a second course of pulse methylprednisolone, or start monthly doses of intravenous cyclophosphamide [53, 57]. Oral prednisone is continued in the latter two protocols. *Intravenous cyclophosphamide* is given as 0.5–1.0 g/m^2 over 60 minutes, one dose monthly for six months. The 0.5 g/m^2 dose is used initially if the GFR is less than 33 ml/min. The dose is raised to 1 g/m^2, as long as white blood cell counts do not drop below 2500/mm^3 on days 7 to 14 after treatment; the dose is lowered if white counts do drop below 2500/mm^3. The infusion of cyclophosphamide is followed by 2 L/m^2 of 0.45% saline over 24 hours. Antiemetics, such as ondansetron hydrochloride, should be employed as necessary. After six monthly doses, some recommend a dose every three months to prevent exacerbations [57].

In 1989 Lin et al. reported nine children with lupus nephritis and azotemia refractory to oral prednisone, pulse methylprednisolone and eight weeks of oral cyclophosphamide [58]. A five day course of intravenous human γ-globulin, 400 mg/kg/day, was administered. Scr fell within one to two weeks in all cases. The mean Scr was 3.6 ± 1.7 mg/dL before γ-globulin and 1.2 ± .7 mg/dL afterwards; minimal toxicity was noted. Although, ideally one should await confirmatory studies, given the impressive results and minimum toxicity reported here, one might consider this treatment in some cases of refractory lupus nephritis with azotemia.

The third therapeutic problem in individuals with azotemia due to lupus nephritis is the long-term *prevention of end stage renal failure*. Most patients who progress to end stage fit into two groups [59–61]. One group has little extrarenal lupus activity, chronic inactive renal histology and slowly progressive renal failure. The second group has active extrarenal disease, active lupus nephritis, and rapidly progressive renal failure. Some of this latter group require long-term dialysis, while others recover renal function. This recovery of GFR may be observed with either an increase [59] or decrease [60] in immunosuppressive therapy.

Controlled studies from the National Institutes of Health (N.I.H.) suggested that combining oral prednisone with cyclophosphamide – intravenously, orally or together with azathioprine – preserves renal function over the long term better than does oral prednisone alone [62]. Complications occurred in all groups, but were most common with oral cyclophosphamide [55, 57, 62]. The authors concluded that the benefit of the cytotoxic drugs outweigh their risk. These findings have been accepted by most practicing nephrologists and rheumatologists, who commonly incorporate cytotoxic drugs into the management of lupus nephritis. Nevertheless, due to flaws in the studies, reservations exist as to whether the data from the N.I.H. justify the authors' conclusions [54, 63, 64].

Inadequacies in the studies are: (1) The groups are not histologically homogeneous; 27% of cases either do not have a renal biopsy or do not have a proliferative class of lupus nephritis and should have been excluded. (2) There are only 12 patients with diffuse- or membrano-proliferative histology in the prednisone control group; if one or two of these patients had had better outcomes, the study might have had a different conclusion. (3) The initial mean Scr in all the groups was normal, which reduces the value of the study in drawing conclusions about the drug treatment of azotemic patients. (4) The intravenous cyclophosphamide protocol initially described in 1982 [65] was later made more aggressive [62], and still later more aggressive again [57]; only time will fully reveal the long–term toxicity and overall benefit of this recent protocol. (5) It is possible that patients who respond promptly to oral prednisone are generally not referred to the N.I.H. for study, which would obscure the fact that many individuals with lupus nephritis do well with prednisone alone. (6) The authors do not seem to fully weigh the toxicity of the cytotoxic agents in drawing their conclusions about their overall benefits. (7) There are not enough cases to perform subgroup analysis in order to adjust the results for characteristics that affect the prognosis of lupus nephritis, such as hypertension and race.

Also, in disagreement with the N.I.H. results is a study from the Mayo Clinic, which showed no reduction in end stage renal disease with the addition of oral cyclophosphamide to oral prednisone [54]. Finally, although the N.I.H. study found no benefit of adding azathioprine to prednisone [62], an analysis of pooled data from several studies showed that azathioprine preserved renal function when combined with oral prednisone [66].

In summary, the N.I.H. results suggest that *long-term cyclophosphamide* reduces the occurrence of chronic renal failure in lupus nephritis. However, due to weaknesses in the studies, the risks of cyclophosphamide and lack of confirmation by the Mayo Clinic group one cannot justify the automatic use of cyclophosphamide to obtain or maintain a remission of lupus nephritis. If one is to employ cytotoxic drugs, it seems prudent to reserve them for those cases not easily controlled with corticosteroids. Many patients respond to oral prednisone and then may be managed with nonsteroidal anti-inflammatory drugs or low dose oral prednisone for flares of extrarenal lupus activity. Acute relapses of lupus nephritis with azotemia should be retreated with oral prednisone, 60 mg per day. If this second episode does not respond easily to corticosteroids or if the patient has a third episode, one may consider adding oral *azathioprine*, 1 mg/kg per day, or intravenous cyclophosphamide, given as described above [57]. Before agreeing to cytotoxic treatment, the patient should be informed about the toxicity of these drugs, and the lack of clear evidence of their efficacy. Azathioprine's main danger is bone marrow suppression and increased risk of infection; it appears safer than cyclophosphamide, which has these plus several additional adverse effects (see above). Patients who have slowly progressive renal insufficiency in the absence of clinical lupus activity should not receive immunosuppressive treatment, since the histologic picture is unlikely to show acute treatable lesions. In questionable cases repeat renal biopsy may be performed to distinguish patients with extensive glomerular scarring and tubular atrophy from those with reversible changes, such as glomerular hypercellularity, immune complex deposition or active interstitial nephritis. It is thought that some non-immunologic mechanisms responsible for progression of chronic renal failure may be ameliorated by control of hypertension, use of converting enzyme inhibitors and other means; these modalities should be used as appropriate (see Chapter 17).

The probability of patients with lupus nephritis progressing to end stage renal disease is increased by male sex, young age, hypertension, overall clinical activity of lupus, elevated Scr at presentation, severity of serologic and renal histologic abnormalities, and perhaps by black race, although not all studies show this [67]. The diffuse proliferative and membranous histologic classes have a worse prognosis, and progress to end stage in about 20% of patients (Table 18.6).

Regarding the prognosis of lupus nephritis complicated by renal failure, about 80% of patients respond initially to treatment with an improvement in GFR, and a lack of response predicts progression to end stage [52, 69]. About half of responsive patients have a prompt fall in Scr, while the other half have a fall in Scr only after a month or more, even with pulse methyprednisolone [69]. Life table analysis shows that after five years of disease 40–72% of patients initially having azotemia progress to end stage renal disease [54, 70, 71].

Polyarteritis Nodosa. Ideally, the physician should manage patients with this condition together with a rheumatologist. Polyarteritis nodosa is treated with corticosteroids. With more severe renal disease, (Scr higher than 3 mg/dL or crescents involving more than 30% of glomeruli) *pulse methylprednisolone* followed by oral prednisone should be used [2], and oral prednisone alone can be used in less severe cases (for administration and adverse effects of methylprednisolone and prednisone see above – *Idiopathic Crescentic GN*) [2, 72–74].

> The literature concerning if or when to use additional treatment is conflicting. On the one hand, there are some reports of patients that have not responded to corticosteroids alone who improve following addition of cyclophosphamide or other immunosuppressives [75–79]. On the other hand, most studies comparing corticosteroids as initial treatment to corticosteroids plus an adjunctive modality show little advantage of adding cyclophosphamide

Table 18.6. Influence of histologic class on progression to ESRD after a mean of 8 to 12 years of observation [67, 68]

	Total patients	Patients with ESRD (%)
Mesangial	26	4
Focal proliferative	24	0
Diffuse proliferative	128	19
Membranous	26	23

ESRD – end stage renal disease.

[72, 80–85] or plasmapheresis [7, 80, 84, 85]. One of these studies found that adding cyclophosphamide reduced the chance of relapses, but without improving survival [81], and another study found that plasmapheresis together with oral immunosuppression led to an improvement in Scr in more dialysis-dependent patients than did oral immunosuppression alone [84]. However, compared with plasmapheresis, pulse methylprednisolone followed by oral prednisone may be equally or more effective in dialysis-dependent patients [2].

In patients with unrelenting vasculitis or acute nephritic syndrome after several weeks of corticosteroid therapy, one should consider adding *cyclophosphamide*. Cyclophosphamide is given orally starting with 2 mg/kg per day, and the dose is adjusted to avoid thrombocytopenia and white blood cell counts below $4,000/mm^2$. When disease activity has stopped, the prednisone and cyclophosphamide should be tapered over several months and discontinued, although low doses of one drug may be needed to maintain the remission in some cases. Some physicians may wish to add *plasmapheresis* to cyclophosphamide in dialysis-dependent patients. This typically consists of an exchange of one plasma volume for an equivolumic amount of albumin and saline, three times a week for three weeks. However, the risk and high cost of plasmapheresis probably outweigh its benefit, since an advantage over pulse methylprednisolone has not been shown. In patients in whom the principal threat of the vasculitis is end stage renal failure, dialytic management may be more prudent than aggressive measures to suppress the immune system. This is especially so if the renal biopsy shows extensive irreversible glomerular scarring and tubular atrophy. In such cases, one should give only enough immunosuppressives to control extrarenal manifestations.

When polyarteritis nodosa is associated with hepatitis B viral infections, antiviral therapy with *ribavirin* or *interferon alfa* should be considered [86].

The prognosis of the microscopic and classic forms of polyarteritis nodosa taken together is for about 75 to 80% of treated patients to undergo a remission within the first three to six months [78, 87]. Unfortunately about a quarter of these individuals experience a relapse, which may involve worsening renal function, between 5 and 68 months after diagnosis [78, 87]. Relapses occur when immunosuppressive drugs have been reduced in dose or stopped. They are managed by intensifying or reintroducing treatment – with good results in a majority of cases [78, 87]. After a few years of follow-up, the mortality rate in polyarteritis nodosa is between 20 and 40%. Many deaths are from lung hemorrhage and infarction of tissues, such as myocardium and bowel, and about a third of deaths are caused by infectious complications of therapy [78, 84, 87–89]. Renal failure usually improves with treatment, but a minority of individuals have irreversible renal failure and require chronic hemodialysis [78, 84, 87, 89].

Wegener's Granulomatosis. Physicians who oversee the management of this condition often coordinate the care of the patient with a rheumatologist, nephrologist, or pulmonologist, depending on which organ systems are involved. Wegener's granulomatosis should be treated with oral *prednisone*, 60 mg per day (or 1 mg/kg per day in larger individuals), and oral *cyclophosphamide*, 2 mg/kg per day, with the dose adjusted to avoid thrombocytopenia and white blood cell counts below 4,000/mm^3. Pulse methylprednisolone should be added if the Scr is higher than 3 mg/dL or crescents involve more than 30% of non-sclerosed glomeruli on biopsy (for administration and adverse effects of pulse methylprednisolone and prednisone – see above *Idiopathic Crescentic GN*). In patients with fulminant disease an increase in the cyclophosphamide dose to 3 to 5 mg/kg per day might be considered [90], but if worsening renal failure is the major problem, it should be managed with dialysis rather than escalation of immunosuppression given the risks of cyclophosphamide (see below). After four to eight weeks at 60 mg per day the dose of oral prednisone is gradually tapered and discontinued over three or more months, if the disease is quiescent. Once a remission is achieved, the cyclophosphamide is continued for one year as maintenance therapy, and then tapered by 25 mg decrements every two months until it is stopped or the disease recurs.

Cyclophosphamide may produce nausea, malaise and other complications (Table 18.7). If any of these side effects becomes a problem or fear of them is an issue, the physician may wish to consider an alternative to long-term cyclophosphamide therapy. *Azathioprine* is not effective in pro-

ducing remissions, but in some cases can maintain the remission once it is achieved [91, 92]. Therefore, once disease activity disappears cyclophosphamide may be stopped, and azathioprine, 1 to 2 mg/kg per day, may be started. It is continued for one year and then gradually tapered in 25 mg decrements and discontinued.

Relapses of Wegener's granulomatosis are managed by intensifying or reintroducing prednisone and cyclophosphamide.

An initial response to treatment of Wegener's granulomatosis may be seen in 5 to 10 days, and up to 90% of patients experience a partial or more often, a complete remission within one to two years of therapy [87, 90, 91, 93]. The majority of patients with renal failure have improvement of azotemia with treatment. While the Scr falls to normal in many cases, recovery of function is often incomplete in patients with severe renal failure [84, 89, 91, 93, 94]. Relapses of disease, often with renal deterioration, occur in about half of patients anytime from 3 months to 16 years after diagnosis [87, 90]. Between fulminant nephritis unresponsive to therapy and gradual loss of GFR over several years, 10 to 20% of patients develop end stage renal failure [87, 89, 90, 93]. Deaths may be associated with initial treatment failure and continue to occur due to relapsing or smoldering disease, so that by eight years after the diagnosis, mortality reaches between 20 and 50% of patients [87, 90, 95].

Table 18.7. Complications of cyclophosphamide reported in patients with Wegener's granulomatosis [90]

Complication	Incidence (%)
Ovarian failure	57
Serious infection*	46
Cystitis	43
Alopecia	17
Pulmonary insufficiency	17
Bladder cancer	3
Lymphoma/myelodysplasia	2

* Infection requiring hospitalization – glucocorticoids are also contributory.

Henoch-Schönlein Purpura. Nonsteroidal anti-inflammatory drugs are recommended for joint symptoms but, because of their potential adverse renal vasomotor effect, ought not be used in the presence of azotemia. Oral *prednisone*, 40 mg per day, may dramatically improve arthralgias and abdominal pain, and bloody diarrhea and hematuria may also subside [96]. Rarely gastrointestinal hemorrhage or perforation will require surgery. Therapy of the renal lesions is not recommended in most cases, because of the low probability of progression to end stage renal disease, and because of the adverse effects and lack of demonstrated benefit of the various treatments. Nevertheless, azotemic patients with extensive glomerular necrosis and crescents are at higher risk to go on to chronic renal failure [97], and based on anecdotal evidence may respond to *pulse methylprednisolone therapy* [96, 98]. Therefore, unless the Scr is improving, azotemia should be evaluated with a renal biopsy. In patients with more than 25% glomeruli involved by segmental necrosis or crescents, pulse methylprednisolone followed by oral prednisone is recommended (for administration of methylprednisolone and prednisone see above – *Idiopathic Crescentic GN*).

Non-renal manifestations of Henoch-Schönlein purpura typically fluctuate for one to six weeks before disappearing, but occasionally recurrences of the rash and other symptoms can be seen over several months or years [97, 99]. At follow-up evaluation, half of patients presenting with azotemia improve to normal renal function, although continued urinary abnormalities are common [96, 100–102]. Patients initially exhibiting more than 50% crescents on renal biopsy have a 35% chance of end stage renal disease [97]. Chronic renal failure mainly occurs in individuals who initially present with azotemia, but initially non-azotemic patients may be affected [101, 102]. End stage renal disease may develop during the acute phase of the disease or anytime over the ensuing years [97, 102].

Essential Mixed Cryoglobulinemia. Palpable purpura requires no therapy. Arthralgias may be treated with high-dose *aspirin* or *nonsteroidal anti-inflammatory drugs*; these agents should, however, be avoided in azotemia. Patients with neurologic involvement, extensive purpura, cutaneous necrosis or an acute nephritic syndrome require aggressive measures. Since the natural history of the disease is characterized by flares and spontaneous remissions, the adverse effects of therapy should be minimized by treating only at times of severe renal or extrarenal disease activity [103]. *Pulse methylprednisolone* followed by oral prednisone is generally recommended [104] (for administration and adverse effects of methylprednisolone and prednisone see above – *Idiopathic Crescentic GN*). A dramatic improvement in purpura and other extrarenal symptoms usually occurs within the first week of therapy, and Scr can fall significantly over a few weeks [104, 105]. Recurrence of renal failure may be treated with a second course of pulse and oral corticosteroids. For patients with failure to respond to or with a contraindication to corticosteroids, a trial of *plasmapheresis* may be undertaken. This consists of an exchange of one plasma volume for an equal volume of albumin and saline, three times a week for three weeks [106, 107]. To reduce the chance of recurrence, some physicians would also add oral *cyclophosphamide*, 2 mg/kg per day, for 1 to 6 months with dose reduction for thrombocytopenia or white blood cell counts below 4,000/mm^3.

For patients with essential mixed cryoglobulinemia associated with chronic hepatitis C virus infection a trial of *interferon alfa* should be considered. This treatment is based on reports of 23 patients with essential mixed cryoglobulinemia and renal involvement; another patient had membranoproliferative GN and a positive test for hepatitis C viral RNA, but cryoglobulin was undetectable [108, 109]. The usual dose of interferon alfa was 3×10^6 units subcutaneously three times weekly for 6 to 12 months. Most of these individuals became hepatitis C viral RNA negative, and showed improvement in skin lesions and renal function after interferon alfa treatment. Unfortunately, viremia and clinical disease recurred within a year after treatment in almost all cases. Retreatment was again effective in three of four cases [109]. Since new studies on the use of interferon alfa continue to be published, the physician should learn the current recommendations.

Azotemic patients with essential mixed cryoglobulinemia typically respond to therapy with a fall in Scr, but may subsequently experience one or more renal exacerbations [110]. Later in the disease, some degree of chronic renal failure is not unusual, but fewer than 10% of cases go on to end stage renal disease [110]. After ten years of disease a mortality rate of 30% has been reported [110]. However, many of the causes of death, such as uncontrolled hypertension, and fatal renal failure and infection [110], should occur infrequently nowadays with the availability of dialysis, modern anti-hypertensive drugs, and restraint in the use of immunosuppressive drugs.

Goodpasture's Syndrome and Anti-GBM-Mediated Crescentic GN. The goal of therapy in both these conditions is to arrest pulmonary hemorrhage, if present, and prevent further glomerular damage. Since tobacco smoking is a cofactor in lung hemorrhage, cessation of smoking may reduce or prevent this complication [111, 112]. The major therapeutic measure, however, is to reduce the plasma levels of anti-GBM antibodies to zero through immunosuppression and plasmapheresis. Thus, anti-GBM antibody levels should be measured weekly to gauge the effectiveness of therapy. Pulmonary hemorrhage should be followed with chest X-rays and hemoglobin levels.

Treatment varies with the severity of renal disease. Patients with no pulmonary hemorrhage and *milder renal disease* (slowly rising Scr less than 3 mg/dL (265 μmol/L) and crescent formation less than 30% of non-sclerosed glomeruli) should receive oral *prednisone*, 60 mg per day or 1 mg/kg per day in larger individuals, and oral *cyclophosphamide*, 2 mg/kg per day, with the latter drug dose adjusted downward to avoid white blood cell counts less than 4,000/mm^3 and platelet counts less than 100,000/mm^3. Treatment is continued for eight weeks or until the anti-GBM antibody disappears. Then the cyclophosphamide is stopped and the prednisone dose is gradually changed to an alternate-day schedule and reduced to zero over several weeks (for adverse effects of corticosteroids and recommended precautions see above – *Idiopathic Crescentic GN*).

The addition of plasmapheresis to immunosuppression speeds the fall in anti-GBM antibody levels [113, 114]. However, two small controlled studies did not show a clinical advantage of adding plasmapheresis to immunosuppression in patients with milder disease [115]. Given the additional risk associated with the procedure [10], plasmapheresis should probably only be used if Scr is rising rapidly or if it goes above 3 mg/dL.

Patients with *more severe renal disease* (Scr 3.0 to 7.0 mg/dL (265 to 620 μmol/L) and 30% crescents or

more), should additionally receive *plasmapheresis* (with albumin and saline replacement) until anti-GBM antibodies are twice the background level. Schedules used have varied from daily [113] to every third day [114]. Three daily plasmaphereses of one plasma volume each followed by three plasmaphereses per week is a resonable protocol.

Patients with the *most severe renal failure* (Scr greater than 7 mg/dL (620 μmol/L) or dialysis-dependence) are very unlikely to recover renal function with therapy [2, 111, 113, 116]. Since there is a risk of infection, in some cases fatal, associated with immunosuppression [8, 113, 114, 117], it is prudent to treat these patients [113] in only two situations. First, even when renal failure is irreversible, pulmonary hemorrhage responds in most cases to intravenous *methylprednisolone*, 1 g per day for three days, or *plasmapheresis*, oral prednisone and cyclophosphamide (described above). In patients with pulmonary hemorrhage, 300 to 400 ml of fresh frozen plasma should be included in the volume of replacement fluid. Second, plasmapheresis plus immunosuppression has been reported to partially reverse renal failure in a few patients on dialysis [114, 117–119], and should be considered in cases without extensive irreversible lesions on renal biopsy. Typically, such individuals have preserved urine output, rapidly progressive renal failure, and biopsies showing some preserved glomerular capillaries. Also, crescents involve less than 85% of glomeruli, and are small and cellular rather than circumferential and fibrotic [111, 114, 117, 119].

With plasmapheresis and immunosuppressive treatment anti-GBM antibodies usually disappear from the blood by ten weeks and remain undetectable [113, 114]; recurrences of the disease are unusual. The prognosis of anti-GBM antibody-mediated disease (Goodpasture's syndrome and crescentic GN) is indicated by the combined results of seven recent reports representing 202 cases with azotemia: 27% of patients improved or stabilized without dialysis, 57% had end stage renal disease and 16% died; early deaths were mostly caused by pulmonary hemorrhage and late deaths by infection associated with the treatment [2, 9, 111, 113, 114, 116, 117].

Complications of Nephrotic Diseases

Rapid progression of underlying disease
The various diseases in this category (Table 11.12) do not have specific therapy and should be managed with general measures for chronic renal failure as discussed in Chapter 17. Two exceptions are diabetic nephropathy and light chain deposition disease.

Diabetic Nephropathy. In order to slow the progression of renal disease, patients with this condition should be treated with *captopril*, 25 mg three times a day, regardless of whether they have hypertension [120]. Once a day angiotensin converting enzyme (ACE) inhibitors are also likely to be effective, but they have not been studied. For control of hypertension one may use higher captopril doses, or add diuretics or calcium channel blockers. Hyperkalemia may be a complication of either diabetic nephropathy or ACE inhibitors, and should be managed with a low potassium diet. Note that serum potassium levels over 5.5 mEq/L are a contraindication to ACE inhibitor therapy.

Light Chain Deposition Disease. Patients with this condition have either an asymptomatic monoclonal gammopathy or multiple myeloma. The latter cases should be treated for myeloma by a specialist in hematology or oncology. Individuals without multiple myeloma but with Scr less than 4 mg/dl should also be treated as if they had myeloma with *melphalan* and *prednisone* in a cyclic fashion. Treatment can be stopped if the monoclonal light chain disappears from the urine, if the renal failure progresses to end stage, or at the end of two years there is no improvement.

Individuals with Scr less than 4 mg/dl at presentation often stabilize or even improve their renal function, compared with untreated patients who usually require dialysis within one to two years [121, 122]. Patients with Scr higher than 4 mg/dl at presentation typically progress to end stage renal failure despite treatment [122]. Patients with multiple myeloma often die of its complications, while other patients may succumb to light chain deposition of the heart or other organs [121–123].

Sequela of the nephrotic pathophysiology

Tubulointerstitial Nephritis in Lipoid Nephrosis. This complication also occurs in focal segmental glomerulosclerosis and IgM nephropathy. Edema may be managed with *diuretics* and a diet restricted to 2g (88 mEq) of sodium per day. A high dosage of furosemide or combination with a thiazide is often necessary, since both nephrotic syndrome and low GFR produce resistance to diuretics. Because of malabsorption caused by bowel edema, intravenous furosemide may be necessary in patients with anasarca. The underlying glomerular disease should be treated with *oral prednisone*, 60 mg per day (for administration and adverse effects of oral prednisone see above – *Idiopathic Crescentic GN*). When the proteinuria disappears, the drug should be gradually switched to an alternate-day schedule, tapered and discontinued over about two months. If there is a partial remission of the proteinuria, the physician may also gradually stop the prednisone after eight weeks of treatment at the full dosage. For patients with continued nephrotic syndrome at the end of eight weeks, prednisone may be continued at full dosage for a total of four months followed by gradual discontinuation over two months [124–127]. Treatment beyond six months may produce a remission in rare cases [126, 127], but is probably not justified given the adverse effects of corticosteroids. Patients with intolerable adverse effects or lack of response to corticosteroids, may be given a trial of *chlorambucil* [128] or *cyclophosphamide* [125, 129, 130].

About 80% of patients will experience a remission of the nephrotic syndrome and acute renal failure over one to five weeks [131, 132]. Most of the remaining individuals have irreversible renal failure and will require renal replacement therapy.

Hypovolemia from Severe Hypoalbuminemia. Hypotension in this situation is likely to be multifactorial with hypoalbuminemia, excess diuretics, gastrointestinal fluid loss, sepsis or other mechanisms contributing in various cases. Management must be tailored to the specific causes in each patient. Volume repletion with *normal saline* is appropriate, especially when fluid losses have eliminated most or all the nephrotic edema. On the other hand, the need for volume repletion is not clear in the hypotensive nephrotic patient with massive edema. *Albumin* infusions, in one or repeated 25g doses, may be used in such patients as a way to draw in interstitial fluid and refill the vascular tree. This is a temporary measure, since the administered albumin will be lost in the urine over a day or so. In cases with poorly understood hypotension, consideration should be given to placing a Swan-Ganz catheter, and making a hemodynamic diagnosis of the low blood pressure.

Renal Vein Thrombosis. (See above at end of the Vascular Causes part of this chapter.)

REFERENCES

1. Weusten B, Jacobs JWG and Bijlsma JWJ. Complications of corticosteroid pulse therapy in rheumatoid arthritis. Br J Rheumatol 1992; 31:S2:125.
2. Bolton KW and Sturgill BC. Methylprednisolone therapy for acute crescentic rapidly progressive glomerulonephritis. Am J Nephrol 1989; 9:368–75.
3. Ballow JE. Complications of therapy. In: Boumpas DT, moderator. Glucocorticoid therapy for immune mediated diseases: basic and clinical correlates. Ann Intern Med 1993; 119:1205–7.
4. Vervoort GMM, Wetzels JFM, Jansen JLJ, Gerlag PGG, Hoorntje SJ, Assmann KJM and Berden JHM. Factors determining therapeutic response and long-term outcome in patients with extracapillary glomerulonephritis. Kidney Int 1988; 33:1035.
5. Glassock RJ. Intensive plasma exchange in crescentic glomerulonephritis: help or no help? Am J Kidney Dis 1992; 20:270–5.
6. Levine JS, Lieberthal W, Bernard DB and Salant DJ. Acute renal failure associated with renal vascular disease, vasculitis, glomerulonephritis, and nephrotic syndrome. In: Lazarus JM, Brenner BM, editors. Acute renal failure. Churchill Livingstone, New York, 1993:3rd ed., 247–355.
7. Glockner WM, Sieberth HG, Wichmann HE, Backes E, Bambauer R, Boesken WH et al. Plasma exchange and immunosuppression in rapidly progressive glomerulonephritis: a controlled, multi-center study. Clin Nephrol 1988; 29:1–8.
8. Bruns FJ, Adler S, Fraley DS and Segel DP. Long-term follow-up of aggressively treated idiopathic rapidly progressive glomerulonephritis. Am J Med 1989; 86:400–6.
9. Keller F, Oehlenberg B, Kunzendorf U, Schwarz A and Offermann G. Long-term treatment and prognosis of rapidly progressive glomerulonephritis. Clin Nephrol 1989; 31:190–7.
10. Cole E, Cattran D, Magil A, Greenwood C, Churchill D, Sutton D et al. A prospective randomized trial of plasma exchange as additive therapy in idiopathic crescentic glomerulonephritis. Am J Kidney Dis 1992; 20:261–9.
11. Nicholls KM, Fairley KF, Dowling JP and Kincaid-Smith P. The clinical course of mesangial IgA associated nephropathy in adults. Quart J Med 1984; 53:227–50.
12. Wyatt RJ, Julian BA, Bhathena DB, Mitchell BL, Holland NH and Malluche HH. IgA nephropathy: presentation, clinical course, and prognosis in children and adults. Am J Kidney Dis 1984; 4:192–200.
13. Rodicio JL. Idiopathic IgA nephropathy. Kidney Int 1984; 25:717–29.
14. Clarkson AR, Seymour AE, Thompson AJ, Haynes WDG, Chan Y-L and Jackson B. IgA nephropathy: a syndrome of uniform morphology, diverse clinical features and uncertain prognosis. Clin Nephrol 1977; 8:459–71.
15. Praga M, Gutierrez-Millet V, Navas JJ, Ruilope LM, Morales JM, Alcazar JM, Bello I and Rodicio JL. Acute worsening of renal function during episodes of macroscopic hematuria in IgA nephropathy. Kidney Int 1985; 28:69–74.
16. Hill PA, Davies DJ, Kincaid-Smith P and Ryan GB. Ultrastructural changes in renal tubules associated with glomerular bleeding. Kidney Int 1989; 36:992–7.
17. Abuelo, JG, Esparza AR, Matarese RA. Endreny RG, Carvalho JS and Allegra SR. Crescentic IgA nephropathy. Medicine 1984; 63:396–406.
18. Welch TR, McAdams J and Berry A. Rapidly progressive IgA nephropathy. Am J Dis Child 1988; 142:789–93.
19. Morrin PAF, Hinglais N, Nabarra B and Kreis H. Rapidly progressive glomerulonephritis. Am J Med 1978; 65:446–60.
20. Hirsch DJ, Jindal KK, Trillo A and Cohen AD. Acute renal failure in Crohn's disease due to IgA nephropathy. Am J Kidney Dis 1992; 20:189–90.
21. Mousa DH, Al-Sulaiman MH and Al-Khader AA. Crescentic glomerulonephritis secondary to IgA nephropathy treated with plasma exchange. Saudi Kidney Dis and Transplant Bull 1993; 4:234–7.
22. D'Amico G and Ferrario F. Mesangiocapillary glomerulonephritis. J Am Soc Nephrol 1992; 2:S159–S166.
23. Ferraris JR, Gallo GE, Ramirez J, Iotti R and Gianantonio C. "Pulse" methylprednisolone therapy in the treatment of acute crescentic glomerulonephritis. Nephron 1983; 34:207–8.
24. Beaufils M, Morel-Maroger L, Sraer J-D, Kanfer A, Kourilsky O and Richet G. Acute renal failure of glomerular origin during visceral abscesses. N Engl J Med 1976; 295:185–9.
25. Rifkinson-Mann, Rifkinson N and Leong T. Shunt nephritis. J Neurosurg 1991; 74:656–9.
26. Melby PC, Musick WD, Luger AM and Khanna R. Poststreptococcal glomerulonephritis in the elderly. Am J Nephrol 1987; 7:235–40.
27. Neild GH, Cameron JS, Ogg CS, Turner DR, Williams DG, Brown CB et al. Rapidly progressive glomerulonephritis with extensive glomerular crescent formation. Quart J Med 1983; 52:395–416.
28. Rovzar MA, Logan JL, Ogden DA and Graham AR. Immunosuppressive therapy and plasmapheresis in rapidly progressive glomerulonephritis association with bacterial endocarditis. Am J Kidney Dis 1986; 7:428–33.
29. McKinsey DS, McMurray TI and Flynn JM. Immune complex glomerulonephritis associated with Staphylococcus aureus bacteremia: response to corticosteroid therapy. Rev Infect Dis 1990; 12:125–7.

29a. Keller CK, Andrassy K, Waldherr R and Ritz E. Postinfectious glomerulonephritis – is there a link to alcoholism? Quart J Med 1994; 87:97–102.

30. Nissenson AR, Baraff LJ, Fine RN and Knutson DW. Poststreptococcal acute glomerulonephritis: fact and controversy. Ann Intern Med 1979; 91:76–86.

31. Lien JWK, Mathew TH and Meadows R. Acute poststreptococcal glomerulonephritis in adults: A long-term study. Quart J Med 1979; 48:99–111.

32. Vogl W, Renke M, Mayer-Eichberger D, Schmitt H and Bohle A. Long-term prognosis for endocapillary glomerulonephritis of poststreptococcal type in children and adults. Nephron 1986; 44:58–65.

33. Ferrario F, Kourilsky O and Morel-Maroger L. Acute endocapillary glomerulonephritis in adults: a histologic and clinical comparison between patients with and without initial acute renal failure. Clin Nephrol 1983; 19:17–23.

34. Chugh KS, Malhotra HS, Sakhuja V, Bhusnurmath S, Singhal PC, Unni VN et al. Progression to end stage renal disease in post-streptococcal glomerulonephritis (PSGN) – Chandigarh Study. Int J Artif Org 1987; 10:189–94.

35. Hinglais N, Garcia-Torres R and Kleinknecht D. Long-term prognosis in acute glomerulonephritis. Am J Med 1974; 56:52–60.

36. A clinico-pathologic study of crescentic glomerulonephritis in 50 children. A report of the Southwest Pediatric Nephrology Study Group. Kidney Int 1985; 27:450–8.

37. Dajan AS, Bisno AL, Chung KJ et al. Prevention of bacterial endocarditis: recommendations of the American Heart Association. JAMA 1990; 264:2919–2.

38. Simmons NA. Antibiotic prophylaxis and infective endocarditis. Lancet 1992; 339:1292–3.

39. Neugarten J, Gallo GR and Baldwin DS. Glomerulonephritis in bacterial endocarditis. Am J Kidney Dis 1984; 3:371–9.

40. Narchi H, Taylor R, Azmy AF, Murphy AV and Beattie TJ. Shunt nephritis. J Pedi Surg 1988; 23:839–41.

41. Arze RS, Rashid H, Morley R, Ward MK and Kerr DNS. Shunt nephritis: report of two cases and review of the literature. Clin Nephrol 1983; 19:48–53.

42. Patrono C and Pierucci A. Renal effects of nonsteroidal anti-inflammatory drugs in chronic glomerular disease. Am J Med 1986; 81 (suppl 2B):71–83.

43. Kimberly RP, Bowden RE, Keiser HR and Plotz PH. Reduction of renal function by newer nonsteroidal anti-inflammatory drugs. Am J Med 1978; 64:804–7.

44. Schwartz MM, Kawala K, Roberts JL, Humes C and Lewis EJ. Clinical and pathological features of membranous glomerulonephritis of systemic lupus erythematosus. Am J Nephrol 1984; 4:301–11.

45. Pasquali S, Banfi G, Zucchelli A, Moroni G, Ponticelli C and Zucchelli P. Lupus membranous nephropathy: long-term outcome. Clin Nephrol 1993; 39:175–82.

46. Pollak VE, Pirani CL and Schwartz FD. The natural history of the renal manifestations of systemic lupus erythematosus. J Lab and Clin Med 1964; 63:537–50.

47. Cathcart ES, Scheinberg MA, Idelson BA and Couser WG. Beneficial effects of methylprednisolone "pulse" therapy in diffuse proliferative lupus nephritis. Lancet 1976; i:163–6.

48. Kimberly RP, Lockshin MD, Sherman RL, McDougal JS, Inman RD and Christian CL. High-dose intravenous methylprednisolone pulse therapy in systemic lupus erythematosus. Am J Med 1981; 70:817–24.

49. Ponticelli C, Zucchelli P, Moroni G, Cagnoli L, Banfi G and Pasquali S. Long-term prognosis of diffuse lupus nephritis. Clin Nephrol 1987; 28:263–71.

50. Barron KS, Brewer EJ Jr., Beale MG and Robson AM. Pulse methylprednisolone therapy in diffuse proliferative lupus nephritis. J Pediatr 1982; 101:137–41.

51. Mackworth-Young CG, David J, Morgan SH and Hughes GRV. A double blind, placebo controlled trial of intravenous methylprednisolone in systemic lupus erythematosus. Ann Rheum Dis 1988; 47:496–502.

52. Donadio JV Jr., Holley KE, Ferguson RH and Ilstrup DM. Progressive lupus glomerulonephritis. Treatment with prednisone and combined prednisone and cyclophosphamide. Mayo Clin Proc 1976; 51:484–94.

53. McCune WJ, Golbus J, Zeldes W, Bohlke P, Dunne R and Fox DA. Clinical and immunologic effects of monthly administration of intravenous cyclophosphamide in severe systemic lupus erythematosus. N Engl J Med 1988; 318:1423–31.

54. Donadio JV Jr. and Glassock RJ. Immunosuppressive drug therapy in lupus nephritis. Am J Kidney Dis 1993; 21:239–50.

55. Austin HA III, Klippel JH, Balow JE, Le Riche NGH, Steinberg AD, Plotz PH et al. Therapy of lupus nephritis. Controlled trial of prednisone and cytotoxic drugs. N Engl J Med 1986; 314:614–9.

56. Carette S, Klippel JH, Decker JL, Austin HA, Plotz PH, Steinberg AD et al. Controlled studies of oral immunosuppressive drugs in lupus nephritis. A long-term follow-up. Ann Intern Med 1983; 99:1–8.

57. Boumpas DT, Austin HA III, Vaughn EM, Klippel JH, Steinberg AD, Yarboro CH and Balow JE. Controlled trial of pulse methylprednisolone versus two regimens of pulse cyclophosphamide in severe lupus nephritis. Lancet 1992; 340:741–5.

58. Lin C-Y, Hsu H-C and Chiang H. Improvement of histological and immunological change in steroid and immunosuppressive drug-resistant lupus nephritis by high-dose intravenous gamma globulin. Nephron 1989; 53:303–10.

59. Kimberly RP, Lockshin MD, Sherman RL, Mouradian J and Saal S. Reversible "end-stage" lupus nephritis. Analysis of patients able to discontinue dialysis. Am J Med 1983; 74:361–8.

60. Coplon NS, Diskin CJ, Petersen J and Swenson RS. The long-term clinical course of systemic lupus erythematosus in end-stage renal disease. N Engl J Med 1983; 308:186–90.

61. Correia P, Cameron JS, Ogg CS, Williams DG, Bewick M and Hicks JA. End-stage renal failure in systemic lupus erythematosus with nephritis. Clin Nephrol 1984; 22:293–302.

62. Steinberg AD and Steinberg SC. Long-term preservation of renal function in patients with lupus nephritis receiving treatment that includes cyclophosphamide versus those

treated with prednisone only. Arth Rheum 1991; 34:945–50.

63. Ponticelli C and Banfi G. Systemic lupus erythematosus (clinical). In: Cameron S, Davison AM, Grunfeld J-P, Kerr D and Ritz E, editors. Oxford textbook of clinical nephrology. Oxford University Press, Oxford, 1992; 646–67.

64. Wallace DJ. A critique of the NIH lupus nephritis survey. Arth Rheum 1992; 35:605.

65. Dinant HJ, Decker JL, Klippel JH, Balow JE, Plotz PH and Steinberg AD. Alternative modes of cyclophosphamide and azathioprine therapy in lupus nephritis. Ann Intern Med 1982; 96:728–36.

66. Felson DT and Anderson J. Evidence for the superiority of immunosuppressive drugs and prednisone over prednisone alone in lupus nephritis. Results of a pooled analysis. N Engl J Med 1984; 311:1528–33.

67. Esdaile JM, Levinton C, Federgreen W, Hayslett JP and Kashgarian M. The clinical and renal biopsy predictors of long-term outcome in lupus nephritis: a study of 87 patients and review of the literature. Quart J Med 1989; 72:779–833.

68. Neumann K, Wallace DJ and Klinenberg JR. Influence of clinical variables, biopsy and treatment on the outcome of 150 patients with lupus nephritis seen at a single center in the 1980s. Arth Rheum 1993; 36:5229.

69. Ponticelli C, Zucchelli P, Banfi G, Cagnoli L, Scalia P, Pasquali S et al. Treatment of diffuse proliferative lupus nephritis by intravenous high-dose methylprednisolone. Quart J Med 1982; 51:16–24.

70. Kimberly RP, Lockshin MD, Sherman RL, Beary JF, Mouradian J and Cheigh JS. "End-stage" lupus nephritis: clinical course to and outcome on dialysis. Medicine 1981; 60:277–87.

71. Magil AB, Ballon HS, Chan V, Lirenman DS, Rae A and Sutton RAL. Diffuse proliferative glomerulonephritis. Determination of prognostic significance of clinical, laboratory and pathologic factors. Medicine 1984; 63:210.

72. Falk RJ, Hogan S, Carey TS, Jennette C and The Glomerular Disease Collaborative Network. Clinical course of anti-neutrophil cytoplasmic autoantibody-associated glomerulonephritis and systemic vasculitis. Ann Intern Med 1990; 113:656–63.

73. Droz D, Noel LH, Leibowitch M and Barbanel C. Glomerulonephritis and necrotizing angiitis. Adv Nephrol 1979; 8:343–63.

74. Levine JS, Lieberthal W, Bernard DB and Salant DJ. Acute renal failure associated with renal vascular disease, vasculitis, glomerulonephritis, and nephrotic syndrome. In: Lazarus JM and Brenner BM, editors. Acute renal failure. Churchill Livingstone Inc., New York, 1993:3rd ed., 247–355.

75. Hollingworth P, Tyndall ADV, Ansell BM, Platts-Mills T, Gumpel JM, Mertin J and Smith DS. Intensive immunosuppression versus prednisolone in the treatment of connective tissue diseases. Ann Rheum Dis 1982; 41:557–62.

76. Fort JG and Abruzzo JL. Reversal of progressive necrotizing vasculitis with intravenous pulse cyclophosphamide and methylprednisolone. Arth & Rheum 1988; 31:1194–8.

77. Fauci AS, Katz P, Haynes BF and Wolff SM. Cyclophosphamide therapy of severe systemic necrotizing vasculitis. N Engl J Med 1979; 301:235–8.

78. Guillevin L, Fain O, Lhote F, Jarrousse B, Huong DLT, Bussel A and Leon A. Lack of superiority of steroids plus plasma exchange to steroids alone in the treatment of polyarteritis nodosa and Churg-Strauss syndrome. Arth & Rheum 1992; 35:208–15.

79. Mathieson PW, Cobbold PS, Hale G, Clark MR, Oliviera DB, Lockwood CM et al. Monoclonal antibody therapy in systemic vasculitis. N Engl J Med 1990; 323:250–4.

80. Guillevin L, Du LTH, Godeau P, Jais P and Wechsler B. Clinical findings and prognosis of polyarteritis nodosa and Churg-Strauss angiitis: a study in 165 patients. Br J Rheum 1988; 27:258–64.

81. Guillevin L, Jarrousse B, Lok C, Lhote F, Jais JP, Du LTH et al. Longterm followup after treatment of polyarteritis nodosa and Churg-Strauss angiitis with comparison of steroids, plasma exchange and cyclophosphamide to steroids and plasma exchange. A prospective randomized trial of 71 patients. J Rheum 1991; 18:567–74.

82. Cohen RD, Conn DL and Ilstrup DM. Clinical features, prognosis, and response to treatment in polyarteritis. Mayo Clin Proc 1980; 55:146–55.

83. Scott DGI, Bacon PA, Elliott PJ, Tribe CR and Wallington TB. Systemic vasculitis in a district general hospital 1972–1980: clinical and laboratory features, classification and prognosis of 80 cases. Quart J Med 1982; 51:292–311.

84. Pusey CD, Rees AJ, Evans DJ, Peters DK and Lockwood CM. Plasma exchange in focal necrotizing glomerulonephritis without anti-GBM antibodies. Kidney Int 1991; 40:757–63.

85. Guillevin L, Leclercq P, Cohen P, Lhote F, Jarrousse B, Gayraud M et al. Treatment of severe polyarteritis nodosa without HBV infection and Churg-Strauss syndrome: a prospective trial in 57 patients comparing prednisone, pulse cyclophosphamide with and without plasma exchange. Clin Exp Immunol 1993; 93(S1):38.

86. Guillevin L, Lhote F, Leon A, Fauvelle F, Vivitski L and Trepo C. Treatment of polyarteritis nodosa related to hepatitis B virus with short term steroid therapy associated with antiviral agents and plasma exchanges. A prospective trial in 33 patients. J Rheumatol 1993; 20:289–98.

87. Gordon M, Luqmani RA, Adu D, Greaves I, Richards N, Michael J et al. Relapses in patients with a systemic vasculitis. Quart J Med 1993; 86:779–89.

88. Adu D, Howie AJ, Scott DGI, Bacon PA, McGonigle RJS and Michael J. Polyarteritis and the kidney. Quart J Med 1987; 62:221–37.

89. Bindi P, Mougenot B, Mentre F, Noel L-H, Peraldi M-N, Vanhille P et al. Necrotizing crescentic glomerulonephritis without significant immune deposits: a clinical and serological study. Quart J Med 1993; 84:55–68.

90. Hoffman GS, Kerr GS, Leavitt RY, Hallahan CW, Lebovics RS, Travis WD et al. Wegener granulomatosis: an analysis of 158 patients. Ann Intern Med 1992; 116:488–98.

91. Pinching AJ, Lockwood CM, Pussell BA, Rees AJ, Sweny P, Evans DJ et al. Wegener's granulomatosis: observations on 18 patients with severe renal disease. Quart J Med 1983; 52:435–60.

92. Fauci AS, Haynes BF, Katz P and Wolff SM. Wegener's granulomatosis: prospective clinical and therapeutic experi-

ence with 85 patients for 21 years. Ann Intern Med 1983; 98:76-85.

93. Grotz W, Wanner C, Keller E, Bohler J, Peter HH, Rohrbach R et al. Crescentic glomerulonephritis in Wegener's granulomatosis: morphology, therapy, outcome. Clin Nephrol 1991; 35:243-51.

94. Andrassy K, Erb A, Koderisch J, Waldherr R and Ritz E. Wegener's granulomatosis with renal involvement: patient survival and correlations between initial renal function, renal histology, therapy and renal outcome. Clin Nephrol 1991; 35:139-47.

95. Anderson G, Coles ET, Crane M, Douglas AC, Gibbs AR, Geddes DM et al. Wegener's granuloma. A series of 265 British cases seen between 1975 and 1985. A report by a Sub-Committee of the British Thoracic Society Research Committee. Quart J Med 1992; 83:427-38.

96. Roth DA, Wilz DR and Theil GB. Schonlein-Henoch syndrome in adults. Quart J Med 1985; 55:145-52.

97. Austin HA III and Balow JE. Henoch-Schonlein nephritis: prognostic features and the challenge of therapy. Am J Kidney Dis 1983; 2:512-20.

98. Ferraris JR, Gallo GE, Ramirez J, Iotti R and Gianantonio C. "Pulse" methylprednisolone therapy in the treatment of acute crescentic glomerulonephritis. Nephron 1983; 34:207-8.

99. Meadow SR, Glasgow EF, White RHR, Moncrieff MW, Cameron JS, Ogg CS. Schonlein-Henoch nephritis. In: Kincaid-Smith P, Mathew TH and Becker EL, editors. Glomerulonephritis: morphology, natural history, and treatment. John Wiley & Sons, London, 1973:1089-1104.

100. Lee HS, Koh HI, Kim MJ and Rha HY. Henoch-Schonlein nephritis in adults: a clinical and morphological study. Clin Nephrol 1986; 26:125-30.

101. Faull RJ, Aarons I, Woodroffe AJ and Clarkson AR. Adult Henoch-Schonlein nephritis. Aust NZ J Med 1987; 17:396-401.

102. Fogazzi GB, Pasquali S, Moriggi M, Casanova S, Damilano I, Mihatsch MJ et al. Long-term outcome of Schonlein-Henoch nephritis in the adult. Clin Nephrol 1989; 31:60-6.

103. Montagnino G. Reappraisal of the clinical expression of mixed cryoglobulinemia. Springer Semin Immunopathol 1988; 10:1-19.

104. De Vecchi A, Montagnino G, Pozzi C, Tarantino A, Locatelli F and Ponticelli C. Intravenous methylprednisolone pulse therapy in essential mixed cryoglobulinemia nephropathy. Clin Nephrol 1983; 19:221-7.

105. Tarantino A, De Vecchi A, Montagnino G, Imbasciati E, Mihatsch MJ, Zollinger HU et al. Renal disease in essential mixed cryoglobulinaemia. Long term follow-up of 44 patients. Quart J Med 1981; 50:1-30.

106. Valbonesi M. Plasmapheresis in the management of cryoglobulinemia. In: Kasprison DO and MacPherson JL, editors. Therapeutic hemapheresis. CRC Publishers, Boca Raton, 1985; 89-96.

107. Ferri C, Moriconi L, Gremignai G, Migliorini P, Paleologo G, Fosella PV et al. Treatment of the renal involvement in mixed cryoglobulinemia with prolonged plasma exchange. Nephron 1986; 43:246-53.

108. Johnson RJ, Gretch DR, Yamabe H, Hart J, Bacchi CE, Hartwell P et al. Membranoproliferative glomerulonephritis associated with hepatitis C virus infection. N Engl J Med 1993; 328:465-70.

109. Misiani R, Bellavita P, Fenili D, Vicari O, Marchesi D, Sironi PL et al. Interferon alfa-2a therapy in cryoglobulinemia associated with hepatitis C virus. N Engl J Med 1994; 330:751-6.

110. D'Amico G, Colasanti G, Ferrario F and Sinico RA. Renal involvement in essential mixed cryoglobulinemia. Kidney Int 1989; 35:1004-14.

111. Heroday M, Bobrie G, Gouarin C, Grunfeld JP and Noel LH. Anti-GBM disease: predictive value of clinical, histological and serological data. Clin Nephrol 1993; 40:249-55.

112. Donaghy M and Rees AJ. Cigarette smoking and lung haemorrhage in glomerulonephritis caused by autoantibodies to glomerular basement membrane. Lancet 1983; ii:1390-3.

113. Savage COS, Pusey CD, Bowman C, Rees AJ and Lockwood CM. Antiglomerular basement membrane antibody mediated disease in the British Isles 1980-4. Brit Med J 1986; 292:301-4.

114. Johnson JP, Moore J Jr., Austin HA III, Balow JE, Antonovych TT and Wilson CB. Therapy of anti-glomerular basement membrane antibody disease: analysis of prognostic significance of clinical, pathologic and treatment factors. Medicine 1985; 64:219-27.

115. Couser WG. Rapidly progressive glomerulonephritis: classification, pathogenetic mechanisms, and therapy. Am J Kidney Dis 1988; 11:449-64.

116. Heilman RL, Offord KP, Holley KE and Velosa JA. Analysis of risk factors for patient and renal survival in crescentic glomerulonephritis. Am J Kidney Dis 1987; 9:98-107.

117. Walker RG, Scheinkestel C, Becker GJ, Owen JE, Dowling JP and Kincaid-Smith P. Clinical and morphological aspects of the management of crescentic antiglomerular basement membrane antibody (Anti-GBM) nephritis/Goodpasture's syndrome. Quart J Med 1985; 54:75-89.

118. Salvidio G, Garibotto G, Saffioti S and Pontremoli R. Good therapeutical response of Goodpasture's syndrome with severe renal failure. Nephron 1989; 52:285.

119. Praga M, Gutierrez Rodero, Andres A, Oliet A, Lumbreras C, Morales JM, Gutierrez-Millet V and Bello I. Anti-glomerular basement membrane antibody (Anti-GBM) glomerulonephritis (GN): Should patients with renal insufficiency be treated? Kidney Int 1988; 34:297.

120. Lewis EJ, Hunsicker LG, Bain R, Rohde RD, for the Collaborative Study Group. The effect of angiotensin-converting-enzyme inhibition on diabetic nephropathy. N Engl J Med 1993; 329:1456-62.

121. Ganeval D, Noel L-H, Preud'Homme J-L, Droz D and Grunfeld J-P. Light-chain deposition disease: its relation with AL-type amyloidosis. Kidney Int 1984; 26:1-9.

122. Heilman RL, Velosa JA, Holley KE, Offord KP and Kyle RA. Long-term follow-up and response to chemotherapy

in patients with light-chain deposition disease. Am J Kidney Dis 1992; 20:34–41.

123. Buxbaum JN, Chuba JV, Hellman GC, Solomon A and Gallo GR. Monoclonal immunoglobulin deposition disease: light chain and light and heavy chain deposition diseases and their relation to light chain amyloidosis. Ann Intern Med 1990; 112:455–64.

124. Pei Y, Cattran D, Delmore T, Katz A, Lang A and Rance P. Evidence suggesting under-treatment in adults with idiopathic focal segmental glomerulosclerosis. Am J Med 1987; 82:938–44.

125. Nolasco F, Cameron JS, Heywood EF, Hicks J, Ogg C and Williams DG. Adult-onset minimal change nephrotic syndrome: a long-term follow-up. Kidney Int 1986; 29:1215–23.

126. Korbet SM, Schwartz MM and Lewis EJ. Minimal-change glomerulopathy of adulthood. Am J Nephrol 1988; 8:291–7.

127. Banfi G, Moriggi M, Sabadini E, Fellin G, D'Amico G and Ponticelli C. The impact of prolonged immunosuppression on the outcome of idiopathic focal-segmental glomerulosclerosis with nephrotic syndrome in adults. A collaborative retrospective study. Clin Nephrol 1991; 36:53–9.

128. Williams SA, Makker SP, Ingelfinger JR and Grupe WE. Long-term evaluation of chlorambucil plus prednisone in the idiopathic nephrotic syndrome in childhood. N Engl J Med 1980; 302:929–33.

129. Geary DF, Farine M, Thorner P and Baumal R. Response to cyclophosphamide in steroid-resistant focal segmental glomerulosclerosis: a reappraisal. Clin Nephrol 1984; 22:109–13.

130. Fujimoto S, Yamamoto Y, Hisanaga S, Morita S, Eto T and Tanaka K. Minimal change nephrotic syndrome in adults: response to corticosteroid therapy and frequency of relapse. Am J Kidney Dis 1991; 17:687–92.

131. Smith JD and Hayslett JP. Reversible renal failure in the nephrotic syndrome. Am J Kidney Dis 1992; 19:201–13.

132. Jennette JC and Falk RJ. Adult minimal change glomerulopathy with acute renal failure. Am J Kidney Dis 1990; 16:432–7.

TUBULAR CAUSES

DOUGLAS SHEMIN

Tubular Cell Necrosis

Acute tubular necrosis due to ischemia
Ischemic ATN occurs in severely ill patients and is a result of sepsis, volume depletion, hypotension, or left ventricular dysfunction. It is generally impossible to prevent, except in the setting of suprarenal aortic reconstructive surgery or coronary artery surgery, when renal ischemia is expected. *Minimization of aortic cross-clamping time* to less than 50 minutes and of *cardiopulmonary bypass time* to less than 160 minutes lowers the risk of renal failure [1, 2]; intraoperative perfusion of the kidneys with hypothermic irrigant has also been shown to be protective in these settings [3]. Prophylactic therapy with mannitol [4], atrial natriuretic factor [5], and calcium antagonists [6] have been demonstrated to be helpful in averting ischemic renal failure in experimental models, but the benefit of these agents has not been shown to be clinically effective. From a practical standpoint, *maintenance of intravascular volume*, with intravenous saline if necessary, should precede aortic or renal vascular surgery, or any major surgery, for that matter, and *potential nephrotoxins should be avoided.*

Treatment of ischemic acute tubular necrosis is supportive, involving the management of acute renal failure (Chapter 16) and the treatment of any underlying and contributory infection, volume depletion, anemia, hypotension, and left ventricular dysfunction. When renal failure is accompanied by oligoanuria, the volume status should be assessed, and *hypovolemia should be corrected* with intravenous saline. Once any hypovolemia has been corrected, there is some clinical evidence that *high doses of intravenous loop diuretics* (400 to 1000 mg/day of furosemide, as a continuous infusion or in divided doses) and *low doses of constant infusion dopamine* (1–3 mcg/kg/min), either singly or in combination, may convert patients to a nonoliguric state, with a urine flow of more than 1500 cc/day [7–10]. If the output rises, furosemide should be continued for 48 to 72 hours. Dopamine only seems to have an effect and should only be initiated within the *first 24 hours of oliguria*; if after 24 hours of therapy there is no clinical response it should be withdrawn. Dopamine and diuretics appear only to increase renal sodium and water excretion and do not improve GFR. However, patients with a high urine output are less likely to become fluid overloaded when given intravenous medications, and enteral or parenteral nutrition; there is also a lower risk of hyperkalemia.

Now that dialysis is readily available, patients with acute tubular necrosis no longer die of renal failure, but of the precipitating illness and its complications. Therefore, prognosis, both for renal improvement and for survival, is dependent upon underlying clinical conditions. Mortality in renal failure attributed to renal hypoperfusion ranges from 25 to 75 percent [11–14], with prognosis poorest in cardiogenic shock and sepsis. In patients who survive, chronic renal failure requiring maintenance dialysis is uncommon, occurring in less than 5% of patients [14]. Even in severe ischemic injury when dialytic support for up to two months is necessary, most patients recover enough renal function to eventually discontinue dialysis, although residual renal insufficiency is common [15].

Acute tubular necrosis due to exogenous toxins

Aminoglycosides. Nephrotoxicity is to some extent, of course, preventible with judicious use of these agents; they should be discontinued if bacterial cultures and sensitivity testing do not justify their use. Prolonged therapy should be discouraged if possible; almost half of all patients treated for more than two weeks develop renal failure [16].

Two studies support the notion that gentamicin or tobramycin *trough levels of above 2.0 mg/L* predict nephrotoxicity [17, 18], and one study associates high peak levels with renal failure [19]; but as aminoglycosides are handled, like inulin, principally via glomerular filtration, it is possible that high levels are a result rather than a cause of renal failure [20]. A recent large study showed no correlation between nephrotoxicity and either peak or trough levels [16].

A number of *formulae* have been devised to calculate aminoglycoside dose alterations in renal insufficiency, using the serum creatinine as a measure of renal function. These formulae are inaccurate if the Scr is unstable or if it overestimates the GFR, as in advanced age or decreased muscle mass. In those circumstances, frequent measurements of aminoglycoside levels and dose adjustments are necessary. In some studies, single daily doses have been shown to have less nephrotoxicity than thrice daily dosing, and to have equal clinical efficacy [21, 22].

It is generally accepted that in order to prevent aminoglycoside induced renal failure, *volume depletion should be corrected* and the *use of other nephrotoxins avoided.*

There is experimental evidence that prevention of potassium and magnesium depletion and administration of polyamino acids, particularly polyaspartic acid, decrease the risk of nephrotoxicity [23–25]. This has not been studied in human subjects.

Treatment of aminoglycoside-induced acute tubular necrosis is supportive. If aminoglycoside concentrations are in the toxic range, the drugs should be held until the levels fall. Then, the dose interval should be prolonged. In most patients who develop renal failure, aminoglycosides are discontinued, although there is experimental evidence that renal function will spontaneously improve even with continued administration of the drug [26]. The overall renal prognosis in aminoglycoside nephrotoxicity is quite good, probably because of the regenerative capacity of the renal tubular cell. [25] In a large study, only one of fifty patients with acute aminoglycoside-induced renal failure did not recover renal function [16].

Amphotericin B. Nephrotoxicity can be prevented by a number of measures. First, since toxicity is dose related, the minimal effective dose should be used. Early studies suggested that a total dose of more than 4000 mg led to renal failure in most patients [27]. In a later study, a daily dose of greater than 0.6 mg/kg/day markedly increased the risk of renal failure [28]. Concomitant volume depletion and use of diuretics also increased the risk [28]. Both one to two liters of *intravenous saline* prior to each amphotericin dose, or a *high sodium diet* (150–300 mEq/day) during therapy have been shown to be effective in preventing renal failure [29, 30].

There is some evidence that amphotericin B, when administered incorporated in phospholipid vesicles, may be less nephrotoxic, but this formulation is currently not commercially available [31].

Treatment of amphotericin-induced renal failure is primarily supportive. Renal prognosis is dose-dependent, with irreversible renal failure tending to occur with total doses of 5000 mg or greater [27]. In one study of fifty patients receiving less than a total dose of 4000 mg amphotericin, renal function was not significantly impaired two months after treatment [32]. There is evidence that renal failure is reversible if amphotericin is discontinued [33] and volume deficits are restored [29].

Cisplatin. Nephrotoxicity is dose dependent, and the incidence increases in patients receiving doses above 2 mg/kg or 75 mg/m^2 [34]. To help prevent nephrotoxicity, *high urine flows* should be induced *with intravenous saline* at a dose of 200 cc/hour for the 12 hours prior to treatment and the 24 hours afterwards. The drug itself should be diluted in a two liter solution of 0.45% saline, with 18 grams mannitol/L [34].

> Concurrent administration of *probenecid*, at a dose of one gram every six hours for a 48 hour period surrounding the cisplatin dose, has been shown to decrease the risk of platinum nephrotoxicity; the mechanism is due to inhibition of tubular secretion of platinum [35]. *Thiosulfate*, at a dose of 3.3 g/m^2 prior to cisplatin and 6.6 g/m^2 afterwards, has also been shown to decrease nephrotoxicity in a clinical setting [34]. Neither of these agents have gained acceptance to date. Atrial natriuretic factor analogs [36] and adenosine antagonists [37] have prevented cisplatin nephrotoxicity experimentally.

Treatment is supportive, and most patients recover renal function, especially when concomitant volume expansion is prescribed.

The long term prognosis is to a great extent dependent upon dose. In one group of patients treated with a mean dose of 450 mg/m^2, GFR dropped in 17 of 22 patients and dropped by a mean of 17% overall; these decreases were sustained one year after treatment [38]. In a review of a number of series of patients receiving lower cumulative doses, the incidence of persistent renal failure ranged from 10 to 20% [39].

Acute tubular necrosis due to myoglobin

Most patients with myoglobinuric renal failure present to medical attention after rhabdomyolysis has occurred. Nevertheless, there is evidence that some prophylactic measures may prevent the development of renal failure in the setting of severe muscle injury. Early infusions of hypertonic *mannitol* will shift fluid from cells to the intravascular volume, and may decrease intracompartmental pressure and prevent muscle damage [40]. Because myoglobin is less soluble and dissociates to nephrotoxic metabolites at a maximally acidic urine pH, and because low urine flow rates will in-

crease the risks of myoglobin-induced tubular damage, early *treatment with an intravenous isotonic saline-bicarbonate solution* may prevent renal failure. Systemic alkalinization will also protect against hyperkalemia. In a study of patients trapped in collapsed buildings with severe crush injuries, immediate administration of intravenous saline even before extrication from the collapsed buildings, followed by a saline/bicarbonate infusion containing mannitol, prevented myoglobinuric renal failure even in patients with severe rhabdomyolysis [41]. Experience indicates that about twelve liters of intravenous saline-bicarbonate solution per day is optimal; this is ideally administered as 0.45% saline with a 50 mEq ampule of NaHCO3 added to each liter, at a rate of 500 cc/hour for a 72 hour period. Mannitol, at a dose of ten gms/L, has been suggested if diuresis is less than 300 cc/hour; this requires caution and close monitoring, as there is an obvious risk of administering high doses of intravenous fluid or mannitol in oliguria. If volume overload develops, alkalinizing fluids and mannitol should be discontinued and intravenous loop diuretics should be given.

If myoglobinuric renal failure does occur despite attempts at prevention, treatment is primarily supportive. In nonoliguric states, intravenous saline and bicarbonate should be administered as above, with close attention to fluid balance. In oliguria, diuretics may be administered in an attempt to convert to a nonoliguric state, but *hemodialysis and ultrafiltration* should be immediately available in case of refractory volume overload. Similarly, cation exchange resins (Kayexalate) may be used to treat hyperkalemia, but dialysis is the second line of therapy. *Beta agonists and insulin*, which shift potassium intracellularly, may be less effective with the diffuse loss of muscle cell membrane integrity that occurs with rhabdomyolysis [42]; beta agonists in excess dosage have actually been implicated as a cause of rhabdomyolysis and myoglobinuria [43].

Hypocalcemia in the syndrome is due to hyperphosphatemia and influx of calcium into damaged muscle cells, and does not reflect total body calcium depletion. Hypocalcemia should not be treated with calcium unless tetany, cardiac arrhythmias, or QT prolongation is present. Exogenously infused calcium may enter muscle cells, worsening rhabdomyolysis [40, 42]. Oral phosphate binders (aluminum hydroxide, with an initial dose of 30 cc three times daily) should be used for severe hyperphosphatemia [42].

The prognosis of myoglobinuric acute renal failure is fairly good. Permanent renal failure or death occurs in less than ten percent of patients in some series [44–46]. The prognosis worsens in the setting of multiple comorbid conditions, however. Mortality reached 40% in a series of patients in which myoglobinuric renal failure was complicated by multiple factors such as burns, sepsis, and systemic hypotension [47].

Tubular Obstruction

Tubular obstruction due to light chains (myeloma kidney)
It is generally not possible to prevent the development of intratubular obstruction and acute renal failure in multiple myeloma, since a majority of patients will present with renal failure as an initial symptom of myeloma kidney [48, 49]. Volume depletion, hypercalcemia, and infection have been shown to exacerbate azotemia [50], and as part of a general attempt to improve renal function, volume deficits should be intravenously replaced, infection diagnosed and treated, and hyperuricemia and hypercalcemia identified and corrected. The use of intravenous bicarbonate to alkalinize the urine is of uncertain efficacy and is not recommended [51]. Radiocontrast agents have been linked to renal failure in myeloma kidney, and an attempt should be made to minimize exposure to contrast media in patients with myeloma.

The pharmacologic treatment of multiple myeloma is beyond the scope of this chapter, but *melphalan, corticosteroids, vincristine, and cyclophosphamide* in various combinations have been shown to improve renal function in some patients with renal failure due to myeloma [52–54]. *Plasmapheresis* was found to be helpful in one controlled trial and did not improve on standard therapy in another [54, 55]; it is probably best used in patients with large urine light chain concentrations who do not respond to chemotherapy. Colchicine has been shown to prevent light chain cast formation in an experimental model but it has not been tested in a clinical setting [56].

The prognosis for untreated myeloma renal failure is poor; most patients die within one month

[57]. While early data demonstrated only a slightly better course in treated patients, two recent studies have been more optimistic. Renal failure actually resolved in about half of myeloma patients treated with chemotherapy, although renal recovery might have been due in part to the reversal of hypercalcemia and volume depletion [58, 59]. The one year survival rate in treated patients ranges from 25 to 70% [52–55, 58, 60].

Tubular obstruction due to tumor lysis syndrome
The risk of tumor lysis syndrome can be minimized by surgical removal of tumor bulk prior to induction chemotherapy [61]. However, this exposes the patient to the risks of general anesthesia and a surgical procedure unnecessary for tumor eradication given the success of chemotherapy in susceptible non-Hodgkin lymphomas. A more rational treatment involves decreasing uric acid production with the xanthine oxidase inhibitor *allopurinol*, at doses of 600–900 mg. daily for two to three days prior to induction of chemotherapy, followed by a dose of 300 mg daily for a week after induction [62]. Additionally, patients should receive three to four liters of *intravenous saline* daily for one to two days prior to and during chemotherapy to increase urinary tubular flow and prevent intratubular deposition of urate and phosphate. *Alkalinization of the urine* with intravenous sodium bicarbonate will prevent intratubular urate deposits, but *promote intratubular phosphate deposits*; its use is controversial, but indications include the presence of uric acid crystals on urinalysis, metabolic acidosis, hyperkalemia, and serum levels of uric acid above 20 mg/dL [62, 63].

Treatment, apart from ongoing allopurinol and intravenous fluids, is principally directed at *correction of metabolic abnormalities*. The serum potassium level may rise more rapidly than in other forms of renal failure due to cell breakdown. It should be checked frequently and sodium polystyrene sulfate (Kayexalate), at a dose of 30 to 60 gms orally or rectally, should be administered if the level rises above 6.0 mEq/L, especially in the case of oliguria. This dose can be given repeatedly. Intravenous calcium, sodium bicarbonate, and insulin are used if the hyperkalemia is associated with cardiotoxicity (see Chapter 16), but emergency hemodialysis may be necessary as well. Hyperphosphatemia should be treated with aluminum or calcium containing phosphate binders. This generally increases the low serum calcium concentration as well, but patients with tetany, cardiac arrhythmias, or conduction abnormalities due to hypocalcemia should be given intravenous calcium. Patients with renal failure will also have decreased renal synthesis of calcitriol as an additional cause for hypocalcemia and may require treatment with oral or parenteral calcitriol if hypocalcemia is sustained [64].

The prognosis in acute renal failure due to the tumor lysis syndrome is quite good, especially in the context of non-Hodgkin lymphoma; there was universal renal recovery in a recent series [62]. Mortality, whether due to acute renal failure, the underlying neoplastic process, or infectious or hematological complications of chemotherapy, tends to be much greater in tumor lysis syndrome associated with leukemias and solid tumors [65–70].

Intratubular obstruction due to miscellaneous etiologies

Oxalic Acid. It may be possible to prevent acute renal failure due to intratubular oxalate formation in the setting of ethylene glycol overdose, even though patients present after ingestion has occurred. *Gastric lavage*, followed by *activated charcoal and sorbitol* to decrease gastrointestinal absorption of ethylene glycol should be initiated if the patient presents soon after ingestion. The enzymatic breakdown of ethylene glycol to oxalic acid and other toxic metabolites by alcohol dehydrogenase can be prevented by administration of *ethanol*, which has a greater affinity for the enzyme than ethylene glycol. A 0.8 to 1.0 gm/kg loading dose is given, followed by a 80–130 mg/kg/hour continuous intravenous infusion [71, 72]. Target blood ethanol levels should be between 100 and 200 mg/dL. The alcohol dehydrogenase inhibitor *4-methylpyrazole* has been used successfully to prevent acute renal failure in this setting, but it is not yet commercially available in the United States [73].

Metabolic acidosis should be treated with *intravenous sodium bicarbonate*. If ethylene glycol levels rise above 50 mg/dL, metabolic acidosis worsens, or renal failure occurs, *hemodialysis* is necessary. Hemodialysis is quite effective at clearing ethylene glycol and its metabolites, which are water soluble and have low molecular weights. Ethanol should be added to dialysate at a concentration of 100 mg/dL and should be continued intravenously during and after dialysis [72]. Glucose levels should be checked frequently during ethanol infusion.

While fatalities do occur in ethylene glycol overdoses, early aggressive treatment can be expected to lead to a favorable outcome and recovery of renal function, even with massive ingestions [72]. Permanent renal failure can rarely occur [71].

Enteric hyperoxaluria due to fat malabsorption or ileal resection. There is evidence that oxalate absorption and renal oxalate excretion may be partially prevented with the use of a *low fat, low oxalate diet and oral calcium supplements*, at an initial dose of 650 mg three times daily. Induction of high urine volumes with three to four liters of oral fluids daily is recommended [74]. *Reversal of jejunoileal bypass*, in patients treated for morbid obesity, will also reverse hyperoxaluria and has been reported to improve renal failure [75].

Methotrexate Nephrotoxicity. This is generally thought to be prevented by administration of *leucovorin* (48 mg every six hours for ten days following the dose), *maintenance of high urine volumes*, and *urinary alkalinization*, with three to four liters daily of 0.45% saline with 50 mEq NaHCO₃/L [76]. *Nonsteroidal antiinflammatory agents* potentiate methotrexate nephrotoxicity [76–78] and should be avoided.

Treatment is primarily supportive. Methotrexate is cleared more efficiently by hemodialysis than peritoneal dialysis or plasma exchange [79, 80], but neither method clears the drug well, and dialysis is not recommended for methotrexate toxicity.

As acute renal failure due to intratubular obstruction by *sulfonamides*, *triamterene*, and *rifampin* occurs rarely, prevention, treatment, and prognosis of these entities has not been extensively described.

REFERENCES

1. Myers BD, Miller DC, Mehigan JT et al. Nature of the renal injury following total renal ischemia in man. J Clin Invest 1984; 73:329–41.
2. Hilberman M, Myers BD, Carrie BJ et al. Acute renal failure following cardiac surgery. J Thor Cardiovasc Surg 1979; 77:880–8.

3. Svensson LG, Crawford ES, Hess KR et al. Thoracoabdominal aortic aneurysms associated with celiac, superior mesenteric, and renal artery occlusive disease: methods and analysis of results in 271 patients. J Vasc Surg 1992; 16:378–90.

4. Hanley MJ and Davidson K. Prior mannitol and furosemide infusion in a model of ischemic acute renal failure. Am J Physiol 1981; 241:F556–F564.

5. Lieberthal W, Sheridan AM and Valeri CR. Protective effect of atrial natriuretic factor and mannitol following renal ischemia. Am J Physiol 1990; 258:F1266–F1272.

6. Epstein M. Calcium antagonists and renal protection. Arch Intern Med 1992; 152:1573–84.

7. Lindner A. Synergism of dopamine and furosemide in diuretic-resistant, oliguric acute renal failure. Nephron 1983; 33:121–6.

8. Davis RF, Lappas DG, Kirklin JK et al. Acute oliguria after cardiopulmonary bypass: renal functional improvement with low-dose dopamine infusion. Crit Care Med 1982; 10:852–6.

9. Brown CB, Ogg CS and Cameron JS. High dose frusemide in acute renal failure: a controlled trial. Clin Neph 1981; 15:90–6.

10. Graziani G, Cantaluppi A, Casati S et al. Dopamine and frusemide in oliguric acute renal failure. Nephron 1984; 37:39–42.

11. Hou SH, Bushinsky DA, Wish JB et al. Hospital-acquired renal insufficiency: a prospective study. Am J Med 1983; 74:243–48.

12. McMurry SD, Luft FC, Maxwell DR et al. Prevailing patterns and predictor variables in patients with acute tubular necrosis. Arch Intern Med 1978; 138:950–5.

13. Kaufman J, Dhakal M, Patel B et al. Community-acquired acute renal failure. Am J Kidney Dis 1991; 17:191–8.

14. Corwin HL and Bonventre JV. Factors influencing survival in acute renal failure. Sem Dialysis 1989; 2:220–5.

15. Spurney RF, Fulkerson WJ and Schwab SJ. Acute renal failure in critically ill patients: prognosis for recovery of kidney function after prolonged dialysis support. Crit Care Med 1991; 19:8–11.

16. Leehey DJ, Braun BI, Thall DA et al. Can pharmacokinetic dosing decrease nephrotoxicity associated with aminoglycoside therapy? J Am Soc Nephrol 1993; 4:81–90.

17. Jaresko GS, Boucher BA, Dole EJ et al. Risk of renal dysfunction in critically ill trauma patients receiving aminoglycosides. Clin Pharm 1989; 8:43–8.

18. Boucher BA, Coffey BC, Kuhl DA et al. Algorithm for assessing renal dysfunction risk in critically ill trauma patients receiving aminoglycosides. Am J Surg 1990; 160:473–80.

19. Moore RD, Smith CR, Lipsky JJ et al. Risk factors for nephrotoxicity in patients treated with aminoglycosides. Ann Intern Med 1984; 100:352–7.

20. Cronin RE. Aminoglycoside nephrotoxicity: pathogenesis and prevention. Clin Neph 1979; 11:251–6.

21. Prins JM, Buller HR, Kuijper EJ et al. Once versus thrice daily gentamicin in patients with serious infections. Lancet 1993; 341:335–9.

22. Gilbert DN. Once-daily aminoglycoside therapy. Antimicrob Agents Chemother 1991; 35:399–405.

23. Williams RD, Hottendorf GH and Bennett DB. Inhibition of renal membrane binding and nephrotoxicity of aminoglycosides. J Pharm Exp Ther 1986; 237:919–25.

24. Ramsammy LS, Josepovitz C, Lane BP et al. Polyaspartic acid protects against gentamicin toxicity in the rat. J Pharmacol Exp Ther 1989; 250:149–53.

25. Humes HD. Aminoglycoside nephrotoxicity. Kidney Int 1988; 33:900–11.

26. Bennett WM. Aminoglycoside nephrotoxicity. Nephron 1983; 35:73–7.

27. Butler WT, Bennett JE, Alling DW et al. Nephrotoxicity of amphotericin B. Ann Intern Med 1964; 61:175–87.

28. Fisher MA, Talbot GH, Maislin G et al. Risk factors for amphotericin B-associated nephrotoxicity. Am J Med 1989; 87:547–52.

29. Heidemann HT, Gerkens JF, Spickard WA et al. Amphotericin B nephrotoxicity in humans decreased by salt depletion. Am J Med 1983; 75:476–81.

30. Llanos A, Cieza J, Bernardo J et al. Effect of salt supplementation on amphotericin nephrotoxicity. Kidney Int 1991; 40:302–8.

31. Lopez-Berestein G, Bodey GP, Fainstein V et al. Treatment of systemic fungal infections with liposomal amphotericin B. Arch Intern Med 1989; 149:2533–6.

32. Miller RP and Bates JH. Amphotericin B toxicity. Ann Intern Med 1969; 71:1089–95.

33. Sacks P and Fellner S. Recurrent reversible acute renal failure from amphotericin. Arch Intern Med 1987; 147:593–5.

34. Erlanger H and Cutler RE. Cisplatin nephrotoxicity. Dial Transplant 1992; 21:559–66.

35. Jacobs C, Kaubisch S, Halsey J et al. The use of probenicid as a chemoprotector against cisplatinum nephrotoxicity. Cancer 1991; 67:1518–24.

36. Pollock DM, Holst M and Opgenorth TJ. Effect of the ANF analog A68828 in cisplatin-induced acute renal failure. J Pharm Exp Ther 1991; 257:1179–83.

37. Knight RJ, Collis MG, Yates MS et al. Amelioration of cisplatinum-induced acute renal failure with 8-cyclopentyl-1,3-dipropylxanthine. Br J Pharmacol 1991; 104:1062–8.

38. Fjeldborg P, Sorenson J and Helkjaer PE. The long-term effect of cisplatin on renal function. Cancer 1986; 58:2214–7.

39. Madias NE and Harrington JT. Platinum nephrotoxicity. Am J Med 1978; 65:307–14.

40. Better OS and Stein JH. Early management of shock and prophylaxis of acute renal failure in traumatic rhabdomyolysis. N Engl J Med 1990; 322:825–9.

41. Ron D, Taitelman U, Michaelson M et al. Prevention of acute renal failure in traumatic rhabdomyolysis. Arch Intern Med 1984; 144:277–80.

42. Honda N. Acute renal failure and rhabdomyolysis. Kidney Int 1983; 23:888–98.

43. Blake PG and Ryan F. Rhabdomyolysis and acute renal failure after terbutaline overdose. Nephron 1989; 53:76–7.

44. Koffler A, Freidler RM and Massry SG. Acute renal failure due to nontraumatic rhabdomyolysis. Ann Intern Med 1976; 85:23–8.

45. Grossman RA, Hamilton RW, Morse BM et al. Non-

traumatic rhabdomyolysis and acute renal failure. N Engl J Med 1974; 291:807–11.

46. Gabow PA, Kaehny WD and Kelleher SP. The spectrum of rhabdomyolysis. Medicine 1982; 61:141–50.

47. Ward MM. Factors predictive of acute renal failure in rhabdomyolysis. Arch Intern Med 1988; 1553–7.

48. Kyle RA. Multiple myeloma: review of 869 cases. Mayo Clin Proc 1975; 50:29–39.

49. Heilman RL, Velosa JA, Holley KE et al. Long-term follow-up and response to chemotherapy in patients with light-chain deposition disease. Am J Kidney Dis 1992; 20:34–41.

50. Cohen DJ, Sherman WH, Osserman EF et al. Acute renal failure in patients with multiple myeloma. Am J Med 1984; 76:247–56.

51. Smolens P. The kidney in dysproteinemic states. AKF Nephrology Letter 1987; 4:27–42.

52. Misiani R, Tiraboschi G, Mingardi G et al. Management of myeloma kidney: an anti-light chain approach. Am J Kidney Dis 1987; 10:28–33.

53. Rota S, Mougenot B, Baudouin B et al. Multiple myeloma and severe renal failure: a clinicopathologic study of outcome and prognosis in 34 patients. Medicine 1987; 66:126–37.

54. Johnson WJ, Kyle RA, Pineda AA et al. Treatment of renal failure associated with multiple myeloma. Arch Intern Med 1990; 150:863–9.

55. Zucchelli P, Pasquali S, Cagnoli L et al. Controlled plasma exchange trial in acute renal failure due to multiple myeloma. Kidney Int 1988; 33:1175–80.

56. Sanders PW. Myeloma kidney. The Kidney 1993; 4:1–7.

57. Wahlin A, Lofvenberg E and Holm J. Improved survival in multiple myeloma with renal failure. Acta Med Scand 1987; 221:205–9.

58. Pozzi C, Pasquali S and Donini U. Prognostic factors and effectiveness of treatment in acute renal failure due to multiple myeloma: a review of 50 cases. Clin Nephrol 1987; 28:1–9.

59. Alexanian R, Barlogie B and Dixon D. Renal failure in multiple myeloma: pathogenesis and prognostic implications. Arch Intern Med 1990; 150:1693–5.

60. Pasquali S, Casanova S, Zucchelli A et al. Long-term survival patients with acute and severe renal failure due to multiple myeloma. Clin Neph 1990; 34:247–54.

61. Tsokos GC, Balow JE, Spiegel RJ et al. Renal and metabolic complications of undifferentiated and lymphoblastic lymphomas. Medicine 1981; 60:218–29.

62. Hande KR and Garrow GC. Acute tumor lysis syndrome in patients with high-grade non-Hodgkin lymphoma. Am J Med 1993; 94:133–9.

63. Cohen LF, Balow JE, Magrath IT et al. Acute tumor lysis syndrome: a review of 37 patients with Burkitt's lymphoma. Am J Med 1980; 68:486–91.

64. Dunlay RW, Camp MA, Allon M et al. Calcitriol in prolonged hypocalcemia in the tumor lysis syndrome. Ann Intern Med 1989; 110:162–4.

65. Stark ME, Dyer MC and Coonley CJ. Fatal acute tumor lysis syndrome with metastatic breast carcinoma. Cancer 1987; 60:762–4.

66. Dirix LY, Prove A, Becquart D et al. Tumor lysis syndrome in a patient with metastatic Merkel cell carcinoma. Cancer 1991; 67:2207–10.

67. Vogelzang NJ, Nelimark RA and Kath KA. Tumor lysis syndrome after induction chemotherapy of small-cell bronchogenic carcinoma. JAMA 1983; 249:513–4.

68. Vogler WR, Morris JG and Winton EF. Acute tumor lysis in T-cell leukemia induced by amsacrine. Arch Intern Med 1983; 143:165–6.

69. Thomas MR, Robinson WA, Mughal TI et al. Tumor lysis syndrome following VP-16-213 in chronic myeloid leukemia in blast crisis. Am J Hematol 1984; 16:185–8.

70. Fer MF, Bottino GC, Sherwin SA et al. Atypical tumor lysis syndrome in a patient with T cell lymphoma treated with recombinant leukocyte interferon. Am J Med 1984; 77:953–6.

71. Verrilli MR, Deyling CL, Pippenger CE et al. Fatal ethylene glycol intoxication: report of a case and review of the literature. Cleve Clin J Med 1987; 54:289–95.

72. Curtin L, Kraner J, Wine H et al. Complete recovery after massive ethylene glycol ingestion. Arch Intern Med 1992; 152:1311–3.

73. Baud FJ, Galliot M, Astier A et al. Treatment of ethylene glycol poisoning with intravenous 4-methylpyrazole. N Engl J Med 1988; 319:97–100.

74. Williams HE. Oxalic acid and the hyperoxaluric syndromes. Kidney Int 1978; 13:410–7.

75. Ehlers SM, Posalaky Z, Strate RG et al. Acute reversible renal failure following jejuno-ileal bypass for morbid obesity: a clinical and pathological (EM) study of a case. Surgery 1977; 82:629–34.

76. Maiche AG, Lappalainen K and Teerenhovi L. Renal insufficiency in patients treated with high dose methotrexate. Acta Oncol 1988; 27:73–4.

77. Maiche AG. Acute renal failure due to concomitant action of methotrexate and indomethacin. Lancet 1986; 1:1390.

78. Singh RR, Malavita AN, Pandey JN et al. Fatal interaction between methotrexate and naproxen. Lancet 1986; 1:1390.

79. Ahmad S, Shen F and Bleyer WA. Methotrexate-induced renal failure and ineffectiveness of peritoneal dialysis. Arch Intern Med 1978; 138:1146–7.

80. Thierry FX, Vernier I, Dueymes JM et al. Acute renal failure after high-dose methotrexate therapy. Nephron 1989; 51:416–7.

INTERSTITIAL CAUSES

AARON SPITAL

Acute Interstitial Nephritis

The most important step in the management of acute interstitial nephritis is early recognition and, if possible, removal of the underlying cause [1–3]. When this can be achieved, the prognosis for recovery of renal function is good. On the other hand, when diagnosis and treatment are delayed, permanent renal dysfunction may ensue [4–6].

While improvement may occur even after a pro-longed course [4], the chances for complete recovery diminish as the duration of disease increases [1, 2]. Therefore, it is imperative that this frequently reversible condition be considered early in all patients with unexplained acute renal failure.

Drug-induced acute interstitial nephritis

Prevention of drug-induced acute interstitial nephritis is difficult, since there are few known risk factors. Exceptions include: (1) patients who have had a previous episode of drug-induced interstitial nephritis are at risk for recurrence when rechallenged with an agent of the same class [7–9]; (2) patients receiving discontinuous therapy with rifampin [10]; (3) patients with renal insufficiency receiving allopurinol [7, 11]; and (4) possibly elderly people receiving NSAIDs [12]. If possible, these high risk situations should be avoided; when they are unavoidable, the Scr and urinalysis should be followed serially.

When drug-induced acute interstitial nephritis does occur, the most important therapeutic measure is to stop the offending agent [1, 2, 6–9]. Often this is all that is necessary to restore normal renal function. However, in some cases renal dysfunction may persist even after the responsible drug has been discontinued. For these refractory patients, a short course of steroids is recommended [1, 2, 6, 13, 14].

> Although there are no well-done controlled studies which prove that steroids are beneficial in the management of drug-induced interstitial nephritis, the anecdotal evidence supporting their efficacy is strong [1, 2, 6, 13, 14]. There are several reports of patients with persistent renal failure despite discontinuing the suspected responsible medication, who improved dramatically when given a course of steroid therapy. Uncontrolled data suggest that steroids may also hasten the rate of recovery [15]. Presumably these agents act by inhibiting the underlying immunological mechanisms of disease.

Steroids should be considered for biopsy-proven cases of acute interstitial nephritis in the following situations [1, 2, 9, 13]: (1) when renal function does not improve spontaneously within 7 to 10 days of stopping the offending drug; and (2) in severe cases presenting with acute oliguric renal failure.

The optimal dose, route of administration and duration of therapy have yet to be established. Short courses of *oral prednisone* and brief pulses of *intravenous methylprednisolone* [13, 14] have been used successfully, though most experience has been with the oral approach. One commonly recommended regimen is to treat with prednisone at a dose of 1.0 mg/kg/day for up to several weeks, followed by rapid tapering regardless of the outcome [1, 2]. This regimen is generally well tolerated. Improvement usually begins quickly, often within 1 to 2 days. If after two weeks there is no sign of recovery and there is little fibrosis and nephron loss on renal biopsy, *cyclophosphamide* may be considered [1, 2]. However, such therapy may be complicated by alopecia, leukopenia, infection, hemorrhagic cystitis, gonadal toxicity and neoplasia and its use is based solely on limited anecdotal experience. Therefore, when considering cyclophosphamide a careful assessment of the potential risks and benefits should be made.

In general, with appropriate early therapy, the prognosis for recovery from drug-induced interstitial nephritis is quite good, with most patients returning to their previous level of renal function within weeks [6–9, 13, 16]. However, a few patients will be left with residual renal dysfunction despite early diagnosis and treatment.

Acute interstitial nephritis associated with infections

Systemic Infection. There is no way to predict the few patients who will develop interstitial nephritis during the course of a systemic infection and prevention is not possible. Therefore, renal function should be monitored in all systemically infected patients as this will facilitate early recognition of renal involvement.

The most important step in the management of interstitial nephritis due to infection is to treat the underlying disease [1, 13, 17, 18]. In general, if the infectious process resolves, renal function will improve spontaneously and recovery is usually complete. However, on occasion renal dysfunction may persist despite seeming resolution of the causal infection. In a few of these cases, *steroids* have been used successfully [13, 19], though there is much less experience with this approach than in drug-induced disease. In the absence of definitive data and contraindications, it seems reasonable to use the same indications and protocol for steroid therapy for interstitial nephritis secondary to systemic infections as is recommended for drug-induced disease [13].

Acute Pyelonephritis. There is no way to identify those few patients with acute pyelonephritis who, in the absence of sepsis, will develop acute renal failure. Therefore, renal function should be monitored in all cases. The concomitant use of NSAIDs may be a risk factor and should be avoided [20]. When renal failure does occur, therapy is directed primarily at eradicating the bacterial infection with appropriate *antimicrobial agents.* Steroids have no role in this condition. With appropriate treatment renal function improves in most patients, although recovery is often slow and incomplete [20–22]. This has led some to suggest that antibiotic therapy should be prolonged [21].

Acute interstitial nephritis caused by systemic disease

Sarcoidosis. *Steroids* appear to be quite effective in the treatment of granulomatous interstitial nephritis secondary to sarcoidosis. Most patients have been treated with prednisone (or its equivalent) beginning at a dose of 1.0 mg/kg/day [23–25]. The response is often dramatic, with renal function improving within the first several weeks. However, few patients recover completely and the majority are left with residual renal impairment [23, 24, 26]. Prolonged therapy with tapering over several months is recommended to avoid relapses, which are not uncommon; when relapses do occur they often respond to repeat courses of steroids [23, 24].

Other Systemic Diseases. Experience in treating interstitial nephritis secondary to SLE, Sjogren's syndrome and primary biliary cirrhosis is very limited and anecdotal. Nonetheless, *steroids* have been used with success in each of these conditions and are recommended [27–30]. The optimal regimen is unknown, but 1.0 mg/kg/day of prednisone is a frequently used dose. In patients who respond, it may be necessary to continue therapy for several months to maintain optimal renal function. Careful long term follow-up is indicated to detect recurrences early.

Idiopathic acute interstitial nephritis

Although some patients with idiopathic acute interstitial nephritis recover spontaneously, *steroids* appear to be very effective in this condition and are recommended at an initial dose of 1.0 mg/kg/day for patients with and without uveitis [31–35]. Dramatic responses with improved renal function are often seen within the first few weeks following short courses of high dose oral prednisone. In patients presenting with proximal tubular dysfunction, markers such as glycosuria should be monitored during and after therapy, in addition to the Scr and urinalysis. Persistence of such abnormalities signals the need for close observation and perhaps continued therapy, even if the Scr has returned to normal [32].

When treated early the prognosis for most patients is good and many, though not all, recover completely. Even when therapy is delayed, improved renal function may still occur. One patient with initially unrecognized acute interstitial nephritis had a dramatic response to steroids with marked improvement in renal function after several months of dialysis [4]. Occasional patients have relapsed when steroids were withdrawn, yet responded to another course of therapy [31, 32].

Chronic Interstitial Nephritis

Xanthogranulomatous pyelonephritis

In diffuse xanthogranulomatous pyelonephritis, *antibiotics* followed by *nephrectomy* of the diseased kidney is the treatment of choice and is usually curative [36, 37]. In those few cases where the process is focal, a more conservative approach may be taken with limited resection combined with antimicrobial therapy [37, 38].

Renal malacoplakia

Unilateral renal malacoplakia is also treated by *nephrectomy* [39, 40]. However, this process is often bilateral and when it is, there is no satisfactory treatment. There are occasional reports of improvement following prolonged antibiotic therapy, with or without limited renal resection [39, 41–43]. Bethanechol, a cholinergic agonist which increases monocytic cyclic-GMP levels and bactericidal activity, has also been used with some success [38, 42, 44]. Nevertheless, in most of these severely affected patients the prognosis is quite poor and the mortality rate is high [39, 40].

Neoplastic Interstitial Infiltration

When acute renal failure develops as a consequence of neoplastic infiltration of the interstitium, renal *radiation* or appropriate systemic *chemotherapy* often results in a reduction in renal size and a dramatic improvement in renal function, sometimes to normal, within 1 to 4 weeks [45–47]. Nevertheless, because of the usually aggressive nature of the underlying disease, the ultimate prognosis of these patients is poor and most die within several months [45, 47].

REFERENCES

1. Clayman MD and Neilson EG. Acute tubulointerstitial nephropathy. Curr Ther Allergy Immunol Rheumatol 1985; 2:197–201.
2. Neilson EG. Pathogenesis and therapy of interstitial nephritis. Kidney Int 1989; 35:1257–70.
3. Ten RM, Torres VE, Milliner DS, Schwab TR, Holley KE and Gleich GJ. Acute interstitial nephritis: immunologic and clinical aspects. Mayo Clin Proc 1988; 63:921–30.
4. Frommer P, Uldall R, Fay WP and Deveber GA. A case of acute interstitial nephritis successfully treated after delayed diagnosis. Can Med Assoc J 1979; 121:585–91.
5. Kida H, Abe T, Tomosugi N, Koshino Y, Yokoyama H and Hattori N. Prediction of the long-term outcome in acute interstitial nephritis. Clin Nephrol 1984; 22:55–60.
6. Linton AL, Clark WF, Driedger AA, Turnbull DI and Lindsay RM. Acute interstitial nephritis due to drugs. Ann Intern Med 1980; 93:735–41.
7. Appel GB and Kunis CL. Acute tubulo-interstitial nephritis. In: Cotran RS, Brenner BM and Stein JH, editors. Tubulo-interstitial nephropathies. Churchill Livingstone, New York, 1983; 151–85.
8. Grunfeld JP, Kleinknecht D and Droz D. Acute interstitial nephritis. In: Schrier RW and Gottschalk C, editors. Diseases of the kidney. Little, Brown and Company, Boston, 1993; 1331–53.
9. Toto RD. Review: acute tubulointerstitial nephritis. Am J Med Sci 1990; 299:392–410.
10. Davis CE, Carpenter JL, Ognibene AJ and McAllister CK. Rifampin-induced acute renal failure. South Med J 1986; 79:1012–5.
11. Singer JZ and Wallace SL. The allopurinol hypersensitivity syndrome: unnecessary morbidity and mortality. Arthritis Rheum 1986; 29:82–7.
12. Abraham PA and Keane WF. Glomerular and interstitial disease induced by nonsteroidal anti-inflammatory drugs. Am J Nephrol 1984; 4:1–6.

13. Buysen JGM, Houthoff HJ, Krediet RT and Arisz L. Acute interstitial nephritis: a clinical and morphological study in 27 patients. Nephrol Dial Transplant 1990; 5:94–9.
14. Pusey CD, Saltissi D, Bloodworth L, Rainford DJ and Christie JL. Drug associated acute interstitial nephritis: clinical and pathological features and the response to high dose steroid therapy. Quart J Med 1983; 52:194–211.
15. Galpin JE, Shinaberger JH, Stanley TM, Blumenkrantz MJ, Bayer AS, Friedman GS et al. Acute interstitial nephritis due to methicillin. Am J Med 1978; 65:756–65.
16. Laberke HG. Treatment of acute interstitial nephritis. Klin Wochenschr 1980; 58:531–2.
17. Cameron JS. Immunologically mediated interstitial nephritis: primary and secondary. Adv Nephrol 1989; 18:207–48.
18. Revert L and Montoliu J. Acute interstitial nephritis. Semin Nephrol 1988; 8:82–8.
19. Arm JP, Rainford DJ and Turk EP. Acute renal failure and infectious mononucleosis. J Infect Dis 1984; 9:293–7.
20. Jones SR. Acute renal failure in adults with uncomplicated acute pyelonephritis: case reports and review. Clin Infect Dis 1992; 14:243–6.
21. Jones BF, Nanra RS and White KH. Acute renal failure due to acute pyelonephritis. Am J Nephrol 1991; 11:257–9.
22. Thompson C, Verani R, Evanoff G and Weinman E. Suppurative bacterial pyelonephritis as a cause of acute renal failure. Am J Kidney Dis 1986; 8:271–3.
23. Casella FJ and Allon M. The kidney in sarcoidosis. J Am Soc Nephrol 1993; 3:1555–62.
24. Hannedouche T, Grateau G, Noel LH, Godin M, Fillastre JP, Grunfeld JP et al. Renal granulomatous sarcoidosis: report of six cases. Nephrol Dial Transplant 1990; 5:18–24.
25. Korzets Z, Schneider M, Taragan R, Bernheim J and Bernheim J. Acute renal failure due to sarcoid granulomatous infiltration of the renal parenchyma. Am J Kidney Dis 1985; 6:250–3.
26. Singer DRJ and Evans DJ. Renal impairment in sarcoidosis: granulomatous nephritis as an isolated cause (two case reports and review of the literature). Clin Nephrol 1986; 26:250–6.
27. Emlen W, Steigerwald JC and Arend WP. Rheumatoid arthritis, Sjogren's syndrome, and dermatomyositis-polymyositis. In: Schrier RW and Gottschalk C, editors. Diseases of the kidney. Little, Brown and Company, Boston, 1993; 2049–61.
28. Rayadurg J and Koch AE. Renal insufficiency from interstitial nephritis in primary Sjogren's syndrome. J Rheumatol 1990; 17:1714–8.
29. Macdougall IC, Isles CG, Whitworth JA, More IAR and MacSween RNM. Interstitial nephritis and primary biliary cirrhosis: a new association? Clin Nephrol 1987; 27:36–40.
30. Tron F, Ganeval D and Droz D. Immunologically-mediated acute renal failure of nonglomerular origin in the course of systemic lupus erythematosus (SLE). Am J Med 1979; 67:529–32.
31. Enriquez R, Gonzalez C, Cabezuelo JB, Lacueva J, Ruiz JA, Tovar JV et al. Relapsing steroid-responsive idiopathic acute interstitial nephritis. Nephron 1993; 63:462–5.
32. Spital A, Panner BJ and Sterns RH. Acute idiopathic

tubulointerstitial nephritis: report of two cases and review of the literature. Am J Kidney Dis 1987; 9:71–8.

33. Hirano K, Tomino Y, Mikami H, Ota K, Aikawa Y, Shirato I et al. A case of acute tubulointerstitial nephritis and uveitis syndrome with a dramatic response to corticosteroid therapy. Am J Nephrol 1989; 9:499–503.

34. Lessard M and Smith JD. Fanconi syndrome with uveitis in an adult woman. Am J Kidney Dis 1989; 13:158–9.

35. Cacoub P, Deray G, Lehoang P, Baumelou A, Beaufils H, DeGroc F et al. Idiopathic acute interstitial nephritis associated with anterior uveitis in adults. Clin Nephrol 1989; 31:307–10.

36. Chuang CK, Lai MK, Chang PL, Huang MH, Chu SH, Wu CJ et al. Xanthogranulomatous pyelonephritis: experience in 36 cases. J Urol 1992; 147:333–6.

37. Goodman M, Curry T and Russell T. Xantho-granulomatous pyelonephritis (XGP): a local disease with systemic manifestations. Medicine 1979; 58:171–81.

38. Ronald AR and Nicolle LE. Infections of the upper urinary tract. In: Schrier RW and Gottschalk C, editors. Diseases of the kidney. Little, Brown and Company, Boston, 1993; 973–1006.

39. Hurwitz G, Reimund E, Moparty KR and Hellstrom WJG. Bilateral renal parenchymal malacoplakia: a case report. J Urol 1992; 147:115–7.

40. Long JP and Althausen AF. Malacoplakia: a 25-year experi-ence with a review of the literature. J Urol 1989; 141:1328–31.

41. Cadnapaphornchai P, Rosenberg BF, Taher S, Prosnitz EH and McDonald FD. Renal parenchymal malakoplakia: an unusual cause of renal failure. N Engl J Med 1978; 299:1110–2.

42. Dobyan DC, Truong LD and Eknoyan E. Renal malacoplakia reappraised. Am J Kidney Dis 1993; 22:243–52.

43. Hahn-Pedersen J and Jorgensen D. Renal malacoplakia. Scand J Urol Nephrol 1983; 17:135–7.

44. Abdou NI, NaPombejara C, Sagawa A, Ragland C, Stechschulte DJ, Nilsson U et al. Malakoplakia: evidence for monocyte lysosomal abnormality correctable by cholinergic agonist in vitro and in vivo. N Engl J Med 1977; 297:1413–19.

45. Glicklich D, Sung MW and Frey M. Renal failure due to lymphomatous infiltration of the kidneys: report of three new cases and review of the literature. Cancer 1986; 58:748–53.

46. Lundberg WB, Cadman ED, Finch SC and Capizzi RL. Renal failure secondary to leukemic infiltration of the kidneys. Am J Med 1977; 62:636–42.

47. Truong LD, Soroka S, Sheth AV, Kessler M, Mattioli C and Suki W. Primary renal lymphoma presenting as acute renal failure. Am J Kidney Dis 1987; 9:502–6.

PART SIX

Problem cases

Twenty cases of renal failure are presented for the reader to diagnose. Discussions of the possible etiologies and the subsequent clinical courses are given after the cases.

PART IV

Problems

Problem cases

Case 1

A 74-year-old woman has had night sweats, fever, fatigue, mild cough and a 30 lb. (13.6 kg) weight loss over five months. A myocardial infarction occurred at age 68, and a coronary artery bypass was performed at age 71. Scr was 0.9 mg/dl (80 μmol/L) seven months ago.

Physical examination shows a blood pressure of 110/60 mmHg, a pulse of 84 per minute, respirations 20 per minute, and a temperature of 37.5 °C. There is a soft systolic murmur at the apex of the heart. The chest is clear.

Initial laboratory studies show Scr 2.6 mg/dl (230 μmol/L), BUN 22 mg/dl (7.9 μmol/L), serum sodium 137 mEq/L, potassium 3.9 mEq/L, chloride 100 mEq/L, bicarbonate 22 mEq/L and urinalysis: clear, specific gravity 1.018, pH 6.0, protein 300 mg/dl, glucose and ketones negative, 45 to 50 red blood cells per hpf and 10 to 15 white blood cells per hpf. *Extrarenal tests* show hemoglobin 10 g/dl, hematocrit 29%, white blood cell count 15,100/mm^3, 85 polymorphonuclear neutrophils, 15 lymphocytes, serum albumin concentration 2.7 g/dl and positive ANCA (1 : 40). The patient has negative ANA and anti-GBM antibody, normal chest X-ray, serum and urine protein and immunofixation electrophoreses, liver function tests and normal serum concentrations of glucose, calcium, phosphorus, uric acid, C3, C4 and CH50. *Additional renal tests*: Renal sonography shows kidneys 10.3 cm bilaterally with no hydronephrosis. The 24 hour urine protein is 1.6 g.

Case 2

A 64-year-old man is admitted to the hospital with cough, weakness, nausea, anorexia and increased thirst, which began during an upper respiratory infection two weeks ago. The patient has had hypertension treated with a thiazide diuretic and potassium chloride for thirty years. He has some residual weakness in the left arm from a cerebrovascular accident one year ago. He takes digoxin for atrial fibrillation. One year ago the Scr was 0.7 mg/dl (62 μmol/L).

Physical examination shows a blood pressure of 115/60 mmHg, pulse 80 per minute and irregular, respirations 18 per minute, and temperature 37 °C. The heart rhythm is irregularly irregular, and the lungs have occasional rhonchi.

Initial laboratory studies show Scr 2.8 mg/dl (248 μmol/L), BUN 54 mg/dl (19 mmol/L), serum sodium 135 mEq/L, potassium 3.4 mEq/L, chloride 97 mEq/L, bicarbonate 22 mEq/L, and urinalysis: clear, specific gravity 1.019, pH 6.0, protein, glucose, ketone and sediment negative.

Case 3

A 73-year-old diabetic man was admitted to the hospital with fever, a right foot ulcer and acute arthritis of the right shoulder. On admission, intravenous gentamicin and ticarcillin/clavulanate were given. Cultures of the ulcer, blood and right shoulder grew *S. aureus* on hospital day 2, and the antibiotics were changed to gentamicin and nafcillin. The gentamicin was stopped on day 9, but the nafcillin was continued, during which time the infection clinically resolved. On day 19 during an upper gastrointestinal hemorrhage caused by gastritis, the blood pressure dropped to 85/40 mmHg for several hours. On day 24, the Scr rose to 1.8 mg/dl (159 μmol/L) from 1.3 mg/dl (115 μmol/L) the day before. Urine output fell to 600 ml per day.

The patient has rheumatoid arthritis. The cur-

233

J.G. Abuelo (ed.), Renal Failure, 233–240.
© 1995 *Kluwer Academic Publishers.*

rent medications are nafcillin (day 24 of treatment), glyburide, subcutaneous heparin and cimetidine.

The physical examination shows a blood pressure of 102/62 mmHg, pulse 84 per minute and temperature 36.8 °C. The left lung field has inspiratory crackles at the base. Both hands and feet show changes of rheumatoid arthritis, and there is moderate edema of the torso and lower extremities. A macular rash is present over the chest and abdomen.

Current laboratory studies (hospital day 26) show Scr 4.0 mg/dl (354 μmol/L), BUN 37 mg/dl (13 mmol/L), serum sodium 134 mEq/L, potassium 5.1 mEq/L, chloride 100 mEq/L, bicarbonate 26 mEq/L, and urinalysis: clear, yellow, specific gravity 1.015, pH 5.0, protein 30 mg/dl, glucose moderate and ketones and sediment negative. *Extrarenal tests* show serum albumin concentration 1.6 mg/dl, calcium 6.9 mg/dl (1.7 mmol/L), hemoglobin 9.8 g/dl, hematocrit 28%, white blood cell count 10,100/mm^3 with 73 polymorphonuclear leukocytes, 20 lymphocytes and 7 eosinophils, platelet count 206,000/mm^3, and normal chest X-ray and serum concentrations of glucose, phosphorus, uric acid, bilirubin and liver enzymes. *Additional renal studies.* A renal sonogram shows normal size kidneys (9.9 cm on right, 10.2 cm on left) with Grade I hydronephrosis on the right. The urine protein to creatinine ratio is 0.2 (upper limit of normal).

Case 4

A 47 year-old woman is admitted to the hospital with severe hypertension and newly discovered azotemia. The blood pressure was 115/70 mmHg five years ago, and 150/95 mmHg one year ago in a dentist's office. The patient did not see a physician, as advised. Since then, she has had intermittent headaches, relieved by aspirin. One week ago the blood pressure was 240/120 mmHg in the dentist's office. On the day before admission, the patient saw a physician who found normal fundi and started enalapril. She admitted the patient to the hospital when the Scr was reported to be 3.4 mg/dl (300 μmol/L).

On physical examination in the hospital the blood pressure is 190/120 mmHg, pulse 82 per minute and temperature 36.8 °C. The funduscopic and cardiac examination are normal.

Initial laboratory studies show Scr 3.7 mg/dl (327 μmol/L), BUN 74 mg/dl (26 mmol/L), serum sodium 147 mEq/L, potassium 4.8 mEq/L, chloride 113 mEq/L, bicarbonate 25 mEq/L and urinalysis: clear, yellow, specific gravity 1.010, pH 5.0, protein 30 mg/dl and glucose, ketones and sediment negative. *Extrarenal tests* show serum albumin concentration of 3.3 g/dl, hemoglobin 11.0 g/dl, hematocrit 34%, white blood cell count 6,100/mm^3 and platelet count 191,000/mm^3. A peripheral renin concentration is 0.2 ng/ml/hour (low normal). The red cell morphology, chest X-ray, electrocardiogram, serum protein electrophoresis, computed tomography of the head and serum concentrations of glucose, calcium, phosphorus, uric acid, bilirubin, liver enzymes, iron and iron binding capacity are normal. The 24-hour urinary catecholamines are normal. *Additional renal tests.* The 24-hour urine protein is 300 mg. Urine protein and immunofixation electrophoresis show mostly albumin and no abnormal proteins. Urine sodium concentration is 47 mEq/L and chloride 59 mEq/L. Creatinine clearance is 23 ml/minute. A renal sonogram shows two small kidneys (7.8 cm on the right, 8.1 cm on the left) without hydronephrosis. The Scr remains stable over one week.

Case 5

The patient is a 57-year-old woman admitted to the hospital with nausea and epigastric pain for two days. The patient has congestive heart failure, aortic stenosis, and tricuspid regurgitation due to rheumatic heart disease. She has an artificial mitral valve. Several recent episodes of gastrointestinal bleeding were caused by gastritis and anticoagulants. Two weeks before admission, the patient had a cardiac catheterization which showed a dilated hypokinetic left ventricle with an ejection fraction of 40%. She was started on captopril 12.5 mg t.i.d. One week before the present admission the blood pressure was 125/70 mmHg, the hemoglobin 13.2 g/dl, the BUN 29 mg/dl (10 mmol/L), and the Scr 1.2 mg/dl (106 μmol/L). The dose of captopril was raised to 25 mg t.i.d. Other medications are digoxin, warfarin, furosemide, spironolactone, and potassium chloride.

The physical examination on admission shows a blood pressure of 118/62 mmHg and pulse 92 per minute without orthostatic changes. The neck veins are not distended. The lungs are clear to auscultation. The heart shows a prosthetic valve click, and a Grade III/VI systolic murmur at the aortic area. The abdomen is normal. There is no peripheral edema.

Initial laboratory studies show Scr 3.6 mg/dl (318 μmol/L), BUN 195 mg/dl (70 mmol/L), serum sodium 119 mEq/L, potassium 7.9 mEq/L, chloride 86 mEq/L, bicarbonate 16 mEq/L; urinalysis: clear, straw-colored, specific gravity 1.003, protein, glucose and ketone negative, 3 to 5 red blood cells per hpf, 11 to 20 white blood cells per hpf. *Extrarenal tests* show hemoglobin 11.4 g/dl, hematocrit 34%, white blood cell count 8,100/mm³, polymorphonuclear leukocytes 87, lymphocytes 11, monocytes 2. The chest X-ray shows marked cardiomegaly with atrial enlargement. The lung fields are clear and the vasculature is not congested. An electrocardiogram reveals an old left bundle branch block. Stool is brown; guaiac test is positive. The digoxin level is in the therapeutic range. Serum uric acid concentration is 10.1 mg/dl (601 μmol/L). Serum concentrations of albumin, calcium, phosphorus, bilirubin, AST and alkaline phosphatase are normal. *Additional renal tests* show urine sodium 14 mEq/L, urine chloride 8 mEq/L.

Case 6

The patient is a 73-year-old man who is hospitalized with left flank and abdominal pain of sudden onset a few hours before admission. He is anuric during the first 8 hours in the hospital, despite placement of a Foley catheter. One year ago, he passed a uric acid stone.

Physical examination shows blood pressure 150/70 mmHg, pulse 92 per minute and temperature 36.1 °C. Abdominal examination is normal. There is no abdominal or costovertebral tenderness or mass.

Initial laboratory studies show Scr 6.2 mg/dl (548 μmol/L), BUN 46 mg/dl (16 mmol/L), serum sodium 135 mEq/L, potassium 5.4 mEq/L, chloride 99 mEq/L and bicarbonate 22 mEq/L.

Case 7

The patient is a 68-year-old man with two previous myocardial infarctions who had a cardiac catheterization for worsening dyspnea on exertion, and then was directly admitted to the hospital. The catheterization showed severe coronary artery disease and increased left ventricular filling pressure.

The patient has had diabetes mellitus for five years, and has passed several uric acid stones during his adult life. He has hypertension, hypercholesterolemia, gout, and chronic renal failure with Scr 2.2 mg/dl (194 μmol/L) and BUN 51 mg/dl (18 mmol/L) one week before admission. For the past several months the patient has had decreased force of urinary stream and a feeling of incomplete emptying of the bladder.

Medications on admission were chlorpropamide, isosorbide dinitrate, gemfibrozil, allopurinol, furosemide, sublingual nitroglycerin, enalapril, atenolol and colchicine. They were continued unchanged in the hospital.

Physical examination shows a blood pressure of 150/80 mmHg and pulse 96 per minute. The patient appears comfortable sitting in a chair, and has no abnormal physical findings.

Initial laboratory studies performed three days after admission show Scr 3.7 mg/dl (327 μmol/L), BUN 70 mg/dl (25 mmol/L), serum sodium 133 mEq/L, potassium 5.2 mEq/L, chloride 98 mEq/L, bicarbonate 20 mEq/L and urinalysis: clear, yellow, specific gravity 1.017, pH 5.5, protein 30 mg/dl, red blood cells 3 to 5 per hpf, white blood cells 1 to 3 per hpf. The next day Scr is 3.6 mg/dl (318 μmol/L) and BUN 64 mg/dl (23 mmol/L). The 24-hour urine outputs during the first three hospital days are 825 cc, 790 cc and 1,800 cc.

Case 8

The patient is a 75-year-old woman with ischemic heart disease and a previous coronary artery bypass who was admitted with crescendo angina. The patient complained of an acute bronchitis with blood-tinged sputum for 3 days. She has chronic renal failure with a recent Scr of 2.8 mg/dl (248 μmol/L). A new iron deficiency anemia was also present on admission; hemoglobin was 7.7 g/dl, serum iron concentration 7 mg/dl (1.3 μmol/L) and total iron binding capacity 282 mg/dl (50.5 μmol/L). The stool test for occult blood was negative. Cimetidine, ampicillin/sulbactam, heparin and iron sulfate were started, and a blood transfusion brought the hemoglobin to 10.3 g/dl. Low dose aspirin, metoprolol, isordil and sublingual nitroglycerin, as needed, were continued. A myocardial infarction was excluded, the angina and bronchitis subsided, and no gastrointestinal source of bleeding was found on upper endoscopy or colonoscopy. However, by the fifth hospital day a new rise in Scr had appeared.

Physical examination shows blood pressure 98/62 mmHg, pulse 56, temperature 37.0 °C, and some pallor of the skin.

Current laboratory studies show a Scr of 3.6 mg/dl (318 μmol/L) and BUN 58 mg/dl (21 mmol/L), up from 2.7 (239 μmol/L) and 57 mg/dl (20 mmol/L) on admission. The serum sodium is 138 mEq/L, potassium 4.3 mEq/L, chloride 105 mEq/L, bicarbonate 19 mEq/L and urinalysis clear, yellow, specific gravity 1.010, protein 30 mg/dl and glucose, ketones and sediment negative.

Case 9

A 22-year-old male clerk was locked up and stabbed in the abdomen during a robbery of a convenience store. Several hours later he is found incoherent and brought to the hospital, where the systolic blood pressure is 40 mmHg. In the operating room a lacerated liver and portal vein are repaired. Fluid replacement includes lactated Ringer's solution, frozen plasma and thirty-six units of packed red cells. The blood pressure is 115/60 mmHg following surgery, but several hours later drops below 80 mmHg systolic. The patient goes back to surgery, where a second laceration of the portal vein is located and repaired, and another nineteen units of packed cells are given. The postoperative blood pressure is 110/70 mmHg. The urine output is 10 ml per hour.

Physical examination after the second operation reveals an unconscious white man on a ventilator with an endotracheal tube in place. The blood pressure is 108/64 mmHg, pulse 112 per minute and temperature 36.0 °C. The patient has a midline abdominal incision and two drains in place. The pulmonary capillary wedge pressure is 5 mmHg.

Initial laboratory studies following the second operation show Scr 1.7 mg/dl (150 μmol/L), BUN 21 mg/dl (7 mmol/L), serum sodium 142 mEq/L, potassium 3.6 mEq/L, chloride 108 mEq/L, bicarbonate 19 and urinalysis: clear, yellow, specific

gravity 1.011, pH 5.5, protein trace, glucose and ketones negative and urine sediment: several muddy granular casts per lpf, 1 to 3 red blood cells and 1 to 4 renal tubular cells per hpf.

Case 10

A 70-year-old woman is evaluated because of new azotemia. One year ago the Scr was 0.9 mg/dl (80 μmol/L) at a routine physical examination. She presented four months ago with fatigue, anemia, anorexia and a twelve pound weight loss. The hemoglobin was 10.1 g/dl, Scr 1.2 mg/dl and iron studies, bone marrow examination, chest X-ray, computed tomography of the abdomen, tuberculin skin test, anti-nuclear antibody, and serum protein electrophoresis were negative.

Physical examination is unremarkable except for pallor of the skin and a further weight loss of five pounds. The blood pressure is 122/76 mmHg, pulse 68 per minute and temperature 37.2 °C.

Initial laboratory studies show Scr 2.5 mg/dl (221 μmol/L), BUN 49 mg/dl (17 mmol/L), serum sodium 139 mEq/L, potassium 3.9 mEq/L, chloride 107 mEq/L, bicarbonate 18 mEq/L and urinalysis: clear, yellow, specific gravity 1.012, protein 30 mg/dl, sediment 2 to 5 red blood cells per hpf, occasional hyaline and granular casts. *Extrarenal tests* show hemoglobin 9.1 g/dl, hematocrit 27.4%, rouleaux formation on the blood smear, serum concentrations of calcium 10.2 mg/dl (2.6 mmol/L), phosphorus 4.2 mg/dl (1.4 mmol/L), uric acid 6.2 mg/dl (369 μmol/L), total protein 7.1 g/dl and albumin 2.9 g/dl. Normal studies included chest X-ray, platelet count and serum concentrations of glucose, bilirubin and liver enzymes. *Additional renal tests.* Renal sonogram shows normal size kidneys (10.3 cm on right, 10.6 cm on left) and no hydronephrosis. The 24-hour urine protein is 6.2 g.

Case 11

A 61-year-old white male with mild chronic renal failure has a new rise in Scr. He has a 40-year history of proteinuria, a 15-year history of hypertension and hypercholesterolemia, and an expanding abdominal aortic aneurysm (5 cm diameter). The Scr had been stable at about 2.1 mg/dl (186 μmol/L) one year before (see Table). The urine protein has been 300 to 1,000 mg/dl by dipstick for at least a decade. The patient smoked two packs of cigarettes a day until 15 years ago. The medications are gemfibrozil, enalapril, diltiazem and diazepam, and have been unchanged for five years.

Physical examination shows a blood pressure of 180/80 mmHg and pulse 64. The patient has a low grade systolic murmur at the lower left sternal border, and an abdominal bruit below the umbilicus. Peripheral pulses are normal.

Initial laboratory studies show Scr 2.8 mg/dl (248 μmol/L), BUN 36 mg/dl (13 mmol/L), serum sodium 141 mEq/L, potassium 5.7 mEq/L, chloride 104 mEq/L, bicarbonate 25 mEq/L and urinalysis: clear, amber, specific gravity 1.025, protein 1,000 mg/dl, 0 to 2 red cells per hpf and occasional granular, waxy and hyaline casts.

Table. Previous Scr concentrations

Time (months elapsed)	Scr	
	(mg/dl)	μmol/L
108	1.2	106
96	1.0	88
72	1.6	141
42	1.6	141
19	2.2	194
6	2.1	186

Case 12

A 56-year-old man is noted to have severe hypertension and azotemia on a routine examination. He has been feeling well and had a normal blood pressure one year before. He has been smoking one pack of cigarettes a day for 40 years, but he denies wheezing, cough or shortness of breath on effort.

A physical examination shows a blood pressure of 210/120 mmHg, a pulse of 72 per minute, and slight edema of the ankles. The fundi are normal and peripheral pulses are of normal amplitude.

Initial laboratory studies show Scr 2.2 mg/dl (194 μmol/L), BUN 26 mg/dl (9 mmol/L), serum sodium 137 mEq/L, potassium 3.2 mEq/L, chloride 90 mEq/L, bicarbonate 29 mEq/L and urinalysis: clear, specific gravity 1.009, pH 5.5, protein 300 mg/dl, glucose, ketone and urine sediment negative. *Extrarenal tests* show serum albumin concentration 2.9 g/dl and normal chest X-ray, complete blood count, serum protein and im-

munofixation electrophoreses and normal serum concentrations of glucose, calcium, phosphorus, uric acid, total bilirubin, aspartate aminotransferase (AST), alkaline phosphatase, C3, C4 and CH50 complement. The urine immuno- and protein electrophoreses reveal the urine protein to be mainly albumin with no abnormal proteins. *Additional renal tests*: Renal sonography shows a 12.0 cm kidney on the right and a 10.2 cm kidney on the left without obstruction. The urine sodium concentration is 63 mEq/L and the chloride concentration 72 mEq/L. The 24 hour urine protein is 4.8 g.

Case 13[3]

A 68-year-old white male with a previous myocardial infarction is admitted for an elevated Scr found during pre-admission testing.

The patient felt well until three weeks prior to admission when he started experiencing intermittent chest pains. A thallium stress test was positive for myocardial ischemia, and admission for cardiac catheterization was planned. The patient began to experience episodes of tea-colored urine ten days prior to admission. Two days prior to admission, the patient slipped on ice in a "spread eagle" position and noted pain and tenderness in his left thigh and the neck. He had no history of renal disease. His medications on admission consisted of the following: diltiazem 30 mg po t.i.d., lovastatin 40 mg po b.i.d., nadolol 80 mg po q.d., alprazolam 0.25 mg po b.i.d., niacin 1 g po q.d., lisinopril 20 mg po q.d., hydrochlorothiazide 50 mg po b.i.d., nitroglycerin 0.4 mg p.r.n.

Physical examination shows diffuse muscle tenderness, edema, and absence of any abrasions or ecchymoses. The blood pressure is 150/100 mmHg, pulse 96 per minute, temperature 99 °F.

Initial laboratory studies show Scr 9.2 mg/dl (813 μmol/L), BUN 113 mg/dl (40 mmol/L), Na 134 mEq/L, K 4.6 mEq/L, Cl 88 mEq/L, bicarbonate 21 mEq/L, and urinalysis: cloudy brown, specific gravity 1.016, pH 6.0, 300 mg/dl protein, heme 3+, white blood cells 15 to 18 per hpf. *Extrarenal tests* show white blood cell count 15,200/mm[3], polymorphonuclear leukocytes 81, lymphocytes 18, monocytes 1, serum concentration of calcium 8.3 mg/dl (2.1 mmol/L), phosphorus 6.1 mg/dl (2.0 mmol/L), uric acid 13.1 mg/dl (779 μmol/L), aspartate aminotransferase 2614 IU and alanine aminotransferase 903 IU. The chest X-ray, hemoglobin, hematocrit, platelet count, glucose, total bilirubin and alkaline phosphatase are normal.

Case 14

A 20-year-old woman is admitted to the hospital with abdominal cramps, nausea and vomiting for four days and jaundice for one day. She has had no previous illnesses. Her only medication is an oral contraceptive containing norethindrone and mestranol for two years.

Physical examination shows a blood pressure of 170/90 mmHg, pulse 100 per minute, temperature 37 °C and respirations 20 per minute. The sclerae are icteric. Extremities show a few ecchymoses.

Initial laboratory studies show Scr 8.3 mg/dl (734 μmol/L), BUN 79 mg/dl (28 mmol/L), serum sodium 137 mEq/L, potassium 4.1 mEq/L, chloride 103 mEq/L, bicarbonate 13 mEq/L and urinalysis: clear, yellow, pH 5.0, specific gravity 1.009, protein 100 mg/dl, glucose and ketones negative, occasional red blood cells and white blood cell per hpf. *Extrarenal tests* show hemoglobin 11.9 g/dl, hematocrit 32.0%, white blood cell count 13,800/mm^3, 75 polymorphonuclear leukocytes, 11 lymphocytes, 2 monocyte, platelet count 26,000/mm^3, blood smear-moderate helmet cells and schistocytes, and serum concentrations of total bilirubin 9.0 mg/dl (154 μmol/L) (direct 3.1 mg/dl), AST 627 IU/L, calcium 9.2 mg/dl (2.3 mmol/L), phosphorus 6.2 mg/dl (2.0 mmol/L), and uric acid 15.0 mg/dl (892 μmol/L). The chest X-ray, serum concentrations of glucose, albumin, fibrinogen and fibrin split products were normal. *Additional renal tests* show a 24-hour-urine protein of 1.9 g, urine concentration of sodium 57 mEq/L and chloride 97 mEq/L. On renal sonogram the kidneys are 10.6 cm in length and show Grade I hydronephrosis on the right.

Case 15

A 57-year-old man seeing a physician for a routine examination has a Scr of 2.9 mg/dl (256 μmol/L) compared to 1.4 mg/dl (124 μmol/L) one year earlier. He has taken atenolol and hydrochlorothiazide for hypertension for over ten years. The patient stopped cigarette smoking ten years ago.

Physical examination shows a blood pressure of 160/95 mmHg and pulse 64 per minute. Except for moderate obesity, the examination is unremarkable.

Initial laboratory studies show Scr 2.9 mg/dl (256 μmol/L), BUN 34 mg/dl (12 mmol/L), serum sodium 137 mEq/L, potassium 3.9 mEq/L, chloride 96 mEq/L, bicarbonate 27 mEq/L and urinalysis: clear, yellow, pH 6.0, specific gravity 1.018, protein, glucose, ketones and sediment negative. *Extrarenal tests* show normal chest X-ray, complete blood count, and serum concentrations of glucose, calcium, phosphorus, uric acid, bilirubin, liver enzymes, total protein and albumin. *Additional renal tests* show a urine protein to creatinine ratio of 0.1 (normal) and a normal renal sonogram with a 10.8 cm right kidney and 10.5 cm left kidney. A left renal biopsy shows normal glomeruli, mild sclerosis of the arterioles, and some focal tubular atrophy and interstitial fibrosis. The changes are considered too mild to explain the azotemia.

Case 16

A 69-year-old man was admitted to the hospital with back and right knee pain. The patient has adult onset diabetes mellitus and chronic lymphocytic leukemia, and had a splenectomy following trauma 30 years ago. Mild hypertension had been treated in the past, but recent blood pressures were about 135/85 mmHg without therapy. *S. aureus* was cultured from the blood, the right knee and a right psoas abscess. The infection responded well to nafcillin, but the patient became tachypneic and confused on the ninth hospital day. The temperature was 36 °C, blood pressure 115/62 mmHg, pulse 106 per minute, and respirations 26 per minute. A urine culture grew 100,000 colonies/ml of *E. coli*. Gentamicin and ampicillin were started and the patient improved clinically by the next day. On the twelfth hospital day, the Scr is noted to be 3.1 mg/dl (274 μmol/L) compared with its previous value of 1.1 mg/dl (97 μmol/L) from the ninth hospital day. The patient feels well.

The medications are prednisone, nafcillin, gentamicin, ampicillin, insulin, carafate and docusate.

Physical examination shows a blood pressure of 140/85 mmHg, pulse 72 per minute and temperature 37 °C. The patient is alert and oriented. The inguinal lymph nodes are slightly enlarged and firm.

Current laboratory studies show Scr 3.1 mg/dl (274 µmol/L), BUN 47 mg/dl (17 mmol/L), serum sodium 135 mEq/L, potassium 4.2 mEq/L, chloride 95 mEq/L, bicarbonate 27 mEq/L and urinalysis: clear, yellow, specific gravity 1.009, pH 5.5, protein 100 mg/dl, glucose and ketones negative, red blood cells 6 to 10 per hpf, white blood cells 7 to 12 per hpf and occasional tubular cells.

Case 17

The patient is a 70-year-old diabetic man who is admitted to the hospital with a five-day history of watery diarrhea, abdominal cramps and a rash on the upper extremities. Two days ago transient gross hematuria was noted. He had hematemesis and passed blood per rectum on the day of admission. The patient has chronic atrial fibrillation, and a tracheostomy performed for laryngeal cancer five years ago. He takes digoxin and glipizide.

Physical examination shows a blood pressure of 150/80 mmHg, pulse irregularly irregular at 80 per minute and temperature 37.1 °C. The patient has a tracheostomy, diffuse tenderness of the abdomen and nonpalpable petechiae on both palms and elbows.

Initial laboratory studies show Scr 5.1 mg/dl (451 µmol/L), BUN 56 mg/dl (20 mmol/L), serum sodium 130 mEq/L, potassium 4.0, chloride 99, bicarbonate 13 mEq/L, and urinalysis: cloudy, amber, specific gravity 1.015, pH 5.0, protein 100 mg/dl, glucose and ketones negative, 11 to 20 red blood cells per hpf, 6 to 10 white blood cells per hpf, few squamous epithelial cells. *Extrarenal tests* show white blood cell count 12,800/mm³, hemoglobin 10.6 g/dl, hematocrit 32.2%, platelet count 409,000/mm³, 76 polymorphonuclear leukocytes, 7 lymphocytes, 11 monocytes and 6 eosinophils, sedimentation rate 26 mm/hour, serum concentration of calcium 6.1 mg/dl (1.5 mmol/L), phosphorus 5.0 mg/dl (1.6 mmol/L), uric acid 9.2 mg/dl (547 µmol/L), total protein 3.5 g/dl and albumin 1.8 g/dl. Urine protein electrophoresis shows albumin and no abnormal proteins. ANA, ANCA, cryoglobulins and rheumatoid factor are negative. The chest X-ray, bilirubin, lactic dehydrogenase, liver enzymes, C3, C4 and CH50 are normal. Upper endoscopy shows duodenal ulcers and duodenitis. *Additional renal tests* show 24-hour urine protein 320 mg, and normal size kidneys without hydronephrosis on renal sonogram (10.3 cm length on the right, 10.5 cm on the left).

Case 18

A 70-year-old man is admitted to the hospital with anuria for the past two days. He had recent weight loss of about 8 lbs. A Scr was 0.9 mg/dl (80 µmol/L) two years ago.

Physical examination shows a blood pressure of 140/85 mmHg, pulse 88 per minute and temperature 36.8 °C. The patient is a somewhat wasted elderly man with 1+ edema of the ankles and feet. He is anuric despite placement of an indwelling urethral catheter.

Initial laboratory studies show Scr 8.1 mg/dl (716 µmol/L), BUN 68 mg/dl (24 mmol/L), serum sodium 143 mEq/L, potassium 4.9 mEq/L, chloride 113 mEq/L, bicarbonate 18 mEq/L. *Extrarenal tests* show serum concentration of calcium 8.0 mg/dl (2.0 mmol/L), phosphorus 6.9 mg/dl (2.2 mmol/L), uric acid 7.0 mg/dl (416 µmol/L) and albumin 3.3 g/dl. The chest X-ray, complete blood count, and liver enzymes are normal. *Additional renal tests*. Renal sonography shows Grade I hydronephrosis on the right. The right kidney is 10.3 cm in length, the left is 10.5 cm. A left renal biopsy shows mild interstitial edema and normal glomeruli.

Case 19

The patient is a 46-year-old Hispanic gardener admitted to the hospital with fatigue, anorexia, 20 lb. weight loss and anemia of six months duration. He vomited once on the day of admission. An evaluation of anemia (hemoglobin 11.1 g/dl) two months ago did not reveal a cause; serum and urine protein electrophoreses, bone marrow aspirate, and folate, vitamin B12 and iron studies were normal.

Physical examination shows a thin middle-aged man with a blood pressure of 114/58 mmHg, pulse 82 per minute and temperature 37 °C.

Initial laboratory studies show Scr 2.2 mg/dl (194 µmol/L), BUN 30 mg/dl (11 mmol/L), serum sodium 133 mEq/L, potassium 5.6 mEq/L, chloride 101, bicarbonate 19 mEq/L and urinalysis: clear, yellow, specific gravity 1.012, pH 5.0, ketones 1+, protein, glucose and sediment negative. *Extrarenal tests* show hemoglobin 10.6 g/dl, hematocrit 32%, uric acid 8.1 mg/dl (482 μmol/L), and normal chest X-ray, white blood cell count, platelet count, and serum concentrations of calcium, phosphorus, total protein, albumin, bilirubin and liver enzymes, *Additional renal tests* show urine concentrations of sodium 41 mEq/L, potassium 30 mEq/L, chloride 72 mEq/L and creatinine 48 mg/dl. Renal ultrasound shows normal size kidneys without hydronephrosis.

Case 20

A 24-year-old white man is admitted to the hospital with a 3-day history of uremic symptoms and a one-day history of scant output of dark brown "Coca-Cola" colored urine.

Six weeks before admission, the patient had an upper respiratory tract infection with bronchitis. It was treated for a week with oral amoxicillin and resolved over three days. The patient then felt well until three days before admission when he developed fatigue, hiccoughs and nausea. He had scant output of dark urine for one day before admission.

The physical examination on admission shows a blood pressure of 145/95 mmHg, pulse 82 per minute, and bilateral costovertebral angle tenderness.

Initial laboratory studies shows Scr 10.6 mg/dl (937 μmol/L), BUN 72 mg/dl (26 mmol/L), serum sodium 134 mEq/L, potassium 4.5 mEq/L, chloride 97 mEq/L, bicarbonate 29 mEq/L, and urinalysis: hazy yellow, specific gravity 1.015, pH 5.5, protein 300 mg/dl, heme large amount, glucose and ketones negative, sediment 0 to 2 red cells per hpf, 0 to 5 white cells per hpf, and many pigmented granular casts. *Extrarenal tests* show platelets 59,000 per mm^3, white count 11,500 per mm^3 with 75 polymorphonuclear leukocytes, 18 lymphocytes and 2 eosinophils, serum concentration of uric acid 9.9 mg/dl (589 μmol/L), phosphorus 6.2 mg/dl (2.0 mmol/L), and albumin 3.3 gm/dl. The chest X-ray, hemoglobin, hematocrit, red cell morphology, and the serum concentrations of calcium, bilirubin, creatine phosphokinase and liver enzymes are normal. *Additional renal tests*: renal sonogram shows the kidneys to have increased density bilaterally with normal size and no hydronephrosis. A spot urine protein/creatinine ratio is 2.8 (equivalent to 2.8 g per 24 hours).

Urine output is less than 200 cc per day. The Scr rises more than 1 mg/dl (88 μmol/L) each day to 20 mg/dl (1768 μmol/L) and uremic symptoms worsen.

Problem cases – diagnoses and discussion

Case 1

Diagnosis – idiopathic crescentic GN

The rise in Scr of 1.7 mg/dl over seven months or less, almost a tripling, excludes chronic renal failure. While the low normal blood pressure and concentrated urine (S.G. 1.018) raise the question of prerenal renal failure, the absence of a precipitating cause and of a high BUN to Scr ratio, and the presence of proteinuria and hematuria make this unlikely. The normal sonogram excludes urinary obstruction. Thus, this patient most likely has an intrinsic renal disease.

In making a diagnosis, the physician should try to explain the hematuria, proteinuria, constitutional symptoms and positive ANCA test.

The *hematuria and proteinuria* suggest an acute nephritic picture. In addition, they are sometimes seen in diseases of the small renal vessels, such as atheroembolic renal disease and malignant hypertension. An idiopathic interstitial nephritis could also be associated with this moderate level of hematuria and proteinuria, as well as with the pyuria.

The *constitutional symptoms* are nonspecific. They can be seen in primary GN such as idiopathic crescentic GN, and secondary GN caused by infections and collagen vascular diseases. They also sometimes occur in atheroembolic or other diseases of the small renal vessels, and in idiopathic acute interstitial nephritis.

A *positive ANCA test* is the most specific feature in this case, and is mainly found in idiopathic crescentic GN, polyarteritis nodosa and Wegener's granulomatosis. The absence of clear-cut extrarenal organ involvement makes the latter two conditions less likely, although such multisystem involvement can develop late in these vasculitides.

In summary, idiopathic crescentic GN is the best clinical diagnosis, but other parenchymal diseases need to be ruled out. Since the treatment depends on the specific diagnosis, a renal biopsy should be performed.

Follow-up

The renal biopsy showed a pauci-immune crescentic GN with 50% of glomeruli involved by crescents. The patient was treated by pulse methylprednisolone and then a course of oral prednisone. This was complicated by severe hypertension, but the constitutional symptoms disappeared and the Scr fell to 1.4 mg/dl (124 μmol/L).

> Hematuria, proteinuria, constitutional symptoms and a positive ANCA suggest an idiopathic crescentic GN.

Case 2

Diagnosis – prerenal renal failure

The clues to diagnosing this case are the relatively low blood pressure, the high BUN to Scr ratio and the negative urinary protein and sediment.

The rise in Scr to 2.8 mg/dl (248 μmol/L) may have been associated with the recent two-week illness and is probably new, suggesting an acute process. The blood pressure of 115/60 mmHg represents relative hypotension in a hypertensive individual, and should lead the physician to wonder whether the combination of reduced salt intake due to anorexia, and obligatory urine salt loss due to a thiazide diuretic resulted in volume depletion, and prerenal renal failure. Once this

J.G. Abuelo (ed.), Renal Failure, 241–253.
© 1995 *Kluwer Academic Publishers.*

possibility is considered, one realizes that the thirst may be a sign of volume depletion, and the moderately high urine specific gravity (1.019) and BUN to Scr ratio are evidence for a prerenal cause. (If it were not for the effect of low protein intake on the BUN, the BUN to Scr ratio might have been higher). Confirmation of this diagnosis might include demonstration of orthostatic "signs", improvement of renal function with volume repletion, and verification of a recent drop in weight caused by fluid loss. (A stable weight would be evidence against hypovolemia.)

Follow-up

On questioning the patient about his weakness, he said that weakness and lightheadedness occurred when he was upright and it was relieved on sitting or lying. On standing, the patient's blood pressure fell from 120 mmHg systolic to 85 mmHg, and the pulse rate rose from 84 to 96 per minute. He was weighed; the weight of 159 lb was 10 lb (4.5 kg) less than his normal weight. A chest X-ray and white blood cell count were normal.

The diuretic was stopped and 4 liters of normal saline were given over two days. The patient recovered his appetite and feeling of well being. The blood pressure rose to 140/85 mmHg and the orthostatic change disappeared. The Scr fell to 0.9 mg/dl (80 μmol/L).

> Low normal blood pressure in a patient with chronic hypertension, high BUN to Scr ratio, urine specific gravity > 1.015 and negative urine sediment suggest prerenal azotemia.

Case 3

Diagnosis – acute (allergic) interstitial nephritis
The initial disseminated staphylococcal infection may have produced acute tubular necrosis due to sepsis or an acute immune complex mediated GN. The onset of azotemia well after resolution of the infection excludes the former possibility, and the lack of hematuria rules out an acute nephritic process.

The hypotensive episode, which resolved four or

five days before the rise in Scr, was not concurrent with the onset of azotemia, and could not have caused the renal failure.

The clues to the diagnosis of this patient are the β-lactam exposure (nafcillin), rash, eosinophilia and normoglycemic glycosuria. They are strongly suggestive of a β-lactam-induced allergic interstitial nephritis. In many patients with this condition, a fall in Scr occurs within ten days after discontinuation of the drug, and may be considered confirmatory of the diagnosis. In others azotemia persists longer, and a renal biopsy may be needed to demonstrate the acute interstitial nephritis.

Follow-up

Vancomycin was substituted for nafcillin. A diuresis ensued two days later and the Scr peaked at 5.1 mg/dl (451 μmol/L). The azotemia resolved over two weeks.

Although the Grade I hydronephrosis on one side raises the question of postrenal renal failure, this is probably not the cause of the azotemia. Hydronephrosis would have to be bilateral to raise the Scr from 1.3 to 4.0 mg/dl. Also a large portion of Grade I hydronephroses (up to 50% of cases) is not due to obstruction.[1] Causes of these false positives include vascular structures, a full bladder, high urine flow, renal cysts and dilated calyces. Before pursuing further investigation of urinary obstruction with intravenous pyelography or urologic consultation, the sonogram should be repeated and other diagnostic possibilities evaluated.

> β-lactam exposure, rash, eosinophilia and renal glycosuria suggest allergic interstitial nephritis.

Case 4

Diagnosis – chronic renal failure of unknown etiology
In making a diagnosis, the physician should take into account the severity of the hypertension, the high BUN to Scr ratio and the small kidney size.

The possibility of malignant hypertension is suggested by the headaches, azotemia and the height of the blood pressure (240/120 mmHg).

However, the normal fundi, low normal renin concentration, small kidney size and peak diastolic blood pressure below 130 mmHg tend to exclude this condition.

The most likely diagnosis is chronic renal failure, with *the small kidneys on sonography being prima facie evidence for atrophic and irreversibly damaged kidneys*. The cause is unknown. The duration of hypertension of a few years at most make hypertensive nephrosclerosis unlikely, and the low protein excretion militates against chronic glomerular disease. Reversible causes of progressive renal failure, such as chronic hypercalcemia, obstructive uropathy, and multiple myeloma are excluded by the evaluation.

The azotemia, small kidneys and new onset of hypertension raise the question of bilateral renal artery stenosis with renal atrophy and renal failure caused by ischemia. Since the patient has no evidence of atherosclerosis, one would need to postulate that the patient has fibromuscular hyperplasia, a rare cause of renal artery stenosis and rarer cause of renal failure. The low renin concentration makes renal artery stenosis even less likely. Moreover, there is little benefit in pursuing this diagnosis, since the likelihood of 8 cm kidneys recovering function after revascularization is poor. The hypertension is probably secondary to the chronic kidney disease, and is partly or mainly being mediated by hypervolemia.

Follow-up

The blood pressure was well controlled with nifedipine, furosemide and an 88 mEq sodium diet. Despite the hope that malignant hypertension was causing an acute reversible component of the azotemia, the Scr did not improve over the next several months.

> An azotemic patient with small kidneys has chronic renal failure.

Case 5

Diagnosis – vasomotor type of renal failure caused by captopril
The physician must consider several clues in solving this case: recent cardiac catheterization with use of radiocontrast media, recent increase in captopril dose, high BUN to Scr ratio, pyuria and salt poor urine.

The low urinary salt content suggests prerenal azotemia, but also may be seen in vasomotor types of renal failure, due for example to contrast media or converting enzyme inhibitors, and in ischemic or pigment types of acute tubular necrosis. The congestive heart failure, the fall in blood pressure, the high BUN to Scr ratio and the low urine sodium concentration initially raise the question of prerenal renal failure due to diuretics, gastrointestinal blood loss or worsening cardiac function. But, the slight degree of blood pressure drop over the week before admission, and the lack of signs of heart failure cast doubt on this explanation. Gastrointestinal bleeding may have contributed to the high BUN to creatinine ratio.

The occurrence of renal failure with a low urine sodium concentration following cardiac catheterization raises the question of a vasomotor reaction to contrast media. *In contrast media reactions BUN and Scr usually begin to rise by one day and peak three to five days after the procedure.* The Scr of 1.2 mg/dl (106 μmol/L) one week after catheterization excludes this cause of renal failure.

The occurrence of azotemia two weeks after cardiac catheterization is consistent with atheroembolic renal disease. However, the absence of eosinophilia and ischemic skin changes in the feet make this less likely.

The renal failure is most likely caused by captopril. Captopril, an angiotensin converting enzyme inhibitor, reduces conversion of angiotensin I to angiotensin II. It may impair renal function in the setting of poor renal perfusion where maintenance of glomerular filtration depends on high angiotensin II levels. The patient's underlying low cardiac output places her kidneys in such an angiotensin II dependent state. The development of renal failure coincides with the increase in captopril dose to 25 mg t.i.d. The low urine sodium further supports this diagnosis. The first diagnostic step should be the discontinuation of captopril in anticipation that the BUN and Scr will fall over two to three days. If improvement is not observed, a renal ultrasound should be obtained to exclude obstruction. One might also consider an allergic interstitial nephritis produced by captopril or furosemide, prerenal renal failure due to worsening of the heart disease, and atheroembolic renal disease precipitated by the cardiac catheterization.

The hyperkalemia was caused by captopril, spironolactone, potassium supplements and worsening of renal function.

Follow-up

On admission, the patient was treated with sucralfate, ranitidine and sodium polystyrene sulfonate exchange resin (Kayexalate). The captopril, spironolactone, furosemide and potassium supplements were stopped. The potassium level rapidly fell to 5.2 mEq/L. Endoscopy showed normal esophagus and stomach. The blood pressure rose to 130/70 mmHg. The patient voided 4 liters during the first 24 hours in the hospital. The BUN and Scr fell over 4 days to 25 (9 mmol/L) and 1.3 mg/dl (115 μmol/L). The serum sodium corrected to 135 mEq/L and the potassium to 3.7 mEq/dl. The pyuria was caused by an asymptomatic urinary infection.

> Congestive heart failure, increase in ACE inhibitor dose, salt poor urine and absence of hematuria and proteinuria suggest a vasomotor type of renal failure.

Case 6

Diagnosis – bilateral ureteral obstruction caused by uric acid crystals
The sudden left flank and abdominal pain, history of urolithiasis and anuria despite a urethral catheter, are the keys to the diagnosis.

Flank pain in patients with renal failure raises a number of diagnostic possibilities: acute pyelonephritis, renal artery embolism, renal vein thrombosis, malacoplakia, xanthogranulomatous pyelonephritis, acute GN and acute interstitial nephritis. However, the most common cause is acute ureteral obstruction by a stone. This is the obvious clinical diagnosis in this case, given the history of passage of a stone one year before. A Scr over 2.5 mg/dl (221 μmol/L) indicates involvement of a solitary kidney or both kidneys. The confirmatory

test is usually a renal sonogram showing hydronephrosis, but there are many false negative results within the first day or two of an acute ureteral obstruction. One should obtain an intravenous pyelogram in such patients if the sonogram is normal.

Follow-up

A renal sonogram showed Grade II hydronephrosis on the right side and Grade I hydronephrosis on the left side. The right kidney was 12.2 cm in length and the left 13.0 cm. Cystoscopy revealed a large amount of yellow-orange debris in the bladder, consistent with uric acid crystals. It was thought that this material was probably obstructing both ureters. A stent was placed in the right ureter. Passage of a left ureteral catheter required bypassing a probable calcareous obstruction. A retrograde pyelogram showed a normal left collecting system, and the ureter was not stented.

There was a post-obstructive diuresis of 3 to 4 liters a day for three days. The BUN and Scr fell to 14 (5 mmol/L) and 2.3 mg/dl (203 μmol/L) over ten days. The uric acid was 11.4 mg/dl (678 μmol/L) on admission and went down to 2.3 mg/dl (137 μmol/L) by discharge.

At the time of cystoscopy the cause of the uric acid precipitation was not known. The patient developed delirium tremens in the hospital and then admitted to heavy ethanol use. Also mild anemia was present and after discharge was shown to be caused by myelofibrosis. Since both excess alcohol use and myelofibrosis stimulate uric acid production, greatly increased urine excretion was probably responsible for the massive uric acid precipitation observed.

> Sudden flank pain, anuria and a history of urolithiasis suggest ureteral obstruction by a stone.

Case 7

Diagnosis – contrast media nephrotoxicity
The patient developed acute-on-chronic renal failure during the hospital stay. In diagnosing this

case, the physician must consider many causes. The worsening heart failure suggests the possibility of prerenal azotemia. The cardiac catheterization may have produced radiocontrast nephrotoxicity or atheroembolic renal disease. The history of urolithiasis and the symptoms of prostatism raise the question of obstructive uropathy. In addition, many of the medications occasionally produce renal failure: gemfibrozil (myoglobinuric ATN), furosemide (prerenal renal failure), furosemide and allopurinol (allergic interstitial nephritis), enalapril (vasomotor effect), and excessive dose of colchicine (nephrotoxic ATN).

The investigation of all these possibilities might include urinary electrolytes, renal sonogram, renal biopsy and discontinuation of medications. *However, when acute renal failure seems typical of radiocontrast nephrotoxicity, it is often best to hold off on other studies in order to see if the Scr peaks within three to five days of the procedure and then improves.* Observing the typical abbreviated course of contrast nephrotoxicity confirms the diagnosis, and avoids unnecessary studies.

Patients with radiocontrast nephrotoxicity almost always have underlying chronic renal failure and are over 40 years of age (most are elderly). Diabetes mellitus is another common risk factor. The rise in Scr begins within 24 hours of the procedure, and oliguria may also be noted within the first day or two.

This patient has the three risk factors for contrast nephrotoxicity, and experienced a rise in Scr and probably a fall in urine output following the catheterization. In addition, four days after the procedure the urine output has increased, and Scr has plateaued. It is appropriate to observe the renal function for another day or two before carrying out further studies.

Follow-up

Over the next three days, the Scr fell to 2.1 mg/dl (186 µmol/L) and BUN to 49 mg/dl (17 mmol/L). The dyspnea on exertion improved with an increased dose of furosemide.

> Underlying renal failure, old age, and a rise in Scr within one day of exposure to contrast medium suggest a vasomotor reaction to contrast media.

Case 8

Diagnosis – false renal failure due to cimetidine

This patient developed acute-on-chronic renal failure as crescendo angina, anemia and acute bronchitis improved. The cause of renal failure is not immediately obvious. The patient's atherosclerosis raises the question of renal failure caused by renal artery stenosis or by atheroembolic renal disease. However, the absence of hypertension or recent aortic manipulation make both possibilities unlikely. The recent administration of a β-lactam antibiotic and cimetidine are more worthy of the physician's attention. Both cause allergic interstitial nephritis. Although no rash or fever are present, one should check the differential count for eosinophilia, and, if elevated, one should consider discontinuation or substitution of these medications (in fact, the white count is 3,500 with 5% eosinophils). Cimetidine blocks tubular secretion of creatinine and produces a rise in Scr without a fall in GFR. The renal handling of urea is not effected and BUN does not change. Since this patient had a rise in Scr with little change in BUN, the cimetidine should be substituted by another H2-blocker or discontinued, and the Scr should be observed for two or three days.

Follow-up

The cimetidine was stopped. In three days the Scr fell from 3.6 (318 µmol/L) back to the baseline of 2.7 mg/dl (239 µmol/L) and the BUN rose from 58 to 61 mg/dl (21 to 22 mmol/L).

> Administration of cimetidine followed by a rise in Scr without a rise in BUN suggests false renal failure.

Case 9

Diagnosis – ischemic acute tubular necrosis (ATN)
The clinical picture of severe hypotension followed by oliguria with numerous muddy brown granular casts and renal tubular cells in the urine sediment is a classic one for ischemic acute tubular necrosis. An isotonic urine specific gravity (1.011) shows that the tubules are unable to concentrate the urine in response to the stimulus of hypovolemia.

One can also see prerenal renal failure in the setting of hemorrhage shock, but the urine sediment should be negative or contain a few hyaline or fine granular casts and the urine should be concentrated (specific gravity > 1.015). Similarly, the tubules in prerenal azotemia respond to salt retaining stimuli to produce urine with a low sodium and chloride content, whereas in ATN, the tubules usually fail to respond to these stimuli and the urine has a high salt content.

There is a continuum between ischemic ATN and prerenal azotemia, and patients may have some features of both conditions. The practical test that distinguishes these two ends of the spectrum is the renal response to volume repletion and to restoration of normal hemodynamics. Recovery of normal renal function occurs promptly in prerenal azotemia, but takes several days to a few weeks in ATN.

Follow-up

The urine showed sodium 53 mEq/L, chloride 64 mEq/L, FeNa 3.1% and FeCl 4.9%. With further volume repletion the systolic blood pressure stabilized at 115 to 120 mmHg, but the urine output remained about 200 ml per day. The Scr rose to 13.1 mg/dl (1158 μmol/L) over four days, and hemodialysis was begun. The patient recovered from his surgery without further complication. The urine output increased to over a liter per day after ten hospital days, and two days later the Scr began to fall. Hemodialysis was stopped. The Scr came down to 1.5 mg/dl (133 μmol/L) over two weeks.

> Hypotension, failure to concentrate the urine, and tubular cells and muddy granular casts in the urine sediment suggest ischemic ATN.

Case 10

Diagnosis – myeloma kidney
The diagnosis in this patient may not be immediately obvious. The clues to be considered in this case are the patient's advanced age, weight loss, the high BUN to Scr ratio, heavy proteinuria, uremia and rouleaux formation.

Proteinuria greater than 2.5 g per day is usually presumptive evidence of a glomerular disease, but in patients over 50 years of age must be confirmed by urine protein electrophoresis. In older individuals, such heavy proteinuria may consist mainly of monoclonal light chains produced by a multiple myeloma rather than of albumin. If albumin is the major urinary protein, one would focus on the nephrotic glomerular diseases, since *the absence of hematuria excludes an acute nephritic process.*

In older patients with undiagnosed renal failure, atherosclerotic causes and multiple myeloma must be considered. This patient has no known risks for atherosclerosis and no findings suggestive of renal artery stenosis or atheroembolic renal disease. The normal serum protein electrophoresis, bone marrow examination, serum calcium concentration and absence of bone pain tend to exclude multiple myeloma. However, *other information points towards multiple myeloma: the anemia unexplained by renal failure, the rouleaux formation, a slightly high serum calcium concentration when corrected for hypoalbuminemia and the discrepancy between the slight amount of protein detected by urine dipstick and the massive proteinuria in a 24-hour urine.* The low reading on the dipstick is due to its insensitivity to urine proteins other than albumin. Lysozyme in the urine of patients with monocytic leukemia is one such protein. However, urinary monoclonal light chains produced by myeloma cells are the most common explanation for this discrepancy. A urine protein electrophoresis should be ordered to discriminate urinary albumin from immunoglobulin light chains.

> *The serum protein electrophoresis may not detect light chain multiple myeloma.* Some 20% of multiple myelomas produce only light chains, which are cleared from the plasma by the kidneys. Thus, the light chains are typically seen on protein electrophoresis of the urine, and not on electrophoresis of the serum, unless the clearance of these proteins is impaired by renal failure. *Thus, both a urine and serum protein electrophoresis are needed to rule out multiple myeloma.*

Follow-up

The urine protein electrophoresis revealed scant albumin and an M protein in the beta region, which was a lambda light chain on immunofixation electrophoresis. The hypoalbuminemia may have been caused by poor nutrition. A bone marrow biopsy showed a marked increase in plasma cells. The patient was treated with melphalan, prednisone and normal saline. The Scr fell to 1.5 mg/dl (133 μmol/L) over one month. The high BUN to Scr ratio decreased; it may have reflected mildly hypovolemia caused by decreased salt intake and increased urinary salt excretion due to the hypercalcemia.

> Anemia, fatigue, weight loss, old age and failure of the urine dipstick to detect heavy proteinuria suggest renal failure caused by multiple myeloma.

Case 11

Diagnosis – chronic renal failure

The factors to be considered in diagnosing the worsening azotemia in this patient are the atherosclerosis, the heavy proteinuria, the angiotensin converting enzyme inhibitor and the rate of progression of the chronic renal failure.

The setting of atherosclerosis raises the possibility of renal failure from renal artery stenosis or atheroembolic disease. The longstanding proteinuria is evidence of a chronic glomerulopathy. An acceleration of renal failure in the absence of hematuria suggests a possible renal vein thrombosis complicating the nephrotic syndrome or rapid progression of the underlying glomerular disease. The stable dose of enalapril for five years makes it an unlikely cause of the rise in Scr.

More important than the above considerations is the question of whether the most recent rise in Scr is due to an acute-on-chronic process or is just the change caused by the underlying rate of loss of GFR. The present Scr may be predicted by plotting 1/Scr versus time and drawing the best fitting line through the points as shown in Fig. 1. One sees that the current Scr (2.8 mg/dl) is close to the line. If further values of Scr approximate the line, no search for an acute process is needed.

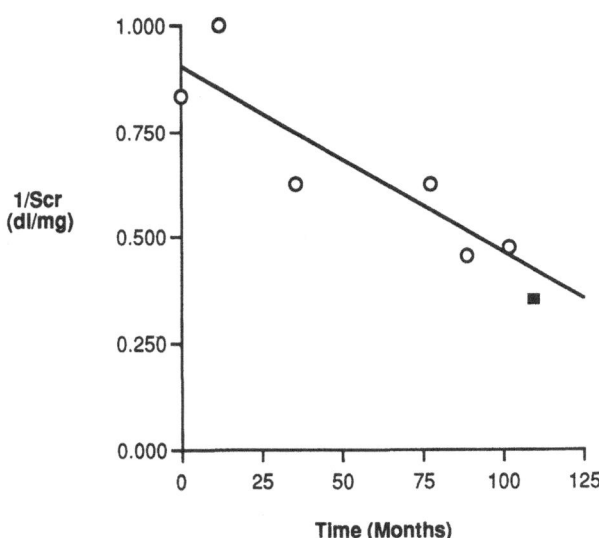

Fig. 1. Plot of 1/Scr (dl/mg) versus time showing that the most recent Scr (■] may well be in keeping with the chronic progressive loss of function.

Follow-up

A repeat Scr one month later was 2.7 mg/dl (239 μmol/L) which further diffused concern about an acute-on-chronic renal failure. An elective repair of the aortic aneurysm was planned. In an added effort to rule out a renal artery stenosis, a magnetic resonance aortography was carried out. Although the renal vessels appeared patent, the image quality was inadequate to completely exclude a renal artery stenosis. The aneurysm repair was successful and had no adverse affect on the Scr, which continued to increase as anticipated.

> A graph of 1/Scr versus time predicts the rise in Scr expected from progression of the chronic renal disease.

Case 12

Diagnosis – renal artery stenosis

Prerenal renal failure is excluded by the hypertension and the urine electrolytes, and postrenal renal failure is excluded by the ultrasound. In the absence of prior Scr values one cannot tell initially if this renal impairment is acute or chronic. In making a diagnosis the physician needs to take into consideration the new onset of severe hypertension in someone over 50 years of age, the nephrotic range proteinuria, the discrepancy in renal size, and the electrolyte abnormalities: hypokalemia and (in the absence of respiratory manifestations) probably metabolic alkalosis.

The heavy proteinuria suggests that a glomerular lesion is responsible for the renal failure. If he has rapidly progressive renal failure without manifestations of a systemic disease, then a primary acute nephritic disease like IgA nephropathy or crescentic glomerulonephritis must be considered.

The absence of hematuria excludes an acute nephritic process. However, progression of a chronic glomerulopathy that normally presents with nephrotic syndrome (like membranous or focal sclerosing glomerulonephritis) is still a possibility, since some of these patients do not have hematuria.

Rarely nephrotic range proteinuria is caused by allergic interstitial nephritis or a disease involving the small or large renal vessel diseases. The fact that the patient took no drugs virtually excludes allergic interstitial nephritis. With regard to vascular diseases, atheroembolic disease would be atypical in the absence of aortic manipulation, eosinophilia and ischemic skin changes in the feet. Malignant hypertension is a possibility, but a distant one, since the diastolic blood pressure is less than 130 mmHg and eye grounds are normal. It would, however, explain the hypokalemic metabolic alkalosis. In malignant hypertension ischemic glomeruli release renin, which stimulates aldosterone production, which increases renal losses of potassium and hydrogen ions.

Heavy proteinuria has been observed in cases of renal artery stenosis and is probably related to extremely high peripheral renin levels (15 to >300 ng/ml/hour) in these patients.[2] Renal artery stenosis is the most likely diagnosis for a number of reasons. *First, atherosclerotic causes of renal failure are more likely in older patients, especially those who smoke. Second, hypertension that starts or escapes from medical control after age 50 is an important clue to renal artery stenosis. Third, a discrepancy in kidney size is another finding suggestive of renovascular disease.* A left renal artery stenosis would account for the small left kidney. Otherwise, one might have to postulate a congenitally hypoplastic kidney or chronic pyelonephritis to explain the discrepancy in size. Fourth, renal artery

stenosis can raise the renin level which produces hypokalemic metabolic alkalosis. Finally, *with mild renal failure, the involvement may be unilateral.* Loss of function on the left side and a doubling of Scr could easily explain the Scr of 2.2 mg/dl (194 μmol/L). Therefore, the physician should look for a left renal artery stenosis with an arteriogram. The risk of precipitating a reversible nephrotoxic reaction with the contrast media is probably outweighed by the anticipated benefit of finding and correcting a stenotic renal artery. The release of cholesterol emboli due to the procedure is of concern, but this is clinically significant in only a small proportion of cases.

Follow-up

In this patient, a peripheral plasma renin activity (interesting, but unnecessary test) was very high at 28 ng/ml/hr, and an abdominal aortogram showed diffuse atherosclerosis of the aorta. An aortic plaque completely occluded the left renal artery orifice, but collateral vessels supplied the left kidney. Bypass surgery reestablished circulation to the left kidney. The serum electrolytes normalized, the urine protein slowly came down to 0.5 g/day and Scr dropped to 1.4 mg/dl (124 μmol/L).

> A history of smoking, discrepancy in kidney size, onset of severe hypertension after age 50 and hypokalemic metabolic alkalosis suggest renal artery stenosis.

Case 13

Diagnosis – myoglobinuric acute tubular necrosis
The history of dark urine and the results of the urinalysis are the key to making the correct diagnosis. The intermittent excretion of a tea-colored urine can be seen in several clinical settings, such as hemoglobinuria, myoglobinuria, bilirubinuria, drug ingestion, beeturia, and porphyria. However, the finding of a urine that is heme positive despite the absence of red blood cells in the urine sediment is suggestive of hemoglobinuria or myoglobinuria. In addition, the elevated transaminases may reflect muscle and not liver injury, since the alkaline phosphatase and bilirubin were normal.

Although there are numerous causes of rhabdomyolysis, trauma is the most common. However, considering the paucity of physical signs of trauma (i.e. no ecchymoses, hematoma) and the fact that significant rhabdomyolysis is mainly seen in moderate to severe injuries, it is unlikely that the fall was cause of the patient's rhabdomyolysis. Second, the patient was intermittently excreting tea-colored urine several days prior to his trauma. The history revealed that he was taking lovastatin (Mevacor), a drug which is known to cause rhabdomyolysis with myoglobinuric acute tubular necrosis.

The mechanism for the acute renal failure secondary to rhabdomyolysis is probably multifactorial and includes renal vasoconstriction secondary to the antagonism of myoglobin to the vasodilating effect of nitric oxide, intratubular obstruction with myoglobin casts, and possibly a direct proximal tubular injury by myoglobin itself. Treatment options include hydration with isotonic saline which enhances renal perfusion and urine flow rate, and a forced alkaline diuresis which decreases the production of toxic breakdown products of myoglobin in the tubule. Early intervention may enhance the success of this maneuver.

Follow-up

Due to the concomitant chest pain that the patient developed during admission, he was transferred to the Coronary Care Unit for further management. High myoglobin levels (1,250 ng/ml) were measured in the urine. A serum creatine phosphokinase was 207,600 IU/L. During the next 48 hours, aggressive intravenous hydration with isotonic sodium bicarbonate was given, but the patient's renal failure worsened and he was then hemodialyzed. The creatine phosphokinase (MM band) rose to a peak of 413,200 IU/L. On the 4th hospital day, the patient developed an acute myocardial infarction and expired. At postmortem examination of the renal histology showed numerous pigmented granular casts within the distal collecting tubules. In addition, the proximal tubules were dilated and contained regenerative tubular epithelium. These findings were consistent with resolving ATN. Finally, histopathology of the muscle tissue showed extensive myofibril degeneration with some evidence of regeneration which again is suggestive of rhabdomyolysis.

> Muscle tenderness, lovastatin use, elevated aminotransferase levels and positive urine heme test in the absence of red blood cells suggest myoglobinuric ATN.

Case 14

Diagnosis – hemolytic uremic syndrome

The clues to the diagnosis in this young woman are the thrombocytopenia and the microangiopathic hemolytic anemia as evidenced by fragmented red blood cells on peripheral blood smear. These findings may occur in scleroderma renal crisis, malignant hypertension and disseminated intravascular coagulation; however, there is no evidence for these entities in the patient's clinical picture. The presentation is more consistent with thrombotic thrombocytopenia purpura or the hemolytic uremic syndrome. These conditions may be the two ends of a continuum. However, this case fits best with hemolytic uremic syndrome because of the association with an oral contraceptive and because of the hypertension, moderately severe renal failure, less severe thrombocytopenia and absence of fever and central nervous systemic manifestations. The clinical picture is characteristic enough to be diagnostic and confirmation by renal biopsy is not needed. The unilateral low-grade hydronephrosis is probably not significant. Appropriate treatment should be initiated.

Follow-up

Hemolytic anemia was further documented with a reticulocyte count of 2.9%, a lactic dehydrogenase concentration >10,000 IU/L, and a haptoglobin of <5 g/dl (normal 12–160 g/dl). The prothrombin time and partial thromboplastic time were normal.

The patient became anuric. The renal failure was managed with hemodialysis. The patient was given aspirin, persantine, high dose prednisone, and plasma exchanges three days in a row. The platelet count then rose rapidly to normal. The LDH gradually fell to under 1,000 IU/L one week after the last plasma exchange. After the last plasma exchange the patient began to make urine and hemodialysis was stopped one week later. The Scr eventually stabilized at 1.8 mg/dl (159 μmol/L).

> Oral contraceptive use, thrombocytopenia, and microangiopathic hemolytic anemia suggest hemolytic uremic syndrome.

Case 15

Diagnosis – left renal artery stenosis
There are few, if any, clues to the diagnosis in this patient. *With an age over 50, the question of myeloma kidney comes up, but the lack of proteinuria by urine protein to creatinine ratio excludes significant amount of urinary light chains.* Although his age and smoking history raise the issue of renal complications of atherosclerosis, no other clinical evidence supports this (i.e. no ischemic toes, eosinophilia, atherosclerotic manifestations or worsening hypertension).

Given the unexplained renal failure a renal biopsy was carried out to look for an intrinsic renal cause, but the non-specific changes seen were insufficient to explain the renal failure.

With parenchymal disease excluded, one must look carefully at the perfusion to the kidneys and the patency of urine outflow. *The absence of any dilatation of the collecting system on the renal sonogram is almost infallible in excluding urinary obstruction.* Since the patient's age and smoking history raise the question of atherosclerosis of the renal arteries, a renal arteriogram should be carried out.

Follow-up

An aortogram and bilateral renal arteriogram showed an insignificant (~25%) stenosis of the right renal artery and a tight stenosis (>90%) of the left renal artery with collateral flow to the segmental arteries. Delayed imaging showed no contrast excretion on the left. The stenosis was dilated successfully by percutaneous transluminal angioplasty. Over the next week, the Scr fell to 1.5 mg/dl (133 μmol/L) and the blood pressure to 135/85 mmHg. Apparently, the underperfused left kidney had minimal function, but sufficient blood supply

via collaterals to remain viable. Correction of the stenosis restored function to the kidney.

> Renal failure "out of the blue" may be caused by volume depletion, intrinsic renal disease, and by vascular or urinary obstruction. Because of the atherosclerotic risk factors, renal artery stenosis ought to be investigated first with an angiogram.

Case 16

Diagnosis – acute tubular necrosis caused by sepsis
The physician must consider a variety of possible causes of renal failure: immune complex GN due to a staphylococcal infection, acute interstitial nephritis due to β-lactam antibiotics or to acute pyelonephritis, and postrenal renal failure due to enlarged retroperitoneal lymph nodes or to two complications of diabetes mellitus: neurogenic bladder and ureteral impaction by a necrotic renal papilla. The use of gentamicin for only three days makes aminoglycoside nephrotoxicity unlikely.

The most significant clinical event, however, from the renal standpoint occurred on the ninth hospital day. The low body temperature, tachypnea, low normal blood pressure, mental confusion and urinary infection are evidence of a septic episode. Also the Scr probably began to rise right after this episode, although intervening Scr values were not measured. *The occurrence of sepsis with a fall in blood pressure at the time when the Scr starts to rise or when the urine output falls is strong evidence for ATN due to sepsis. The systolic blood pressure need not fall below 110 mmHg.* The diagnosis will be confirmed by a spontaneous recovery in renal function in the next week or two. While waiting for a fall in Scr, the physician might investigate the other possible diagnoses by measuring a post void residual urine, and ordering a renal sonogram, serum complement levels and a urine and blood for eosinophils.

Follow-up

Over the next three hospital days, the Scr stabilized

at 3.1 mg/dl (274 µmol/L) and began to fall. One week later the Scr was 1.1 mg/dl (97 µmol/L).

> An episode of sepsis with a fall in blood pressure within the normal range at the time of rise in Scr suggests ischemic ATN.

Case 17

Diagnosis – Henoch-Schonlein purpura
In diagnosing this case, only a few possibilities need to be considered. The abdominal pain, atrial fibrillation, hematuria and proteinuria raise the question of a renal embolism. However, the lactic dehydrogenase is not elevated and there is another likely cause of the abdominal pain (see below). The history of malignancy suggests a possible urinary obstruction from retroperitoneal metastases, but the sonogram shows no hydronephrosis. The key clue is the vasculitis-like picture with a rash, an acute nephritic picture and probable involvement of the gut. Serologic studies were negative. Essential mixed cryoglobulinemia is excluded by the absence of cryoglobulins. Wegener's granulomatosis is unlikely without a positive ANCA test or respiratory involvement. With gastrointestinal involvement, Henoch-Schonlein purpura would be a likely diagnosis, although it is rare in adults, and the rash in this disease is usually on the lower extremities. This diagnosis can often be confirmed on skin biopsy by finding a leukocytoclastic vasculitis with IgA deposition. The physician should obtain this study.

Follow-up

A skin biopsy showed an IgA-mediated leukocytoclastic vasculitis. The Scr rose to 7.1 mg/dl (628 µmol/L) and hemodialysis was initiated. Since treatment of possible glomerular crescent formation should be a consideration in this condition, a renal biopsy was performed. It showed mild mesangial proliferative GN with mesangial deposition of IgA and C3, consistent with IgA nephropathy or Henoch-Schonlein purpura. There were no crescents. After two dialysis treatments, the Scr fell spontaneously and decreased to 2.1

mg/dl (186 µmol/L) over several weeks. Petechial lesions appeared over the lower extremities and were still appearing after six weeks of illness.

> Hematuria, proteinuria, skin rash, GI bleeding and other GI symptoms suggest Henoch-Schonlein purpura.

Case 18

Diagnosis – bilateral ureteral obstruction
This patient presents no clues to the etiology of the renal failure. As a result, his physician performed a renal biopsy to look for parenchymal disease. The biopsy was virtually normal. The next step is to consider the possibility of inadequate renal perfusion or inadequate drainage of urine through the ureters, despite little or no dilatation of the kidneys by sonogram. Grade I hydronephrosis is usually not caused by urinary obstruction and any obstruction would have to be bilateral to produce such severe renal failure. Nevertheless, the low grade dilatation suggests that cystoscopy with retrograde pyelograms should be the next diagnostic step.

Follow-up

Cystoscopy was carried out and urine flow was reestablished after inserting a left ureteral catheter, which was left in place. Retrograde pyelograms showed minimal hydronephrosis bilaterally. The Scr came down to 2.6 mg/dl (230 µmol/L) over four days. Unfortunately, the patient developed sepsis and hypotension, and died two days later. An autopsy showed a carcinoma of the prostate with metastatic invasion of the ureters.

> Renal failure "out of the blue" may be caused by volume depletion, intrinsic renal disease, and by vascular or urinary obstruction. Because of the mild unilateral hydronephrosis ureteral obstruction should be investigated first with a retrograde pyelogram.

Case 19

Diagnosis – prerenal renal failure caused by Addison's disease

The clinical clues that must be considered here are the six-month history of anemia and wasting, the slightly elevated serum potassium concentration and the low normal blood pressure.

The serum potassium level should not be elevated in mild renal failure unless there is an additional problem with potassium handling. For example, aldosterone levels may be low, as in primary adrenal insufficiency, or the renal tubules may be unresponsive to aldosterone as in obstructive uropathy. Obstruction was excluded by the normal renal sonogram. Plasma renin and aldosterone concentrations might be ordered to evaluate this.

The low normal blood pressure raises the question of prerenal azotemia, but the lack of renal salt avidity, a concentrated urine, and of previous fluid loss militate against this. Nevertheless, the physician's concern about prerenal azotemia should not be allayed. If volume depletion has occurred through renal salt losing, no obvious fluid losses will be apparent and the urine will not have a low salt content. The physician should look for orthostatic changes in pulse and blood pressure.

Follow-up

The patient's blood pressure fell to 80/40 mmHg on standing and the pulse rose by 20 per minute. It was speculated that poor salt intake and renal salt wasting had caused volume depletion. Intravenous saline was given at two liters per day. The blood pressure rose to 135/80 mmHg and the Scr fell to 0.9 mg/dl (80 μmol/L) after three days.

Given the unexplained anorexia, wasting, fatigue and anemia, it was postulated that the hyperkalemia and renal salt losing were caused by low aldosterone secretion due to Addison's disease. Primary adrenal insufficiency was diagnosed with a low morning plasma cortisol concentration, a high plasma ACTH level and an abnormal ACTH stimulation test. Cortisol and fludrocortisone were given as hormone replacement. The anemia, anorexia and fatigue gradually improved.

> Renal failure "out of the blue" may be caused by volume depletion, intrinsic renal disease, and by vascular or urinary obstruction. Because of the low normal blood pressure, volume depletion should be investigated first with a trial of volume expansion.

Case 20

Diagnosis – acute interstitial nephritis

In making a diagnosis, the physician should consider the dark urine, the bilateral tenderness over the kidneys, the heavy proteinuria, the granular casts and the thrombocytopenia.

The rapid rise of Scr in the hospital demonstrates that the renal failure is acute, although a chronic component cannot be excluded. Since the history and high blood pressure exclude prerenal renal failure, and the ultrasound rules out obstruction, the patient has an intrinsic renal disease. The granular casts also reflect a parenchymal etiology.

The history of a respiratory infection, the "Coca-Cola" colored urine, and the heavy proteinuria (more than 300 mg/dl on dipstick, more than 2.5 urine protein to creatinine ratio) at first suggest an acute glomerulonephritis. *But, the absence of hematuria excludes an acute nephritic process.*

The history of dark urine and large amount of heme in the urine with scant red blood cells suggest hemoglobinuric or myoglobinuric tubular necrosis. However, the normal hemoglobin, hematocrit and creatine phosphokinase exclude significant hemolysis or rhabdomyolysis.

The low platelet count and proteinuria raise the question of a small vessel disease. However, we can exclude malignant hypertension based on the blood pressure, scleroderma based on the normal skin, and thrombotic thrombocytopenic purpura and hemolytic uremic syndrome based on the absence of hemolytic anemia.

Penicillin analogues like amoxicillin can cause acute allergic nephritis, sometimes with heavy proteinuria. This diagnosis is unlikely since such patients generally present while they are still taking the drug and not weeks later. Finally, there is no hypotension or nephrotoxin exposure to suggest acute tubular necrosis.

In summary, a careful consideration of the findings in this case do not permit us to make a diagnosis or even suggest one. Except for the thrombocytopenia, this is renal failure "out of the blue", which is to say that the evaluation discloses no problem other than the kidney disease. *In cases of renal failure due to undiagnosed intrinsic disease, a renal biopsy should be performed, because it will usually be diagnostic, and treatment is often possible.*

Follow-up

This patient was treated with hemodialysis and underwent a renal biopsy that showed an acute interstitial nephritis. There was patchy tubular destruction, and interstitial edema and infiltration mostly of lymphocytes and histiocytes. Regeneration of tubular epithelium suggested a resolving phase. In fact, urine output rose after the renal biopsy and Scr fell to 3.8 mg/dl (336 μmol/L) over the next five days, at which point the patient was discharged. The low platelet count and heme positive urine resolved and were never explained. Thus, this patient either had an idiopathic acute interstitial nephritis or a delayed allergic interstitial nephritis caused by amoxicillin. Of interest is the costovertebral angle tenderness, which can be seen with acute interstitial nephritis.

> Renal failure "out of the blue" may be caused by volume depletion, intrinsic renal disease, and by vascular or urinary obstruction. Because of the proteinuria and granular casts, intrinsic renal disease should be investigated first with a renal biopsy.

NOTES

1. Scola FH, Cronan JJ and Schepps B. Grade 1 hydronephrosis: pulsed Doppler US evaluation. Radiology 1989; 171:519–20. Ellenbogen PH, Scheible FW, Talner LB and Leopold GR. Sensitivity of gray scale ultrasound in detecting urinary tract obstruction. Am J Roentgenol 1978; 130:731–3.
2. Sato H, Saito T, Kasai Y, Abe K and Yoshinaga K. Massive proteinuria due to renal artery stenosis. Nephron 1989; 51:136–7. Kumar A and Shapiro AP. Proteinuria and nephrotic syndrome induced by renin in patients with renal artery stenosis. Arch Intern Med 1980; 140:1631–4.
3. Case and discussion were contributed by Dr. Fred Tan.

APPENDIX A. MEDICATIONS THAT CAUSE RENAL FAILURE WITH PROPER USE[1]

False renal failure (see Chapter 7)
Impaired tubular secretion of creatinine
    Salicylate
    Cimetidine
    Trimethoprim
Positive interference with creatinine measurement
    Cefoxitin
    Acetohexamide
    Methyldopa
    5-Flucytosine (Ektachem method)

Chronic renal failure
Retroperitoneal fibrosis (see Postrenal renal failure below)
Hemolytic uremic syndrome (see Vascular causes below)
Nephrotoxic tubular damage (see Tubular causes below)
Chronic Interstitial Nephritis (see Interstitial causes below)

Prerenal renal failure
Volume depletion
    Laxatives
    Diuretics
    Renal salt wasting-Cisplatin [1]
    Capillary leak
        Gonadotropins [2]
        All-trans retinoic acid [3]
Reduced vascular resistance
    Antihypertensive
    Coronary vasodilators
        Nitrates
        Calcium channel blockers
    Interleukin-2 [4–6]

Postrenal renal failure
Retroperitoneal fibrosis
    Methylsergide [7]
    Bromocriptine [8]
    Dihydroergotamine [9]
Sloughed papilla[2]
    Nonsteroidal anti-inflammatory drugs [10]
    Aspirin [11]

Ureteral obstruction by clots – ϵ – Aminocaproic acid [12]
Ureteral obstruction by stones – Sulfadiazine [13]
Neurogenic bladder[3]
    Narcotics
    Drugs with anticholinergic activity
        Atropine and related alkaloids
        Antihistamines
        Phenothiazines
        Disopyramide phosphate [14]

Vascular causes of renal failure (see Chapter 10)
Vasomotor disturbance
    Nonsteroidal anti-inflammatory drugs
    Angiotensin converting enzyme inhibitors
    Nifedipine
    Cyclosporin A
    Contrast media
    Interleukin 2/α-interferon [15]
    Demeclocycline [16]
    Flosequinan [17]
    Mannitol [18]
Atheroembolic disease
    Anticoagulation
    Thrombolytic therapy
        Tissue plasminogen activator
        Streptokinase
Hemolytic uremic syndrome
    Mitomycin C
    Oral contraceptives
    Bleomycin
    Conjugated estrogens
    Quinine
Vasculitis – Carbamazepine [19]

Glomerular causes of renal failure
Crescentic glomerulonephritis
    D-Penicillamine [20]
    Hydralazine [21]
    Interleukin–2 [22]
Goodpasture's syndrome – D-penicillamine [23]
Vasculitis
    Hyposensitization treatment [24]
    Penicillin [25]
    Sulfa [26, 27]

J.G. Abuelo (ed.), Renal Failure, 255–267.
© 1995 *Kluwer Academic Publishers.*

Tubular causes of renal failure [28]
Acute tubular necrosis
  Antibiotics
    Aminoglycosides
    Demeclocycline
    Amphotericin B
    Capreomycin [29]
    Pentamidine
    Foscarnet [30]
  Anesthetics
    Methoxyflurane
    Enflurane
    Halothane
  Cancer chemotherapy [31, 32]
    Cisplatin
    Interferon Alfa-2a, Alfa-2b
    Streptozocin
    Pentostatin
    5-azacytidine
    Ifosfamide [33, 34]
    Plicamycin
    Carboplatin [35]
    Asparaginase
    Fludarabine
    Dacarbazine
    Amsacrine
    Mitoxantrone
  Intravascular hemolysis [36]
    Thiopental [37]
    Chloramphenicol
    Chloroquine
    Dapsone
    Aspirin
    Quinine sulfate [38]
  Rhabdomyolysis
    Lipid lowering drugs [39, 40]
    Hypertonic sodium chloride – Therapeutic
    abortion [41]
    Cyclosporine A [42]
  Miscellaneous
    Dextran [43]
    Lithium [46]
    Deferoxamine [44]
    Fumaric acid [47]
    EDTA [45]
    Intravenous immunoglobulin [48]
Chronic tubular atrophy
  Methyl CCNU
  BCNU
  Cyclosporin A

  Lithium
Intratubular Obstruction
  Methotrexate
  Acetazolamide
  Sulfonamides
  Acyclovir
  Tumor lysis syndrome
  Naftidrofuryl oxalate [49]
  Triamterene

Interstitial causes of renal failure [50]
Antibiotics
  Methicillin
  Sulfonamides
  Penicillin G
  Cotrimoxazole
  Ampicillin
  Rifampin
  Amoxicillin
  Ciprofloxacin [53–54]
  Nafcillin
  Norfloxacin [55]
  Carbenicillin
  Polymyxin
  Oxacillin
  Kanamycin
  Piperacillin [51]
  Gentamicin
  Cephalothin
  Colistin
  Cephalexin
  Ethambutol
  Cephalexin
  Ethambutol
  Cefazolin [52]
  Chloramphenicol
  Tetracyclines
  Erythromycin
  Vancomycin
  Acyclovir [56]
Nonsteroidal anti-inflammatory drugs
  Naproxen
  Ibuprofen
  Fenoprofen
  Zomepirac
  Mefenamate
  Phenylbutazone
  Tolmetin
  Indomethacin
  Diflunisal

Diclofenac
Piroxicam
Ketoprofen
Diuretics
Furosemide
Chlorthalidone
Thiazides
Triamterene
Miscellaneous
Diphenylhydantoin
Phenobarbital
Glafenin
Alpha-methyldopa
Phenidione
Gold and bismuth salts
Allopurinol
Diazepam
Cimetidine
D-penicillamine
Sulfinpyrazone
Alpha-interferon
Aspirin
Phenacetin
Carbamazepine
Phenazone
Clofibrate
Antipyrine
Azathioprine
Carbamazepine
Sulfasalazine [57]
Carboplatin [59]
5-Aminosalicylic acid [58]
Intravesical BCG [60]

NOTES

1. Many drugs are listed based on one or few reported cases. Nephrotoxic reactions to such medications may be very rare or may not occur at all, if the reported cases were misdiagnosed.
2. These drugs cause papillary necrosis, but renal failure due to obstruction by a sloughed papilla has not been reported.
3. Renal failure is occasionally observed in clinical practice, but I am not aware of case reports in the literature.

REFERENCES

1. Hutchison FN, Perez EA, Gandara DR, Lawrence HJ and Kaysen GA. Renal salt wasting in patients treated with cisplatin. Ann Intern Med 1988; 108:21–5.
2. Golan A, Ron-El R, Herman A, Soffer Y, Weinraub Z and Caspi E. Ovarian hyperstimulation syndrome: An update review. Obstet and Gynecol Survey 1989; 44:430–40.
3. Frankel SR, Eardley A, Lauwers G, Weiss M and Warrell RP Jr. The "retinoic acid syndrome" in acute promyelocytic leukemia. Ann Intern Med 1992; 117:292–6.
4. Kozeny GA, Nicolas JD, Creekmore S, Sticklin L, Hano JE and Fisher RI. Effects of interleukin-2 immunotherapy on renal function. J Clin Oncol 1988; 6:1170–6.
5. Webb DE, Austin HA III, Belldegrun A, Vaughan E, Linehan WM and Rosenberg SA. Metabolic and renal effects of interleukin-2 immunotherapy for metastatic cancer. Clin Nephrol 1988; 30:141–5.
6. Rosenberg SA, Packard BS, Aebersold PM, Solomon D, Topalian SL, Toy ST et al. Use of tumor-infiltrating lymphocytes and interleukin-2 in the immunotherapy of patients with metastatic melanoma. N Engl J Med 1988; 319:1676–80.
7. Graham JR, Suby JI, LeCompte PR and Sandowsky NL. Fibrotic disorders associated with methysergide therapy for headache. N Engl J Med 1966; 274:359–68.
8. Bowler JV, Ormerod IE and Legg NJ. Retroperitoneal fibrosis and bromocriptine. Lancet 1986; 2:466.
9. Malaquin F, Urban T, Ostinelli J, Ghedira H and Lacronique J. Pleural and retroperitoneal fibrosis from dihydroergotamine. N Engl J Med 1989; 321:1760.
10. O'Brien WM. Pharmacology of nonsteroidal anti-inflammatory drugs. Am J Med 1983; 75:32–8.
11. Wortmann DW, Kelsch RC, Kuhns L, Sullivan DB and Cassidy JT. Renal papillary necrosis in juvenile rheumatoid arthritis. J Pediatr 1980; 97:37–40.
12. Pitts TO, Spero JA, Bontempo FA and Greenberg A. Acute renal failure due to high-grade obstruction following therapy with e-Aminocaproic acid. Am J Kidney Dis 1986; 8:441–4.
13. Kronawitter U, Jakob K, Zoller WG, Rauh G and Goebel FD. Acute renal failure caused by sulphadiazine stones: complication of toxoplasmosis treatment in a patient with AIDS. Dtsch Med Wochenschr 1993; 118:1683–6.
14. Danziger LH and Horn JR. Disopyramide-induced urinary retention. Arch Intern Med 1983; 143:1683–6.
15. Mercatello A, Hadj-Aissa A, Negrier S, Allaouchiche B, Coronel B, Tognet E et al. Acute renal failure with preserved renal plasma flow induced by cancer immunotherapy. Kidney Int 1991; 40:309–14.
16. Perez-Ayuso RM, Arroyo V, Camps J, Jimenez W, Rodamilans M, Rimola A et al. Effect of demeclocycline on renal function and urinary prostaglandin E2 and kallikrein in hyponatremic cirrhotics. Nephron 1984; 36:30–7.
17. Wood SM, Dudley CRK, Devaney AM and Winearls CG. Flosequinan and renovascular disease. Lancet 1993; 341:116–7.
18. Dorman HR, Sondheimer JH and Cadnapaphornchai P. Mannitol-induced acute renal failure. Medicine 1990; 69:153–9.
19. Imai H, Nakamoto Y, Hirokawa M, Akihama T and Miura AB. Carbamazepine-induced granulomatous necrotizing angiitis with acute renal failure. Nephron 1989; 51:405–8.
20. Ntoso KA, Tomaszewski, Jimenez SA and Neilson EG. Penicillamine-induced rapidly progressive glomerulonephritis in patients with progressive systemic sclerosis: Suc-

cessful treatment of two patients and a review of the literature. Am J Kidney Dis 1986; 8:159–63.

21. Thompson CH and Kalowski S. Anti-glomerular basement membrane nephritis due to hydralazine. Nephron 1991; 58:238–9.

22. Chan TM, Cheng IKP, Wong KL, Chan KW and Lai CL. Crescentic IgA glomerulonephritis following interleukin-2 therapy for hepatocellular carcinoma of the liver. Am J Nephrol 1991; 11:493–6.

23. Gavaghan TE, McNaught PJ, Ralston M and Hayes JM. Penicillamine-induced "Goodpasture's syndrome": successful treatment of a fulminant case. Aust N Z J Med 1981; 11:261–5.

24. Phanuphak P and Kohler PF. Onset of polyarteritis nodosa during allergic hyposensitization treatment. Am J Med 1980; 68:479–85.

25. Schrier RW, Bulger RJ and VanArsdel PP Jr. Nephropathy associated with penicillin and homologues. Ann Intern Med 1966; 64:116–27.

26. Mullick FG, McAllister HA Jr, Wagner BM and Fenoglio JJ Jr. Drug related vasculitis. Human Pathol 1979; 10:313–25.

27. Minetti L, diBelgioioso, GB and Busnach G. Immunohistological diagnosis of drug-induced hypersensitivity nephritis. Contr. Nephrol. 1978; 10:15–29.

28. Humes HD and Weinberg JM. Toxic nephropathies. In: Brenner BM and Rector FC Jr, editors. The kidney. W.B. Saunders Company, Philadelphia, 1986:3rd ed., 1491–532.

29. Yue WY and Cohen SS. Toxic nephritis with acute renal insufficiency caused by administration of capreomycin. Diseases of the Chest 1966; 49:549–51.

30. Palestine AG, Polis MA, De Smet MD, Baird BF, Falloon J, Kovacs JA et al. A randomized, controlled trial of foscarnet in the treatment of cytomegalovirus retinitis in patients with AIDS. Ann Intern Med 1991; 115:665–73.

31. Drugs of choice for cancer chemotherapy, The Medical Letter on Drugs and Therapeutics 1993; 35:43–50.

32. Rieselbach RE and Garnick MB. Renal diseases induced by antineoplastic agents. In: Schrier RW and Gottschalk CW, editors. Diseases of the kidney. Little Brown and Company, Boston, 1993:5th ed., 1165–86.

33. Ghosn M. Droz JP, Theodore C, Pico JL, Baume D, Spielmann M et al. Salvage chemotherapy and refractory germ cell tumors with etoposide (VP-16) plus ifosamide and high dose cisplatin. Cancer 1988; 62:24.

34. Patterson WP and Khojasteh A. Ifosfamide-induced renal tubular defects. Cancer 1989; 63:649–51.

35. Smit EF, Sleijfer D Th, Meijer S, Mulder NH and Postmus PE. Carboplatin and renal function. Ann Intern Med 1989; 110:1034.

36. Chugh KS, Singhal PC, Nath IVS, Tewari SC, Muthusethupathy MA, Viswanathan S et al. Spectrum of acute renal failure in north India. J Assoc Phys India 1978; 26:147–54.

37. Habibi B, Basty R, Chodez S and Prunat A. Thiopental-related immune hemolytic anemia and renal failure. N Engl J Med 1985; 312:353–5.

38. Muehrcke RC. Acute renal failure: diagnosis and management. C.V. Mosby Company, St. Louis, 1969: 188.

39. Marais GE and Larson KK. Rhabdomyolysis and acute renal failure induced by combination lovastatin and gemfibrozil therapy. Ann Intern Med 1990; 112:228–30.

40. Bizzaro N, Bagolin E, Milani L, Cereser C and Finco B. Massive rhabdomyolysis and simvastatin. Clin Chem 1992; 38:1504.

41. Dominguez De Villota E, Cavanilles JM, Stein L, Shubin H and Weil MH. Hyperosmolal crisis following infusion of hypertonic sodium chloride for purposes of therapeutic abortion. Am J Med 1973; 55:116–22.

42. Chagnac A, Wisnovitz M, Zevin D, Korzets A, Mittelman M and Levi J. Cyclosporin–associated rhabdomyolysis and anterior compartment syndrome in a renal transplant recipient. Clin Nephrol 1993; 39:351–2.

43. Druml W, Polzleitner D, Laggner AN, Lenz K and Ulrich W. Dextran-40, acute renal failure and elevated plasma oncotic pressure. N Engl J Med 1988; 318:252–3.

44. Koren G., Bentur Y, Strong D, Harvey E, Klein J, Baumal R et al. Acute changes in renal function associated with deferoxamine therapy. Am J Dis Child 1989; 143:1077–80.

45. Moel DI and Kumar K. Reversible nephrotoxic reactions to a combined 2,3-dimercapto-1-propanol and calcium disodium ethylenediaminetetraacetic acid regimen in asymptomatic children with elevated blood lead levels. Pediatrics 1982; 70:259–62.

46. Boton R, Gaviria M and Batlle DC. Prevalence, pathogenesis, and treatment of renal dysfunction associated with chronic lithium therapy. Am J Kidney Dis 1987; 10:329–45.

47. Roodnat JI, Christiaans MHL, Nugteren-Huying WM, Schroeff JG van der, Zouwen P van der, Stricker BHC et al. Akute Niereninsuffizienz bei der behandlung der psoriasis mit fumarsaure-estern. Schweiz Med Wochenschr 1989; 119:826–30.

48. Pasatiempo AMG, Kroser JA, Rudnick M, Hoffman BI. Acute renal failure after intravenous immunoglobulin therapy. J Rheumatol 1994; 21:347–9.

49. Moesch C, Rince M, Daudon M, Aldigier J-C, Leroux-Robert C. Renal intratubular crystallisation of calcium oxalate and naftidrofuryl oxalate. Lancet 1991; 338:1219–20.

50. Cameron JS. Immunologically mediated interstitial nephritis: Primary and secondary. Adv Nephrol 1989; 18:207–48.

51. Dorner O, Piper C, Dienes HP, Berg PA, Egidy HV. Akute interstitielle nephritis nach piperacillin. Klin Wochenschr 1989; 67:682–6.

52. Nemati C, Abuelo JG. Cephalosporin induced hypersensitivity nephritis: Report of a case caused by cefazolin. Rhode Island Med J 1981; 64:91–4.

53. Hootkins R, Fenves AZ, Stephens MK. Acute renal failure secondary to oral ciprofloxacin therapy: a presentation of three cases and a review of the literature. Clin Nephrol 1989; 32:75–8.

54. Rastogi S, Atkinson JLD, McCarthy JT. Allergic nephropathy associated with ciprofloxacin. Mayo Clin Proc 1990; 65:987–9.

55. Boelaert J, de Jaegere PP, Daneels R, Schurgers M, Gordts B, van Landuyt HW. Case report of renal failure during norfloxacin therapy. Clin Nephrol 1986; 25:272.

56. Rashed A, Azadeh B, Abu Romeh SH. Acyclovir-induced

acute tubulo-interstitial nephritis. Nephron 1990; 56:436–8.

57. Dwarakanath AD, Michael J, Allan RN. Sulphasalazine induced renal failure. Gut 1992; 33:1006–7.

58. Mehta RP. Acute interstitial nephritis due to 5-aminosalicylic acid. Can Med Assoc J 1990; 143:1031–2.

59. McDonals BR, Kirmani S, Vasquez M, Mehta RL. Acute renal failure associated with the use of intraperitoneal cor-

boplatin: A report of two cases and review of the literature. Am J Med 1991; 90:386–91.

60. Modesto A, Marty L, Suc J-M, Kleinknecht D, de Fremont J-F, Marsepoil T, et al. Renal complications of intravesical bacillus Calmette-Guérin therapy. Am J Nephrol 1991; 11:501–4.

APPENDIX B. NEPHROTOXINS OTHER THAN PROPERLY USED LEGITIMATE DRUGS

Overdose of legitimate drugs or abuse of illicit drugs

Renal lesion	Drug	Circumstance of administration
Acute interstitial nephritis	Chlorprothixene [1]	Suicide
Chronic glomerulonephritis (Heroin nephropathy)	Heroin [2]	Narcotic addiction
	Pentazocine [3, 4]	Narcotic addiction
Chronic interstitial nephritis (Analgesic nephropathy)	Acetaminophen [5]	Analgesic abuse
	Nonsteroidal anti-inflammatory drugs [6]	Analgesic abuse
Hemoglobinuric ATN	Methyl-tert-butyl ether [7]	Dissolution of gallstones
Hypercalcemia	Vitamin A [8]	Acne treatment
	Vitamin D	Hypoparathyroidism [9], metabolic bone disease [10]
Hyperoncotic state	Albumin [11]	Refractory ascites
Myoglobinuric ATN	Amoxapine [12, 13]	Suicide
	Amphetamines [14]	Drug overdose
	Barbiturates [15]	Drug overdose
	Cocaine [16, 16a]	Drug overdose
	Diazepam [15]	Drug overdose
	Doxepin/nitrazepam [17]	Suicide
	"Ecstasy" [18]	Drug abuse
	Ethanol [14, 15]	Alcoholism
	Glutethemide [14]	Drug overdose
	Heroin [14]	Drug overdose
	Methadone [14]	Drug overdose
	Phencyclidine [14]	Drug overdose
	Phenylpropanolamine [19]	Weight loss, drug overdose
	Strychnine [20]	Mistaken for cocaine
	Terbutaline [21]	Suicide
Necrotizing vasculitis	Methamphetamine [22]	Drug overdose
Nephrotoxic ATN	Acetaminophen [23–25]	Suicide
	Aspirin [26]	Suicide
	Boric acid [27]	Diaper rash
	Bismuth salts [28]	Taken for warts
	Colchicine [29, 30]	Suicide
	Colloidal bismuth [31]	Drug overdose
	Lead [32]	Inadvertently self injected with opium
	Nomifensine [33]	Suicide
	Pennyroyal oil [34]	Attempted abortion
	Paraldehyde [35]	Drug overdose
	Triamterene [36]	Suicide
	Uranium [37]	Clinical investigation
Obstruction (stones)	Magnesium antacid [38]	Antacid abuse
Osmotic nephrosis	Mannitol [39–41]	Excessive dose
Oxalosis	i.v. vitamin C [42–44]	Excessive dose
Tubular obstruction	Ciprofloxacin [45]	Drug overdose
Vasomotor reaction	Ibuprofen [46]	Drug overdose

Ingestion of nephrotoxic chemicals

Probable renal lesion	Chemical	
Acute interstitial nephritis	Endosulfan [47]	
Chronic tubulointerstitial nephritis	Cadmium [48], fluoride [49]	Lead [50, 51]
Hemoglobinuric ATN	Aniline [52]	Ethylene glycol dinitrate [59]
	Bromate salts [53, 54]	Lysol (British) [83]
	Chlorate compounds [55]	Naphthalene [59a]
	Copper sulfate [56]	Paraphenylene diamine [59b, 59c]
	Cresol [57, 58]	Propylene glycol [59]
Myoglobinuric ATN	Copper sulfate [60]	Methanol [91]
	Lindane [61]	Paraphenylene diamine [61a]
	Mercuric chloride [60]	Zinc phosphide [60]
Nephrotoxic ATN	Arsenic salts [62]	Hydrocarbons [78]
	Barium chloride [63]	Mercury salts [79, 80]
	Carbon tetrachloride [64]	Methylene chloride [81]
	Chlordane [65]	Paraquat [82]
	Chloroform [66]	Tartaric acid [83]
	(2,4 di- and methyl-)chlorophenoxyacetic acid [67]	Tetrachloroethylene [59]
	Chromium compounds [68–71]	Thallium [84]
	Diquat [72]	Tetralin [85]
	Ethylene dichloride [66]	Trichloroethylene [86]
	Ethylene dibromide [73, 74]	Triphenyltin acetate [87]
	Germanium compounds [75–77]	Turpentine [88]
		Yellow phosphorus [89]
Oxalosis	Diethylene glycol [90]	Ethylene glycol butyl ether [93]
	Ethylene glycol [91, 92]	Oxalic acid [94, 95]
Pseudoazotemia	Isopropanol [96, 97]	

Ingestion of nephrotoxic foods

Probable renal lesion	Food	Toxin
Chronic interstitial nephritis	Vichy water [49]	Fluoride
	Worcestershire sauce [98]	Unknown
Hypercalcemia (milk-alkali syndrome)	Milk [99, 100]	Calcium
Hemoglobinuric ATN	Fava or broad beans (*Vicia faba L.*) [101]	Divicine and isouramil
Myoglobinuric ATN	Licorice [102]	Glycyrrhizic acid (hypokalemia)
	Wild birds (chaffinch [103], quail [104, 105], European robin [103])	? cicutoxin
Nephrotoxic ATN	Djenkol beans (*Pithecolabium lobatum*) [106]	? Djenkolic acid
	Carp bile (*Ctenopharyngodon idellus* and other species) [107, 108]	? cyprinol
Oxalosis	Rhubarb (*Rheum rhaponticum*) [109]	Oxalic acid

Ingestion of nephrotoxic plants

Plant	Scientific name	Toxic compounds
Autumn crocus [30]	*Colchicum autumnale*	Colchicine
Castor bean [110]	*Ricinus communis*	Ricin and recinine
Chinese herbs for slimming [111]	Exact plants unknown	Unknown
Daphne [112]	*Daphne mezereum*	Daphnin, vesicant resin and mezerenic acid anhydride

(Continued)

Plant	Scientific name	Toxic compounds
Herbal remedies	*Securidaca longipedunculata [106]* and unknown plants *[113]*	Methyl salicylate, saponius, tanins and gaultherin
Impila [106]	*Callilepsis laureola*	Atractyloside
Marking-nut tree [106]	*Semecarpus anacardium*	Phenolic constituents
Poison mushrooms [114]	*Amanita phalloides [115]*, *Cortinarius species [116, 117]* and *Gyromitra species [114]*	Amatoxin cyclopeptides, orellanin, gyromitrin & homologues
Rosary pea [112]	*Abrus precatorius*	Abrin and abric acid
Vascular plant [118]	*Taxus celebica*	Sciadopitysin
Water hemlock [119]	*Cicuta maculata*	Cicutoxin

Inhalation or cutaneous absorption of toxic chemicals

Probable renal lesion	Chemical	
Chronic interstitial nephritis	Mineral spirits [120]	
Glomerulonephritis	Hydrocarbons [120–125]	Silicon [126]
Hemoglobinuric ATN	Arsine gas [127]	
Myoglobinuric ATN	Carbon monoxide [128, 129]	
Nephrotoxic ATN	Boric acid [27]	Lysol (British) [83]
	Cadmium [130]	
	Carbon tetrachloride [59, 131]	Methylchloride or bromide gas [83]
	Chromium [132]	Methylene chloride [138]
	Diethylene glycol [133]	Mycotoxins [139]
	1, 2-dichloropropane [134]	Phenol [83, 140]
	Diesel fuel [135]	Polyethylene glycol [141]
	Dioxane [83]	Povidone-iodine [142]
	Dynamite [136]	Tetrachloroethylene [59]
	Ethylene dibromide [73]	Toluene [143, 144]
	Gasoline [137]	Trichloroethylene [145]
Pseudoazotemia	Acetone (contaminating acetylene) [146]	

Envenomation by poisonous stings or bites

Common name	Scientific name	Location
Arthropods-Arachnids		
Scorpion [147]	*Buthus sauloci*	Iran
Brown recluse spider [148]	*Loxosceles reclusa*	Western hemisphere
South American house spider [149]	*Loxosceles lacta*	Western hemisphere
Arthropods-hymenoptera		
Bees:		
Africanized bee [150, 151]	*Apis mellifera scutellata*	Africa and western hemisphere
Wax bee [149]	*Apis mellificus*	Worldwide
Honey bee [152]	*Apis mellifera*	Worldwide
Wasps:		
Indian hornet [153]	*Vespa affinis*	Asia
Oriental hornet [154]	*Vespa orientalis*	Asia
Yellow jacket (European wasp) [155, 156]	*Vespula germanica*	Europe
Coelenterates		
Portuguese man-of-war [157]	*Pysalia physalis*	North Carolina
Snakes		
Australian brown snake [158]	*Pseudonaja textilis textilis*	Australia

(Continued)

Common name	Scientific name	Location
Black mamba [159]	*Dendroaspis polylepis*	Southern Africa
Boomslang [160]	*Dispholidus typus*	Southern Africa
Small-eyed black snake [161]	*Cryptophis nigrescens*	Australia
Dugite [162]	*Demansia nuchalis affinis*	Australia
Gwardar [162]	*Demansia nuchalis nuchalis*	Australia
Palestinian viper [163]	*Vipera palestinae*	Israel
Pit vipers:		
Copperhead [149]	*Agkistrodon contortrix*	Western hemisphere
Jararaca [164]	*Bothrops jararaca*	South America
Mamushi [165]	*Agkistrodon halys*	Japan
Rattlesnake [149, 166]	*Crotalus terrificus and others*	Western hemisphere
Water moccasin (cotton mouth) [149]	*Agkistrodon piscivorus*	Western hemisphere
Pit viper [167]	*Agkistrodon hypnale*	Sri Lanka
Puff adder [168]	*Bitis arietans*	Africa
Rough scaled snake [169]	*Tropidechis carinatus*	Australia
Russel's viper [170, 171]	*Vipera russelli*	Asia
Saw-scaled sand viper [172, 173]	*Echis carinatus & coloratus*	Africa, India, Mid-east
Seasnake [174]	*Enhydrina schistosa*	Asian waters
Small African snake [149]	*Atracepaspis microlapidata*	Africa
Tiger snake [175]	*Notechis scutatus*	Australia

REFERENCES

1. Scheithauer, W, Ulrich W, Kovarik J and Stummvoll H-K. Acute oliguria associated with chlorprothixene overdosage. Nephron 1988; 48:71–3.
2. Dubrow A, Mittman N, Ghali V and Flamenbaum W. The changing spectrum of heroin-associated nephropathy. Am J Kidney Dis 1985; 5:36–41.
3. Stachura I, Jayakumar S and Pardo M. Talwin addict nephropathy. Clin Nephrol 1983; 19:147–53.
4. May DC, Helderman JH, Eigenbrodt EH and Silva FG. Chronic sclerosing glomerulopathy (Heroin-associated nephropathy) in intravenous T's and Blues abusers. Am J Kidney Dis 1986; 8:404–9.
5. DeBroe ME and Elseviers MM. Analgesic nephropathy – Still a problem? Nephron 1993; 64:505–13.
6. Adams DH, Michael J, Bacon PA, Howie AJ, McConkey B and Adu D. Non-steroidal anti-inflammatory drugs and renal failure. Lancet 1986; i:57–60.
7. Ponchon T, Baroud J, Pujol B, Valette PJ and, Perrot D. Renal failure during dissolution of gallstones by methyl-tert-butyl ether. Lancet 1988; ii:276–7.
8. Fisher G and Skillern PG. Hypercalcemia due to hypervitaminosis A. JAMA 1974; 227:1974.
9. Cardella CJ, Birken BL, Roscoe M and Rapoport A. Role of dialysis in the treatment of severe hypercalcemia: report of two cases successfully treated with hemodialysis and review of the literature. Clin Nephrol 1979; 12:285–90.
10. Schwartzman MS and Franck WA. Vitamin D toxicity complicating the treatment of senile, postmenopausal and glucocorticoid-induced osteoporosis. Am J Med 1987; 82:224–30.
11. Rozich JD and Paul RV. Acute renal failure precipitated by elevated colloid osmotic pressure. Am J Med 1989; 87:358–60.
12. Jennings AE, Levey AS and Harrington JT. Amoxapine – associated acute renal failure. Arch Intern Med 1983; 143:1525–7.
13. Skinazi F, Davous P and Bleichner G. Insuffisance renale aigue apres intoxication volontaire par l'amoxapine. La Presse Med 1991; 20:130.
14. Gabow PA, Kaehny WD and Kelleher SP. The spectrum of rhabdomyolysis. Medicine 1982; 61:141–52.
15. Koffler A, Friedler RM and Massry SG. Acute renal failure due to nontraumatic rhabdomyolysis. Ann Intern Med 1976; 85:23–8.
16. Pogue VA and Nurse HM. Cocaine-associated acute myoglobinuric renal failure. Am J Med 1989; 86:183–6.
16a. Parks JM, Reed G and Knochel JP. Case report: cocaine-associated rhabdomyolysis. Am J Med Sci 1989; 296:334–6.
17. Hojgaard AD andersen PT and Moller-Petersen J. Rhabdomyolysis and acute renal failure following an overdose of doxepin and nitrazepam. Acta Med Scand 1988; 223:79–82.
18. Henry JA, Jeffreys KJ and Dawling S. Toxicity and deaths from 3, 4-methylenedioxy-methamphetamine ("ecstasy"). Lancet 1992; 340:384–7.
19. Swenson RD, Golper TA and Bennett WM. Acute renal failure and rhabdomyolysis after ingestion of phenylpropanolamine-containing diet pills. JAMA 1982; 248:1216.
20. Boyd RE, Brennan PT, Deng J-F, Rochester DF and Spyker DA. Strychnine poisoning. Am J Med 1983; 74:507–12.
21. Blake PG and Ryan F. Rhabdomyolysis and acute renal failure after terbutaline overdose. Nephron 1989; 53:76–7.

22. Citron BP, Halpern M, McCarron M, Lundberg GD, McCormick R, Prucers I et al. Necrotizing angiitis associated with drug abuse. NEJM 1970; 283:1003–11.

23. Kleinman, JG, Acute renal failure associated with acetaminophen ingestion. Report of a case and review of the literature. Clin Nephrol 1980; 14:201–5.

24. Cobden I, Record CO, Ward MK and Kerr DNS. Paracetamol-induced acute renal failure in the absence of fulminant liver damage. BMJ 1982; 284:21–2.

25. Davenport A and Finn R. Paracetamol (acetaminophen) poisoning resulting in acute renal failure without hepatic coma. Nephron 1988; 50:55–6.

26. Rupp DJ, Seaton RD and Wiegmann TB. Acute polyuric renal failure after aspirin intoxication. Arch Intern Med 1983; 143:1237–8.

27. Skipworth GB, Goldstein N and McBride WP. Boric acid intoxication from "medicated talcum powder". Arch Derm 1967; 95:83–6.

28. Urizar R and Vernier RL. Bismuth nephropathy. JAMA 1966; 198:207–9.

29. Murray SS, Kramlinger KG, McMichan JC and Mohr DN. Acute toxicity after excessive ingestion of colchicine. Mayo Clin Proc 1983; 58:528–532.

30. Ellwood MG and Robb GH. Self-poisoning with colchicine. Postgrad Med J 1971; 47:129–38.

31. Huwez F, Pall A, Lyons D and Stewart MJ. Acute renal failure after overdose of colloidal bismuth subcitrate. Lancet 1992; 340:1298.

32. Beattie AD, Briggs JD, Canavan JSF, Doyle D, Mullin PJ and Watson AA. Acute lead poisoning. Quart J Med 1975;44:275–84.

33. Skinner R and Ferner RE. Acute renal failure without acute intravascular haemodialysis after Nomifensine overdosage. Human Toxicol 1986; 5:279–80.

34. Sullivan JB, Rumack BH, Thomas H, Peterson RG and Bryson P. Pennyroyal oil poisoning and hepatoxicity. JAMA 1979; 242:2873–4.

35. Gutman RA and Burnell JM. Paraldehyde acidosis. Am J Med 1967; 43:435–40.

36. Farge D, Turner MW, Roy DR and Jothy S. Dyazide-induced reversible acute renal failure associated with intracellular crystal deposition. Am J Kidney Dis 1986, VIII:445–9.

37. Luessenhop AJ, Gallimore JC, Sweet WH, Struxness EG and Robinson J. The toxicity in man of hexavalent uranium following intravenous administration. AJR 1958; 79:83–100.

38. Millette CH and Snodgrass GL. Acute renal failure associated with chronic antacid ingestion. Am J Hosp Pharm 1981; 38:1352–5.

39. Horgan KJ, Ottaviano YL and Watson AJ. Acute renal failure due to mannitol intoxication. Am J Nephrol 1989; 9:106–9.

40. Weaver A and Sica DA. Mannitol-induced acute renal failure. Nephron 1987; 45:233–5.

41. Rello J, Triginer C, Sanchez JM and Net A. Acute renal failure following massive mannitol infusion. Nephron 1989; 53:377–8.

42. Swartz RD, Wesley JR, Somermeyer MG and Lau K. Hyperoxaluria and renal insufficiency due to ascorbic acid administration during total parenteral nutrition. Ann Intern Med 1984; 100:530–1.

43. McAllister CJ, Scowden EB, Dewberry FL and Richman A. Renal failure secondary to massive infusion of vitamin C. JAMA 1984; 252:1684.

44. Lawton JM, Conway LT, Crosson JT, Smith CL and Abraham PA. Acute oxalate nephropathy after massive ascorbic acid administration. Arch Intern Med 1985; 145:950–1.

45. George MJ, Dew RB III and Daly JS. Acute renal failure after an overdose of ciprofloxacin. Arch Intern Med 1991; 151:620.

46. Perazella MA and Buller GK. Can ibuprofen cause acute renal failure in a normal individual? A case of acute overdose. Am J Kidney Dis 1991; 18:600–2.

47. Segasothy M and Pang KS. Acute interstitial nephritis due to Endosulfan. Nephron 1992; 62:118.

48. Weeden RP. Occupational renal disease. Am J Kidney Dis 1984; 3:241–57.

49. Lantz O, Jouvin M-H, De Vernejoul M-C and Druet P. Fluoride-induced chronic renal failure. Am J Kidney Dis 1987; 10:136–9.

50. Pollock CA and Ibels LS. Lead intoxication in paint removal workers on the Sydney Harbour Bridge. Med J Australia 1986; 145:635–9.

51. Cullen MR, Robbins JM and Eskenazi B. Adult inorganic lead intoxication: presentation of 31 new cases and a review of recent advances in the literature. Medicine 1983; 62:221–47.

52. Lubash GD, Phillips RE, Shields JD and Bonsnes RW. Acute aniline poisoning treated by hemodialysis. Arch Intern Med 1964; 114:530–2.

53. Kutom A, Bazilinski NG, Magana L and Dunea G. Bromate intoxication: Hairdressers' anuria. Am J Kidney Dis 1990; 15:84–5.

54. Lichtenberg R, Zeller W Patrick, Gatson R and Morrison Hurley R. Bromate poisoning. J Pediatr 1989; 114:891–4.

55. Stavrou A, Butcher R and Sakula A. Accidental self-poisoning by sodium chlorate weed-killer. Practitioner 1978; 221:397–9.

56. Chugh KS, Singhal PC, Sharma BK, Das KC and Datta BN. Acute renal failure following copper sulphate intoxication. Postgrad Med J 1977; 53:18–23.

57. Cason JS. Report on three extensive industrial chemical burns. BMJ 1959; 1:827–9.

58. Muehrcke RC. Acute renal failure: diagnosis and management. CV Mosby Company, St. Louis, 1969:214.

59. Schreiner GE and Maher JF. Toxic nephropathy. Am J Med 1965; 38:409–49.

59a. Gidron E and Leurer J. Naphthalene poisoning. Lancet 1956; 1:228–31.

59b. Bourquia A, Jabrane AJ, Ramdani B and Zaid D. Toxicite systemique de la paraphénylène diamine. La Presse Med 1988; 17:1798–800.

59c. Chugh KS, Malik GH and Singhal PC. Acute renal failure following paraphenylene diamine (hair dye) poisoning: report of two cases. J Med 1982; 13:131–7.

60. Chugh KS, Singhal PC, Nath IVS, Pareek SK, Ubroi HS and Sarkar AK. Acute renal failure due to non-traumatic

rhabdomyolysis. Postgrad Med J 1979;55:386–92.

61. Munk ZM and Nantel A. Acute lindane poisoning with development of muscle necrosis. CMA Journal 1977; 117:1050–2.

61a. Averbukh Z, Modai D, Leonov Y, Weissgarten J, Lewinsohn G, Fucs L et al. Rhabdomyolysis and acute renal failure induced by paraphenylenediamine. Human Toxicol 1989; 8:345–8.

62. Sanz P, Corbella J, Nogue S, Munne P and Rodriguez-Pazos M. Rhabdomyolysis in fatal arsenic trioxide poisoning. JAMA 1989; 262:3271.

63. Wetherill SF, Guarino MJ and Cox RW. Acute renal failure associated with barium chloride poisoning. Ann Intern Med 1981; 95:187–8.

64. Alston WC. Hepatic and renal complications arising from accidental carbon tetrachloride poisoning in the human subject. J Clin Path 1970; 23:249–53.

65. Derbes VJ, Forest WW and Johnson MJ. Fatal chlordane poisoning. JAMA 1955; 158:1367–9.

66. Kluwe WM and Hook JB. The nephrotoxicity of low molecular weight halogenated alkane solvents, pesticides and chemical intermediates. In: Hook JB, editor. Toxicology of the kidney. Raven Press, New York, 1981: 179–226.

67. Kancir CB, Andersen C and Olesen AS. Marked hypocalcemia in a fatal poisoning with chlorinated phenoxy acid derivatives. Clin Toxicol 1988; 26:257–64.

68. Kaufman DB, DiNicola W and McIntosh R. Acute potassium dichromate poisoning. Amer J Dis Child 1970; 119:374–6.

69. Sanz P, Nogue S, Munne P, Torra R and Marques F. Acute potassium dichromate poisoning. Human & Exper Toxicol 1991; 10:228–9.

70. Michie CA, Hayhurst M, Knobel GJ, Stokol JM and Hensley B. Poisoning with a traditional remedy containing potassium dichromate. Human & Exper Toxicol 1991; 10:129–31.

71. Picaud JC, Cochat P, Parchoux B, Berthier JC, Gilly J, Chareyre S et al. Acute renal failure in a child after chewing of match heads. Nephron 1991; 57:22506.

72. Vanholder R, Colardyn F, deReuck J, Praet M, Lameire N and Ringoir S. Diquat intoxication. Report of two cases and review of the literature. Am J Med 1981;70:1267–71.

73. Letz GA, Pond SM, Osterloh JD, Wade RL and Becker CE. Two fatalities after acute occupational exposure to ethylene dibromide. JAMA 1984; 2521:2428–31.

74. Olmstead EV. Pathological changes in ethylene dibromide poisoning. AMA Arch Ind Health 1960; 21:525–9.

75. Sanai T, Okuda S, Onoyama K, Oochi N, Oh Y, Kobayashi K et al. Germanium dioxide-induced nephropathy: a new type of renal disease. Nephron 1990; 54:53–60.

76. Takeuchi A, Yoshizawa N, Oshima S, Kubota T, Oshikawa Y, Akashi Y et al. Nephrotoxicity of germanium compounds: report of a case and review of the literature. Nephron 1992; 60:436–42.

77. Hess B, Raisin J, Zimmermann A, Horber F, Bajo S, Wyttenbach A et al. Tubulointerstitial nephropathy persisting 20 months after discontinuation of chronic intake of germanium lactate citrate. Am J Kidney Dis 1993; 21:548–52.

78. Janssen S, van der Geest S, Meijer S and Uges DRA. Impairment of organ function after oral ingestion of refined petrol. Intensive Care Med 1988; 14:238–40.

79. Sauder P, Livardjani F, Jaeger A, Kopferschmitt J, Heimburger R, Waller C et al. Acute mercury chloride intoxication. Effects of hemodialysis and plasma exchange on mercury kinetic. Clin Toxicol 1988; 26:189–97.

80. Kostyniak PJ, Greizerstein HB, Goldstein J, Lachaal M, Reddy P, Clarkson TW et al. Extracorporeal regional complexing haemodialysis treatment of acute inorganic mercury intoxication. Human Toxicol 1990; 9:137–41.

81. Roberts CJC and Marshall FPF. Recovery after "lethal" quantity of paint remover. BMJ 1976; 1:20–1.

82. Van de Vyver FL, Giuliano RA, Paulus GJ, Verpooten GA, Franke JP, De Zeeuw RA et al. Hemoperfusion-hemodialysis ineffective for paraquat removal in life-threatening poisoning? Clin Toxicol 1985; 23:117–31.

83. Gosselin RE, Smith RP, Hodge HC and Braddock JE. Clinical toxicology of commercial products. The Williams & Wilkins Company, Baltimore, 1984:5th ed.

84. Saddique A and Peterson CD. Thallium poisoning: a review. Vet Hum Toxicol 1983; 25:16–22.

85. Drayer DE and Reidenberg MM. Metabolism of tetralin and toxicity of cuprex in man. Drug Metab and Disposition 1973; 1:577–9.

86. Kleinfeld M and Tabershaw IR. Trichloroethylene toxicity: A report of five fatal cases. Arch Ind Hyg Occup Med 1954; 10:134–41.

87. Lin J-L and Hsueh S. Acute nephropathy of organotin compounds. Am J Nephrol 1993; 13:124–8.

88. Chapman EM. Observations of the effect of paint on the kidneys with particular reference to the role of turpentine. J Ind Hyg Toxicol 1941; 23:277–89.

89. McCarron MM and Gaddis GP. Acute yellow phosphorus poisoning from pesticide pastes. Clin Toxicol 1981; 18:693–711.

90. Geiling EMK and Cannon PR. Pathologic effects of elixir of sulfanilamide (diethylene glycol) poisoning. JAMA 1938; 111:919–26.

91. Hall AH. Ethylene glycol and methanol: poisons with toxic metabolic activation. Emergency Med Reports 1992; 13:29–38.

92. Wine H, Savitt D and Abuelo JG. Ethylene glycol intoxication. Sem Dial 1994; 7:338–45.

93. Rambourg-Schepens MO, Buffet M, Bertault R, Jaussaud M, Journe B, Fay R et al. Severe ethylene glycol butyl ether poisoning. Kinetics and metabolic pattern. Human Toxicol 1988; 7:187–9.

94. Winchester J. Methanol, isopropyl alcohol, higher alcohols, ethylene glycol, cellosolves, acetone and oxalate. In: Haddad LM and Winchester JF, editors. Clinical management of poisoning and drug overdose. WB Saunders, Philadelphia, 1983:393–409.

95. Jeghers H and Murphy R. Practical aspects of oxalate metabolism N Engl J Med 1945; 233:208–15.

96. G erard SK and Khayam-Bashi H. Characterization of creatinine error in ketotic patients. Amer J Clin Pathol 1985; 84:659–64.

97. Hawley PC and Falko JM. "Pseudo" renal failure after

isopropyl alcohol intoxication. South Med J 1982; 75:630–1.

98. Douthwaite AH. Pitfalls in medicine. BMJ 1956; 2:958–62.

99. Abreo K, Adlakha A, Kilpatrick S, Flanagan R, Webb R and Shakamuri S. The milk-alkali syndrome. Arch Intern Med 1993; 153:1005–10.

100. Kleinman GE, Rodriquez H, Good MC and Caudle MR. Hypercalcemic crisis in pregnancy associated with excessive ingestion of calcium carbonate antacid (milk-alkali syndrome): successful treatment with hemodialysis. Obstet & Gynecol 1991; 78:496.

101. Symvoulidis A, Voidiclaris S, Mountokalakis T and Pougounias H. Acute renal failure in G-6-PD deficiency. Lancet 1972; 2:819–20.

102. Mourad G, Galley P, Oules R, Mimran A and Mion C. Hypokalemic myopathy with rhabdomyolysis and acute renal failure in the course of chronic licorice ingestion. Kidney Int 1979; 15:452.

103. Rizzi D, Introna F Jr, Gagliano Candela R, Di Nunno C, Ricco R, Recchia R et al. Rabdiomiolisi tossica e tubulonecrosi nell'avvelenamento da cicuta. La Clinica Therapeutica 1988; 124:187–92.

104. Billis AG, Kastanakis S, Giamarellou H and Daikos GK. Acute renal failure after a meal of quail. Lancet 1971; 2:702.

105. Papapetropoulos T, Hadziyannis S and Ouzounellis T. On the pathogenetic mechanism of quail myopathy. JAMA 1980; 244:2263–4.

106. Kibukamusoke J. Renal hazards from plants and plant products. In: Tropical nephrol. Marcel Dekker Inc., New York, 1984:318–32.

107. Park SK, Kim DG, Kang SK, Han JS, Kim SG, Lee JS et al. Toxic acute renal failure and hepatitis after ingestion of raw carp bile. Nephron 1990; 56:188–93.

108. Lim P-S, Lin J-L and Huang C-C. Acute renal failure due to ingestion of the gallbladder of grass carp. Clin Nephrol 1992; 37:104–5.

109. Kalleila H and Kauste O. Ingestion of rhubarb leaves as cause of oxalic acid poisoning. Ann Paediatr Fenn 1964; 10:228–31.

110. Wedin GP, Neal JS, Everson GW and Krenzelok EP. Castor bean poisoning. Amer J Emergency Med 1986; 4:259–61.

111. Vanherweghem J-L, Depierreux M, Tielemans C, Abramowicz D, Dratwa M, Jadoul M et al. Rapidly progressive interstitial renal fibrosis in young women: association with slimming regimen including Chinese herbs. Lancet 1993; 341:387–91.

112. Kunkel DB. Poisonous plants. In: Haddad LM and Winchester JF, editors. Clinical management of poisoning and drug overdose. WB Saunders, Philadelphia, 1983:317–35.

113. Gold CH. Acute renal failure from herbal and patent remedies in blacks. Clin Nephrol 1980; 14:128–34.

114. Koppel C. Clinical symptomatology and management of mushroom poisoning. Toxicon 1993; 31:1513–40.

115. Klein AS, Hart J, Brems JJ, Goldstein L, Lewin K and Busuttil RW. Amanita poisoning: treatment and the role of liver transplantation. Am J Med 1989; 86:187–94.

116. Holmdahl J, Mulec H and Ahlmen J. Acute renal failure after intoxication with cortinarius mushrooms. Human Toxicol 1984; 3:309–13.

117. Delpech N, Rapior S, Cozette AP, Ortiz JP, Donnadieu P andary C et al. Évolution d'une insuffisance rénale aiguë par ingestion volontaire de Cortinarius orellanus. La Presse Med 1990; 19:122–4.

118. Lin J–L and Ho Y–S. Flavonoid-induced acute nephropathy. Am J Kidney Dis 1994; 23:433–40.

119. Carlton BE, Tufts E and Girard DE. Water hemlock poisoning complicated by rhabdomyolysis and renal failure. Clin Toxicol 1979; 14:87–92.

120. Narvarte J, Saba SR and Ramirez G. Occupational exposure to organic solvent causing chronic tubulointerstitial nephritis. Arch Intern Med 1989; 149:154–8.

121. Daniell WE, Couser WG and Rosenstock L. Occupational solvent exposure and glomerulonephritis. JAMA 1988; 259:2280–3.

122. Ravnskov U, Lundstrom S and Norden A. Hydrocarbon exposure and glomerulonephritis: evidence from patient's occupations. Lancet 1983; 2:1214–6.

123. Churchill DN, Fine A and Gault MH. Association between hydrocarbon exposure and glomerulonephritis. An appraisal of the evidence. Nephron 1983; 33:169–72.

124. Bell GM, Gordon ACH, Lee P, Doig A, MacDonald MK, Thomson D et al. Proliferative glomerulonephritis and exposure to organic solvents. Nephron 1985; 40:161–5.

125. Bonzel K-E, Muller-Wiefel DE, Wingen A-M, Waldherr R and Weber M. Anti-glomerular basement membrane antibody-mediated glomerulonephritis due to glue sniffing. Eur J Pediatr 1987; 146:296–300.

126. Arnalich F, Lahoz C, Picazo ML, Monereo A, Arribas JR, Martinez Ara J et al. Polyarteritis nodosa and necrotizing glomerulonephritis associated with long-standing silicosis. Nephron 1989; 51:544–7.

127. Wilkinson SP, McHugh P, Horsley S, Tubbs H, Lewis M, Thould A et al. Arsine toxicity aboard the asiafreighter. BMJ 1975; 3:559–63.

128. Jackson RC, Bunker NV, Elder WJ and O'Conner PJ. Case of carbon monoxide poisoning with complications, successful treatment with an artificial kidney. BMJ 1959; 2:1130–4.

129. Bessoudo R and Gray J. Carbon monoxide poisoning and nonoliguric acute renal failure. CMA J 1978; 119:41–4.

130. Beton DC, Andrews GS, Davies HJ et al. Acute cadmium poisoning: five cases with one death from renal necrosis. Brit J Indust Med 1966; 23:292–301.

131. Folland DS, Schaffner W, Ginn HE, Crofford OB and McMurray DR. Carbon tetrachloride toxicity potentiated by isopropyl alcohol. JAMA 1976; 236:1853–6.

132. Harry P, Mauras Y, Chennebault JM, Allain P and Alquier P. Insuffisance renale aigue apres brulures cutanees par l'acid chromique (chrome VI). La Presse Med 1984; 13:2520.

133. Cantarell MC, Fort J, Camps J, Sans M and Piera L. Acute intoxication due to topical application of diethylene glycol. Ann Intern Med 1987; 106:478–9.

134. Locatelli F and Pozzi C. Relapsing hemolytic uremic syndrome after organic solvent sniffing. Lancet 1982; 2:220.

135. Crisp AJ, Bhalla AK and Hoffbrand BI. Acute tubular necrosis after exposure to diesel oil. BMJ 1979; 2:177–8.

136. Genin R, Ged E, Maddio B and Fen Chong M. Insuffisance renale aigue apres exposition a la dynamite. Nouv Presse Med 1982; 11:2360.

137. Walsh WA, Scarpa FJ, Brown RS, Ashcraft KW, Green VA, Holder TM et al. Gasoline immersion burn. NEJM 1974; 291:830.

138. Miller L, Pateras V, Friederici H and Engel G. Acute tubular necrosis after inhalation exposure to methylene chloride. Arch Intern Med 1985; 145:145–6.

139. DiPaolo N, Guarnieri A, Loi F, Sacchi G, Mangiarotti AM and DiPaolo M. Acute renal failure from inhalation of mycotoxins. Nephron 1993; 64:621–5.

140. Foxall PJD, Bending MR, Gartland KPR and Nicholson JK. Acute renal failure following accidental cutaneous absorption of phenol: application of NMR urinalysis to monitor the disease process. Human Toxicol 1989; 9:491–6.

141. Bruns DE, Harold DA, Rodeheaver GT and Edlich R. Polyethylene glycol intoxication in burn patients. Burns Incl Therm Inj 1982; 9:49–52.

142. Aronoff GR, Friedman SJ, Doedens DJ and Lavelle KJ. Increased serum iodide concentration from iodine absorption through wounds treated tropically with povidone-iodine. Am J Med Sci 1980; 279:173–6.

143. Russ G, Clarkson AR, Woodroffe AJ, Seymour AE and Cheng IKP. Renal failure from "glue sniffing". Med J Aust 1981; 2:121–2.

144. Reisin E, Teicher A, Jaffe R and Eliahou HE. Myoglobinuria and renal failure in toluene poisoning. Brit J Indust Med 1975; 32:163–8.

145. David NJ, Wolman R, Milne FJ and Van Niekerk I. Acute renal failure due to trichloroethylene poisoning. Brit J Industr Med 1989; 46:347–9.

146. Foley RJ. Inhaled industrial acetylene. A diabetic ketoacidosis mimic. JAMA 1985; 254:1066–7.

147. Chadha JS and Leviav A. Hemolysis, renal failure and local necrosis following scorpion sting. JAMA 1979; 240:1038.

148. Wasserman GS and Anderson PC. Loxoscelism and necrotic arachnidism. J Toxicol-Clin Toxicol 1984; 21:451–72.

149. Muehrcke RC. Acute renal failure: diagnosis and management. CV Mosby Company, St. Louis, 1969:190–1.

150. Mejia G, Arbelaez M, Henao JE, Alvaro AS and Arango JL. Acute renal failure due to multiple stings by Africanized bees. Ann Intern Med 1986; 104:210–211.

151. Munoz-Arizpe R, Valencia-Espinoza L, Velasquez-Jones L, Abarca-Franco C, Gamboa-Marrufo J and Valencia-Mayoral P. Africanized bee stings and pathogenesis of acute renal failure. Nephron 1992; 61:478.

152. Sert M, Tetiker T and Paydas S. Rhabdomyolysis and acute renal failure due to honeybee stings as an uncommon cause. Nephron 1993; 65:647.

153. Shilkin KB, BTM Chen and Khoo OT. Rhabdomyolysis caused by hornet venom. BMJ 1972; i:156–7.

154. Sakhuja V, Bhalla A, Pereira BJG, Kapoor MM, Bhusnurmath SR and Chugh KS. Acute renal failure following multiple hornet stings. Nephron 1988; 49:319–21.

155. Bousquet J, Huchard G and Michel F-B. Toxic reactions induced by hymenoptera venom. Ann Allergy 1984; 52:371–4.

156. Nace L, Bauer P, Lelarge P, Bollaert P-E, Larcan A and Lambert H. Multiple European wasp stings and acute renal failure. Nephon 1992; 61:477.

157. Guess HA, Saviteer PL and Morris RC. Hemolysis and acute renal failure following a Portuguese man-of-war sting. Pediatrics 1982; 70:979–81.

158. Shapel GJ, Utley D and Wilson GC. Envenomation by the Australian common brown snake-Pseudonaja (Demansia) textilis. Med J Aust 1971; 1:142–4.

159. Visser J and Chapman DS. Snakes and snakebite. Cape Town:Purnell and Sons, 1978.

160. Lakier JB and Fritz VU. Consumptive coagulopathy caused by a boomslang bite. SA Med J 1969; 43:1052–5.

161. Furtado MA and Lester IA. Myoglobinuria following snakebite. Med J Australia 1968; 20:674–6.

162. Harris ARC, Hurst PE and Saker BM. Renal failure after snake bite. Med J Aust 1976; 2:409–11.

163. Efrati P and Reif L. Clinical and pathological observations on 65 cases of viper bite in Israel. Am J Trop Med Hyg 1953; 2:1085–108.

164. Amaral CFS, Da Silva OA, Godoy P and Miranda D. Renal cortical necrosis following Bothrops Jararaca and B. Jararacussu snake bite. Toxicon 1985; 23:877–85.

165. Otsuji Y, Irie Y, Ueda H, Yotsueda K, Kitahara T, Yokoyama K et al. A case of acute renal failure caused by Mamushi (Agkistrodon halys) bite. Med J Kagoshima Univ (Jpn) 1978; 30:129–35.

166. Azevedo-Marques MM, Cupo P, Coimbra TM, Hering SE, Rossi MA and Laure CJ. Myonecrosis, myoglobinuria and acute renal failure induced by South American rattlesnake (Crotalus durrissus terrificus) envenomation in Brazil. Toxicon 1985; 23:631–6.

167. Varagunam T and Panabokke RG. Bilateral cortical necrosis of the kidneys following snakebite. Postgrad Med J 1970; 46:449–51.

168. Seedat JK, Reddy J and Edington DA. Acute renal failure due to proliferative nephritis from snake bite poisoning. Nephron 1974; 13:455–63.

169. Patten BR, Pearn JH, DeBuse P, Burke J and Covacevich J. Prolonged intensive therapy after snake bite. A probable case of envenomation by the rough-scaled snake. Med J Aust 1985; 142:467–9.

170. Chugh KS. Snake-bite-induced acute renal failure in India. Kidney Int 1989; 35:891–907.

171. Date A, Pulimood R, Jacob CK, Kirubakaran MG and Shastry JCM. Haemolytic uraemic syndrome complicating snake bite. Nephron 1986; 42:89–90.

172. Mittal BV, Kinare SG and Acharya VN. Renal lesions following viper bites. Indian J Med Res 1986; 83:642–51.

173. Porath A, Gilon D, Schulchynska-Castel H, Shalev O, Keynan A and Benbassat J. Risk indicators after envenomation in humans by Echis Coloratus (Mid-east saw scaled viper). Toxicon 1992; 30:25–32.

174. Sitprija V, Sribhibhadh R and Benyajati C. Hemodialysis in poisoning by sea-snake venom. BMJ 1971; 3:218–9.

175. Hood VL and Johnson JR. Acute renal failure with myoglobinuria after snakebite. Med J Aust 1975; 2:638–41.

Index

ANCA (anti-neutrophil cytoplasmic antibody), 35, 36
   in Goodpasture's syndrome, 106
   in idiopathic crescentic GN, 96
   in lupus nephritis, 100
   in polyarteritis nodosa, 101–2
   in Wegener's granulomatosis, 103, 104
accelerated hypertension (see malignant hypertension)
acetaminophen as a cause of chronic renal failure, 51
acetazolamide as a cause of tubular obstruction, 126
acetohexamide as cause of false renal failure, 27
acidosis, management of, 157–8, 179
acute cortical necrosis, 76–7
acute glomerulonephritis (see acute nephritic diseases)
acute interstitial nephritis, 131–7
   drug-induced, 132–5
      prevention, 226
      prognosis, 227
      treatment, 226–7
   idiopathic, 136–7
      treatment, 227
      prognosis, 228
   in systemic diseases, 135–6
      treatment, 227
   infection–induced, 135
      prognosis, 227
      treatment, 227
acute nephritic diseases, 93–107
   causes, 94–5
   clinical picture, 94, 96–7
   definition, 93
   diagnosis, 97
   pathophysiology, 93–4
   primary glomerular diseases, 94–7
   secondary glomerular diseases, 97–107
   urinalysis, 94
acute pyelonephritis, 135
acute renal failure
   complications, 153–4
   dialysis and hemofiltration in management, 162–6
   treatment, 153–68
   nutrition, 159–60
acute tubular necrosis, 117–122
   causes, 117–121
   clinical picture, 118–21
   diagnosis, 119, 121, 123–4
   due to hepatorenal syndrome, 67–68
   due to nephrotic syndrome, 107
   general features, 117
   hemoglobinuric, 120–2
   ischemic, 117–9
   myoglobinuric, 120–2
      prevention, 221

      prognosis, 222
      treatment, 222
   nephrotoxic, 119–20
      prevention, 220–1
      prognosis, 220–1
      treatment, 220–1
   pathology, 118
   pathophysiology, 117, 120
   treatment, 219–22
   urinalysis, 117
   urine sodium, 37, 117
acute-on-chronic renal failure
   definition, 4
   diagnosis, 51–2
   prevention, 172–3
acyclovir as a cause of tubular obstruction, 126
age factor
   in causation of renal failure, 7–8
   in progressive reduction of GFR, 26
alcoholic ketoacidosis as a cause of false renal failure, 26–7
alkalosis, metabolic, 31
"allergic" interstitial nephritis (see drug-induced acute interstitial nephritis)
allopurinol as a cause of interstitial nephritis, 134
aminoglycosides as a cause of acute tubular necrosis, 119
   prevention, 220
   prognosis, 220
   treatment, 220
amyloidosis, 108
amphotericin B as a cause of acute tubular necrosis, 119–20
   prevention, 221
   prognosis, 221
   treatment, 220
analgesic nephropathy, 51
anemia of renal failure, management of, 161, 180
aneurysm, renal artery or dissecting aortic, 80
angiotensin converting enzyme inhibitor
   as a cause of hyperkalemia, 179
   as a cause of vasomotor disturbance, 66–8
   use in hypertension of chronic renal failure, 176
   use in limiting progression of renal failure, 173–4
antifreeze (see ethylene glycol)
anti-glomerular basement membrane antibodies
   in Goodpasture's syndrome, 106
   in idiopathic crescentic GN, 94, 96
antihistamines in management of pruritis, 160, 181
anuric renal failure, definition, 4
arteriography (angiography), 42–3
   in malignant hypertension, 74
   in polyarteritis nodosa, 101
   in renal artery stenosis, 78–9
   in renal infarction, 80–1

J.G. Abuelo (ed.), Renal Failure, 269–276.
© 1995 Kluwer Academic Publishers.

in undiagnosed patients, 149–50
atheroembolic renal disease, 70–1
    prevention, 194–5
    prognosis, 195
    treatment, 194
azotemia, definition, 4

BUN to Scr ratio, 27–8
    in ischemic acute tubular necrosis, 118
    in myoglobinuric acute tubular necrosis, 121
    in postrenal renal failure, 59
    in prerenal azotemia, 56
    in thrombotic thrombocytopenia purpura, 76
bacterial endocarditis, GN due to, 98–99
    prevention, 207
    prognosis, 207
Bence-Jones protein (see immunoglobulin light chains)
beta-blockers as a cause of hyperkalemia, 179
beta-lactam antibiotics as a cause of acute interstitial nephritis,
    132–3
bilateral cortical necrosis (see acute cortical necrosis)
biliary cirrhosis as a cause of acute interstitial nephritis, 136
biopsy, renal, 43
    in undiagnosed patients, 149–50
bladder outlet obstruction, management of, 189–90
bleeding (see platelet dysfunction)
blood pressure (see hypertension or hypotension)
blood urea nitrogen or BUN (see urea)
bone survey, roentgenologic, in chronic renal failure, 51
bumetanide in management of hypervolemia, 161

CAVH/CAVHD/CVVH/CVVHD (see dialysis and hemofil-
    tration)
calcitriol in management of renal osteodystrophy, 177–8
calcium gluconate in management of hyperkalemia, 156
captopril (renography) radionuclide scan
    in renal artery stenosis, 79–80
cefoxitin as a cause of false renal failure, 26–7
chemical nephrotoxins, 15–6, appendix B
    as a cause of nephrotoxic ATN, 119–20
cholesterol emboli (see atheroembolic renal disease)
chronic glomerular diseases, 109
chronic hemodialysis, 181–2
    complications, 182
    prognosis, 182
    vascular access, 182
chronic interstitial nephritis associated with infection, 137
    treatment, 228
chronic peritoneal dialysis, 182–3
chronic renal failure, 49–53
    chronic hemodialysis in management of, 181–2
    consequences, 169–70
    in pregnant women, 174–5
    management of anemia, 180
    management of bleeding, 180–1
    management of hyperkalemia, 179
    management of hyperlipidemia, 176
    management of hypertension, 176
    management of hypervolemia, 178–9

management of metabolic acidosis, 179
management of nausea and vomiting, 181
management of neuromuscular symptoms, 181
management of pruritis, 181
management of renal osteodystrophy, 177–8
progression
    factors in, 170–1
    slowing rate of, 173–5
renal transplantation, 183–4
    complications, 184
    prognosis, 184
cimetidine as a cause of false renal failure, 26–7
cirrhosis
    as a cause of glomerulonephritis, 95
    as a cause of hepatorenal syndrome, 67–9
cisplatin as a cause of acute tubular necrosis, 120
    prevention, 221
    prognosis, 221
    treatment, 220
colic, renal, use of intravenous pyelogram, 42, 61
complement, serum, 36
    in bacterial endocarditis, GN due to, 99
    in atheroembolic renal disease, 70–1
    in essential mixed cryoglobulinemia, 104–6
    in hemolytic uremic syndrome, 74–5
    in lupus nephritis, 100
    in membranoproliferative GN, 97
    in polyarteritis nodosa, 101
    in poststreptococcal GN, 98
    in ventriculoatrial shunts, GN due to, 99
    in visceral abscesses, GN due to, 99
    in Wegener's granulomatosis, 103,104
computed tomography, 43
    in acute cortical necrosis, 76–7
    in renal infarction, 80–1
contrast media nephrotoxicity, 66, 67, 69
    prevention, 194
creatinine, serum concentration, 25–7
    low values, 25–6, 27
    misleading elevation, 26–7
    reciprocal serum creatinine (1/Scr), 51–2, 171–2
crescentic GN (see idiopathic crescentic GN)
cryoglobulin
    definition, 104–5
    in essential mixed cryoglobulinemia, 104–6
    in bacterial endocarditis, GN due to, 99
    in lupus nephritis, 100
    in polyarteritis nodosa, 101
    in poststreptococcal GN, 98
    in ventriculoatrial shunts, GN due to, 99
    in visceral abscesses, GN due to, 99
cyclophosphamide
    intravenous in lupus nephritis, 208
    oral in Goodpasture's syndrome, 213
    oral in idiopathic crescentic GN, 205
    oral in lupus nephritis, 208–9
    oral in polyarteritis nodosa, 210
    oral in tubulointerstitial nephritis due to lipoid nephrosis,
    214–5

oral in Wegener's granulomatosis, 211
cyclosporine A as a cause of vasomotor disturbance, 66–68

DDAVP/deamino-D-arginine vasopressin (see desmopressin acetate)
definitions
    categories of renal failure, 7
    terms qualifying renal failure, 4–5
dense deposit disease, 94, 96
desmopressin acetate in management of platelet dysfunction, 161, 180–1
diabetes mellitus
    diabetic ketoacidosis as a cause of false renal failure, 26–7
    diabetic nephropathy, 49, 108
        effect of pregnancy, 175
        slowing progression of, 174, 214
dialysis and hemofiltration, 162–6
    indications in acute renal failure, 162
    hemodialysis
        acute, 163–4
        chronic, 181–2
    hemofiltration/hemodiafiltration, 165–6
    peritoneal dialysis
        acute, 164–5
        chronic, 182–3
diuretics
    as a cause of acute interstitial nephritis, 134
    for hyperkalemia, 179
    for hypertension in chronic renal failure, 176
    for hypervolemia in acute renal failure, 161
    for hypervolemia in chronic renal failure, 178
dopamine in management of hypervolemia, 161
Doppler (duplex) sonography in renal artery stenosis, 80
drug dosage modification in renal failure, 159

E. coli
    0157:H7 as a cause of hemolytic uremic syndrome, 74
    0157:H7 as a cause of thrombotic thrombocytopenia purpura, 75
    as a cause of acute pyelonephritis, 135
    as a cause of malacoplakia, 137
    as a cause of xanthogranulomatous pyelonephritis, 137
electrolytes, serum, 29, 31
electrophoresis, serum and urine, 36
embolism (see renal infarction)
end-stage renal disease (see chronic renal failure)
eosinophilia/eosinophiluria
    in atheroembolic renal disease, 70–1
    in drug-induced acute interstitial nephritis, 132–5
    urine sediment, 29
erythropoietin in management of anemia, 161, 180
essential mixed cryoglobulinemia, 104–6
    prognosis, 213
    treatment, 212–3
estrogen in management of platelet dysfunction, 161, 181
ethylene glycol ingestion as a cause of tubular obstruction, 125–7
    prevention, 223
    prognosis, 223

treatment, 223
Evan's syndrome (see thrombotic thrombocytopenia purpura)
extrarenal or systemic conditions as causes of renal failure, 16, 95, 148
eye findings, 23

FENa (see urine sodium)
false renal failure, 26–7, 49
fat pad biopsy in diagnosis of amyloidosis, 108
fibromuscular hyperplasia (see renal artery stenosis)
flank or back pain
    history, 14
    in acute cortical necrosis, 77
    in acute interstitial nephritis, 132
    in acute nephritic diseases, 94
    in atheroembolic renal disease, 70
    in idiopathic acute interstitial nephritis, 136
    in malacoplakia, 137
    in rifampin-induced interstitial nephritis, 134
    in xanthogranulomatous pyelonephritis, 137
fludrocortisone acetate for hyperkalemia, 179
fluid "challenge"
    in prerenal azotemia, 56
    in undiagnosed patients, 149–50
fluid loss (see hypovolemia)
5-flucytosine as a cause of false renal failure, 26–7
focal segmental glomerulosclerosis,
    as a cause of chronic renal failure, 49, 107
    as a cause of tubulointerstitial nephritis, 107–8
        treatment, 214–5
    as a rapidly progressive nephrotic disease, 107–8
foscarnet as a cause of acute tubular necrosis, 120
furosemide
    "challenge" in prerenal azotemia, 56
    in management of hypervolemia, 161, 178

gallium scan, 42
    in diagnosis of acute interstitial nephritis, 131–7
glomerular causes of renal failure, classification, 93
glomerular filtration rate (GFR)
    estimate using serum creatinine concentration, 26–4
    high glomerular filtration rate, 25–6
glomerular hypertension causing progression of renal failure, 170–1
Goodpasture's syndrome, 106
    prognosis, 214
    treatment, 213–4

HELLP syndrome mimicking hemolytic uremic syndrome, 74
HIV (see human immune deficiency virus)
Hantavirus as a cause of acute interstitial nephritis, 135
hematuria, gross
    history, 14
    in acute interstitial nephritis due to beta-lactam antibiotics, 133
    in acute nephritic diseases, 94, 96
    in atheroembolic renal disease, 70
    in hemolytic uremic syndrome, 74–5
    in malignant hypertension, 73

in postrenal renal failure, 59
in renal infarction, 80–1
in thrombotic thrombocytopenia purpura, 76
urinalysis, 28
hematuria, microscopic, 29, 147
hemoglobinuria (see acute tubular necrosis, hemoglobinuric)
hemolytic uremic syndrome, 74–5
as a cause of acute cortical necrosis, 76–7
prevention, 197
prognosis, 197–8
treatment, 197
Henoch-Schonlein purpura
as a cause of glomerulonephritis, 103–4
as a cause of postrenal renal failure, 60
prognosis, 212
treatment, 212
hepatitis B as a cause of polyarteritis nodosa, 101–2
hepatitis C
as a cause of essential mixed cryoglobulinemia, 104–6
as a cause of membranoproliferative GN, 97
treatment, 212–3
hepatorenal syndrome, 67, 68–9
prevention, 191–2
prognosis, 192
treatment, 192
urine sodium in diagnosis of, 37–8
hereditary diseases, history, 16
history, 13–9
family, 16
occupational, 16
social, 16
human immune deficiency virus (HIV)
as a cause of HIV nephropathy, 107
as a cause of hemolytic uremic syndrome, 74
as a cause of thrombotic thrombocytopenia purpura, 75
history, 16
hydronephrosis (see postrenal renal failure)
hypercalcemia
as a cause of chronic renal failure, 51
as a cause of vasomotor disturbances, 66–9
associated with myeloma kidney, 123
associated with sarcoidosis, 135–6
treatment, 192–3
hyperkalemia
miscellaneous causes, 29, 31
due to acute interstitial nephritis, 132
due to pentamidine-induced acute tubular necrosis, 120
due to postrenal renal failure, 59
due to tumor lysis syndrome, 124
treatment, 156–7, 79
hyperlipidemia in chronic renal failure, 176
hyperphosphatemia
in acute or chronic renal failure, management of, 158, 177–8
in tumor lysis syndrome, 124–5
hypertension
in acute nephritic syndrome, 94
in atheroembolic renal disease, 70–1
in chronic renal failure, management of, 176
in malignant hypertension, 72–4

treatment, 195–6
in renal artery stenosis, 78
in renal embolism, 81
in scleroderma, 71–2
physical examination, 22
hypervolemia, 21
in acute nephritic diseases, 94
in acute renal failure, management of, 161–2
in chronic renal failure, management of, 178–9
in prerenal azotemia, 55–6
hypocalcemia
in acute renal failure, 158
treatment, 158–9
in myoglobinuric acute tubular necrosis, 121
in tumor lysis syndrome, 124
treatment, 222
hypokalemia
as a cause of myoglobinuric acute tubular necrosis, 120
due to aminoglycosides, 119
due to amphotericin B, 119
due to cisplatin, 120
due to malignant hypertension, 73
due to miscellaneous causes, 31
due to multiple myeloma, 123
due to renal artery stenosis, 78
hyponatremia in acute renal failure, 153–5
treatment, 154–5
hypotension
as a cause of ischemic acute tubular necrosis, 118
as a cause of prerenal azotemia, 56
history, 14
minimal, 14, 56
physical examination, 22
hypovolemia, 14–5, 21–2
as a cause of ischemic acute tubular necrosis, 118
as a cause of prerenal azotemia, 55–6
treatment, 187–8

idiopathic crescentic GN, 94, 96
as a cause of chronic renal failure, 49
prognosis, 206
treatment, 205–6
IgA nephropathy, 94, 96
as a cause of chronic renal failure, 49
treatment, 206
immunoglobulin light chains
as a cause of amyloidosis and light chain deposition disease, 108
as a cause of myeloma kidney, 122
testing serum and urine for, 36
incidence of renal failure
due to different causes, 7–8
factors influencing, 7
overall, 3, 8
infectious mononucleosis as a cause of interstitial nephritis, 135
insulin, use in renal failure, 159
interstitial nephritis (see acute or chronic interstitial nephritis)
intravenous cyclophosphamide (see cyclophosphamide)
intravenous pyelogram, 40–2

in postrenal renal failure, 41–2, 61

Kayexalate (see sodium polystyrene sulfonate)

large vessel diseases, 77–81
leg cramps/restless legs, 181
leptospirosis as a cause of interstitial nephritis, 135
leukemia
    as a cause of neoplastic interstitial infiltration, 138
        treatment, 228
    as a cause of tumor lysis syndrome, 124–5
        treatment, 223
light chain deposition disease, 108
    treatment, 214
lipoid nephrosis as a cause of tubulointerstitial nephritis, 107–8
    treatment, 214–5
lipomatosis, renal sinus, 40
low protein diet
    use in limiting progression of renal failure, 173–4
    use in managing nausea and vomiting, 181
lupus (see systemic lupus erythematosis)
lymphoma
    as a cause of glomerulonephritis, 95
    as a cause of myeloma kidney, 122
    as a cause of neoplastic interstitial infiltration, 138
        treatment, 228
    as a cause of tumor lysis syndrome, 124–5

magnetic resonance angiography in renal artery stenosis, 89
malacoplakia, 137
    treatment, 228
malabsorption as a cause of hyperoxaluria, 125
malignancy (see neoplasm)
malignant hypertension, 72–4
    due to acute nephritic diseases, 94
    due to renal artery stenosis, 78
    due to scleroderma, 71–2
    prognosis, 196–7
    treatment, 195–6
meperidine hydrochloride, use in renal failure, 159
methyldopa as a cause of false renal failure, 27
methylprednisolone (see pulse methylprednisolone)
methotrexate as a cause of tubular obstruction, 126
    prevention, 224
    treatment, 224
metoclopramide for nausea and vomiting, 160, 181
metolazone, use in hypervolemia, 161–2, 178–9
microangiopathic hemolytic anemia
    in hemolytic uremic syndrome, 74–5
    in malignant hypertension, 72–4
    in scleroderma, 71–2
    in thrombotic thrombocytopenia purpura, 75–6
microscopic polyarteritis nodosa (see polyarteritis nodosa)
minimal change disease (see lipoid nephrosis)
mitomycin C (see hemolytic uremic syndrome)
muscle cramps, management of, 181
mycoplasma pneumonia as a cause of interstitial nephritis, 135
myeloma kidney, 122–4
    as a cause of chronic renal failure, 51
    causes, 122

    clinical picture, 122–3
    definition, 122
    diagnosis, 123–4
    pathogenesis, 123
    prevention, 222
    prognosis, 222
    treatment, 222
myoclonic jerks, management of, 181
myoglobinuria (see acute tubular necrosis, myoglobinuric)
narcotic analgesics, use in renal failure, 159
nausea and vomiting, management of, 160, 181
neoplasm
    as a cause of glomerulonephritis, 95
    as a cause of hypercalcemia, 66–9
    as a cause of interstitial infiltration, 138
        treatment, 228
    as a cause of postrenal renal failure, 59–60
    renal failure due to chemotherapy, 119, appendix A
nephrosclerosis, hypertensive (benign arteriolar), 49, 65
nephrotic diseases, 107–9
    as a cause of renal vein thrombosis, 80–1, 107, 108
    as a cause of tubulointerstitial nephritis, 107
        treatment, 214–5
    causes, 107
nephrotic proteinuria/syndrome
    as a cause of renal vein thrombosis, 80–1, 107,108
    as a cause of tubulointerstitial nephritis, 107
    due to acute nephritic syndrome, 94
    due to amyloidosis, 108
    due to diabetic nephropathy, 108
    due to hemolytic uremic syndrome, 75
    due to light chain deposition disease, 108
    due to malignant hypertension, 73
    due to nephrotic diseases, 107–9
    due to nonsteroidal anti-inflammatory drugs, 133–4
    due to renal artery stenosis, 78
    due to thrombotic thrombocytopenia purpura, 76
nephrotoxins
    acute tubular necrosis, 119–20
    appendices A and B
    history, 15–6
neurogenic bladder, 59–60
    treatment, 190
nonsteroidal anti-inflammatory drugs
    as a cause of acute cortical necrosis, 76–7
    as a cause of chronic renal failure, 51
    as a cause of drug-induced acute interstitial nephritis, 132–5
    as a cause of hyperkalemia, 179
    as a cause of vasomotor disturbances, 66–9
nutrition in acute renal failure, 159–60

obstruction/obstructive uropathy (see postrenal renal failure)
oliguric renal failure
    acute tubular necrosis, 117
    definition, 4
osmolal gap in ethylene glycol ingestion, 125–7
osteodystrophy, renal, 176–7
oxalic acid/oxaluria as a cause of tubular obstruction, 125–7
    treatment, 223–4

parathyroidectomy in management of renal osteodystrophy, 177–8
pelvic malignancy causing postrenal renal failure, 59, 60
pentamidine isethionate as a cause of acute tubular necrosis, 120
phenytoin, use in renal failure, 159
plasmapheresis
    in essential mixed cryoglobulinemia, 212
    in Goodpasture's syndrome, 213
    in idiopathic crescentic GN, 205–6
    in myeloma kidney, 222
    in polyarteritis nodosa, 210
platelet dysfunction, management of, 161, 180–1
polyarteritis nodosa
    as a cause of glomerulonephritis, 101–2
    as a cause of postrenal renal failure, 60
    as a cause of renal infarction, 80–1
    prognosis, 211
    treatment, 210–1
postpartum renal failure (see hemolytic uremic syndrome)
postrenal renal failure, 59–63
    as a cause of chronic renal failure, 5
    BUN to Scr ratio, 27, 59
    physiological hydronephrosis of pregnancy, 61
    postobstructive diuresis, 188–9
    prognosis, 191
    treatment, 188–91
    with minimal or no hydronephrosis, 61
poststreptococcal GN, 97–8
    prognosis, 207
    treatment, 206–7
potassium (see hyperkalemia or hypokalemia)
pregnancy
    gravid uterus causing postrenal renal failure, 61
    impact on diabetic nephropathy, 175
    impact on lupus nephritis, 175
    impact on progression of renal failure, 174–5
    physiological hydronephrosis, 61
    prognosis in women with chronic renal failure, 174–5
prerenal azotemia, 55–7
    as distinguished from hepatorenal syndrome, 68–9
    prevention, 187
    treatment, 187–8
    urine sodium, 37–8
prochlorperazine for nausea and vomiting, 160, 181
prostate cancer or hypertrophy
    as a cause of postrenal renal failure, 59, 60
    treatment, 189–90
protein, 24-hour urine, 36–7
protein restricted diet (see low protein diet)
protein to creatinine ratio, urine, 37
proteinuria
    diagnoses suggested, 147
    heavy (see nephrotic proteinuria/syndrome)
    in acute interstitial nephritis, 132, 133–6
    in acute nephritic syndrome, 94
    in chronic renal failure, 50
    in hemolytic uremic syndrome, 74–5
    in interstitial nephritis due to beta-lactam antibiotics, 133
    in interstitial nephritis due to NSAID's, 133–4

    in interstitial nephritis due to rifampin, 134
    in interstitial nephritis due to sarcoidosis, 136
    in interstitial nephritis due to Sjogren's syndrome, 136
    in malignant hypertension, 72–4
    in myeloma kidney, 122–4
    in nephrotic diseases, 107–9
    in postrenal renal failure, 59
    in prerenal azotemia, 56
    in renal artery stenosis, 78
    in renal infarction, 80–1
    in scleroderma, 71–2
    in thrombotic thrombocytopenia purpura, 76
    in vasomotor disturbances, 68
    interpretation, 28, 37
    quantitation, 36–7
    urinalysis, 28
pruritus, management of, 160, 181
pulse methylprednisolone/oral prednisone
    in acute interstitial nephritis, 226
    in essential mixed cryoglobulinemia, 212
    in Goodpasture's syndrome, 214
    in Henoch-Schonlein purpura, 212
    in idiopathic crescentic GN, 205
    in lupus nephritis, 208
    in membranoproliferative GN, 206
    in polyarteritis nodosa, 210
    in poststreptococcal and other postinfectious GN, 205–7
    in Wegener's granulomatosis, 211
pyuria, 29

quinine sulfate in management of muscle cramps, 181

radiation nephritis, 65
radionuclide scan, 42
    captopril radionuclide scan in renal artery stenosis, 79–80
    diuretic renography in postrenal renal failure, 61
    in renal infarction, 81
red cell casts, 29
renal artery thrombosis (see renal infarction)
renal artery stenosis, 77–80
    arteriography, 78–9
    as a cause of malignant hypertension, 73–4
    causes, 78
    pathophysiology, 78
    prognosis, 199
    treatment, 198–200
renal artery embolism (see renal infarction)
renal cortical necrosis (see acute cortical necrosis)
renal infarction, 80–1
    prevention, 200
    treatment, 200
renal osteodystrophy, 176–7
renal vein thrombosis, 80–1
    prevention, 200
    treatment, 200–1
renin, elevation in peripheral vein
    malignant hypertension, 72–4
    renal artery stenosis, 77–9
    scleroderma, 71–2

restless legs, 181
rifampin
    as a cause of acute interstitial nephritis, 134
    as a cause of tubular obstruction, 126
ruptured bladder as a cause of postrenal renal failure, 59–60

salicylate as a cause of false renal failure, 26–7
salt losing kidneys
    as a cause of prerenal azotemia, 56
    history, 14–5
sarcoidosis
    as a cause of acute interstitial nephritis, 135–6
        treatment, 227
    as a cause of glomerulonephritis, 95
scleroderma, renal, 71–2
    prognosis, 195
    treatment, 195
sepsis
    as a cause of acute tubular necrosis, 118
    as a cause of vasomotor disturbances, 66–8
    treatment, 193–4
shunt nephritis (see ventriculoatrial shunts)
Sjogren's syndrome as a cause of acute interstitial nephritis, 136
    treatment, 277
skin biopsy, 35
    in essential mixed cryoglobulinemia, 104–6
    in Henoch-Schonlein purpura, 103–4
    in polyarteritis nodosa, 101–2
    in Wegener's granulomatosis, 103, 104
small vessel disease, 70–7
sodium bicarbonate for hyperkalemia, 156–7
sodium bicarbonate or citrate for metabolic acidosis, 158, 179
sodium polystyrene sulfonate for hyperkalemia, 156–7, 179
sonogram, renal, 39–40
    in chronic renal failure, 51
    in obstruction, 39–40, 61
    in renal atrophy, 40
spiral CT angiography in renal artery stenosis, 80
stones
    as a cause of postrenal renal failure, 59–61
    as a cause of obstruction with false negative renal sonogram, 42, 61
    use of intravenous pyelogram, 42, 61
sulfonamides
    as a cause of acute interstitial nephritis, 134
    as a cause of tubular obstruction, 125
systemic diseases, history, 16
systemic lupus erythematosis
    as a cause of acute interstitial nephritis, 136
    as a cause of lupus nephritis, 99–100
        effect of pregnancy, 175
        prognosis, 210
        treatment, 207–10
systemic sclerosis (see scleroderma)

Takayasu's arteritis (see renal artery stenosis)
theophylline, use in renal failure, 159
thrombotic microangiopathy
    in hemolytic uremic syndrome, 74–5

in malignant hypertension, 73
    in scleroderma, 71
    in thrombotic thrombocytopenia purpura, 75–6
thrombotic thrombocytopenia purpura, 75–6
    prognosis, 198
    treatment, 198
triamterene as a cause of tubular obstruction, 126
trimethoprim as a cause of false renal failure, 26–7
toxoplasmosis as a cause of acute interstitial nephritis, 135
tuberculosis as a cause of chronic interstitial nephritis, 137
tubular obstruction, 122–7
    due to acetazolamide, 126
    due to acyclovir, 126
    due to ethylene glycol, 125–7
    due to methotrexate, 126
    due to myeloma kidney, 122–4
    due to oxalic acid, 125–7
    due to rifampin, 126
    due to sulfonamide, 125
    due to triamterene, 126
    due to tumor lysis syndrome, 124–5
    treatment, 222–4
tubulointerstitial nephritis due to nephrotic syndrome, 107
    treatment, 214–5
tumor lysis syndrome, 124–5
    prevention, 222–3
    prognosis, 223
    treatment, 223

ultrasound (see sonogram, renal)
undiagnosed patient, evaluation of, 149–50
ureteral obstruction, management of, 190–1
uremia
    definition, 5
    management of anemia, 180
    management of bleeding, 180–1
    management of nausea and vomiting, 160, 181
    management of neuromuscular symptoms, 181
    management of pericarditis/tamponade, 160–1
    management of pruritis, 181
    management of renal osteodystrophy, 177–8
    symptoms, 13, 170, 171
urethral catheter in diagnosis of postrenal renal failure, 61
urinalysis, 28–31, 147
urine chloride, 38–9
    prerenal azotemia, 56
urine sediment, 29–30, 147
    prerenal azotemia, 56
urine sodium, 37–8
    in acute tubular necrosis, 117–118
    in contrast media nephrotoxicity, 67, 69
    in hepatorenal syndrome, 67, 68–9
    in hypercalcemia, 67
    in acute interstitial nephritis due to NSAID's, 133–4
    in postrenal renal failure, 59
    in prerenal azotemia, 56
    in renal artery stenosis, 78
    in vasomotor disturbances, 67, 68, 69

valproate, use in renal failure, 159
vascular causes of renal failure, 65–82
    causes, 65
    incidence, 65
vasculitis, renal, 101–6
    capsule description, 101
vasomotor disturbances, 66–9
    causes, 66
    due to angiotensin converting enzyme inhibitor, 66–8
    due to contrast media nephrotoxicity, 66, 67, 69
    due to cyclosporine A, 66–68
    due to hepatorenal syndrome, 67, 68–9
    due to nonsteroidal anti-inflammatory drugs, 66–8
    pathophysiology, 66
venography, renal, in renal vein thrombosis, 108
ventriculoatrial shunts, GN due to, 99

prognosis, 207
    treatment, 207
visceral abscesses, GN due to, 99
    treatment, 206–7
    prognosis, 207
volume status (see hypervolemia or hypovolemia)

Wegener's granulomatosis
    as a cause of glomerulonephritis, 103–4
    as a cause of postrenal renal failure, 60
    prognosis, 211
    treatment, 211–2
Whitaker test for postrenal renal failure, 61

xanthogranulomatous pyelonephritis, 137
    treatment, 228

Developments in Nephrology

1. J.S. Cheigh, K.H. Stenzel and A.L. Rubin (eds.): *Manual of Clinical Nephrology of the Rogosin Kidney Center.* 1981   ISBN 90-247-2397-3
2. K.D. Nolph (ed.): *Peritoneal Dialysis.* 1981 ed.: out of print
   3rd revised and enlarged ed. 1988 (not in this series)   ISBN 0-89838-406-0
3. A.B. Gruskin and M.E. Norman (eds.): *Pediatric Nephrology.* 1981
                ISBN 90-247-2514-3
4. O. Schück: *Examination of the Kidney Function.* 1981   ISBN 0-89838-565-2
5. J. Strauss (ed.): *Hypertension, Fluid-electrolytes and Tubulopathies in Pediatric Nephrology.* 1982   ISBN 90-247-2633-6
6. J. Strauss (ed.): *Neonatal Kidney and Fluid-electrolytes.* 1983   ISBN 0-89838-575-X
7. J. Strauss (ed.): *Acute Renal Disorders and Renal Emergencies.* 1984
                ISBN 0-89838-663-2
8. L.J.A. Didio and P.M. Motta (eds.): *Basic, Clinical, and Surgical Nephrology.* 1985
                ISBN 0-89838-698-5
9. E.A. Friedman and C.M. Peterson (eds.): *Diabetic Nephropathy.* Strategy for Therapy. 1985   ISBN 0-89838-735-3
10. R. Dzúrik, B. Lichardus and W. Guder: *Kidney Metabolism and Function.* 1985
                ISBN 0-89838-749-3
11. J. Strauss (ed.): *Homeostasis, Nephrotoxicy, and Renal Anomalies in the Newborn.* 1986   ISBN 0-89838-766-3
12. D.G. Oreopoulos (ed.): *Geriatric Nephrology.* 1986   ISBN 0-89838-781-7
13. E.P. Paganini (ed.): *Acute Continuous Renal Replacement Therapy.* 1986
                ISBN 0-89838-793-0
14. J.S. Cheigh, K.H. Stenzel and A.L. Rubin (eds.): *Hypertension in Kidney Disease.* 1986
                ISBN 0-89838-797-3
15. N. Deane, R.J. Wineman and G.A. Benis (eds.): *Guide to Reprocessing of Hemodialyzers.* 1986   ISBN 0-89838-798-1
16. C. Ponticelli, L. Minetti and G. D'Amico (eds.): *Antiglobulins, Cryoglobulins and Glomerulonephritis.* 1986   ISBN 0-89838-810-4
17. J. Strauss (ed.) with the assistence of L. Strauss: *Persistent Renalgenitourinary Disorders.* 1987   ISBN 0-89838-845-7
18. V.E. Andreucci and A. Dal Canton (eds.): *Diuretics.* Basic, Pharmacological, and Clinical Aspects. 1987   ISBN 0-89838-885-6
19. P.H. Bach and E.H. Lock (eds.): *Nephrotoxicity in the Experimental and Clinical Situation*, Part 1. 1987   ISBN 0-89838-997-1
20. P.H. Bach and E.H. Lock (eds.): *Nephrotoxicity in the Experimental and Clinical Situation*, Part 2. 1987   ISBN 0-89838-980-2
21. S.M. Gore and B.A. Bradley (eds.): *Renal Transplantation.* Sense and Sensitization. 1988   ISBN 0-89838-370-6
22. L. Minetti, G. D'Amico and C. Ponticelli: *The Kidney in Plasma Cell Dyscrasias.* 1988
                ISBN 0-89838-385-4
23. A.S. Lindblad, J.W. Novak and K.D. Nolph (eds.): *Continuous Ambulatory Peritoneal Dialysis in the USA.* Final Report of the National CAPD Registry 1981–1988. 1989
                ISBN 0-7923-0179-X

Developments in Nephrology

24. V.E. Andreucci and A. Dal Canton (eds.): *Current Therapy in Nephrology.* 1989
ISBN 0-7923-0206-0
25. L. Kovács and B. Lichardus: *Vasopressin.* Disturbed Secretion and its Effects. 1989
ISBN 0-7923-0249-4
26. M.E. de Broe and J.W. Coburn (eds.): *Aluminum and Renal Failure.* 1990
ISBN 0-7923-0347-4
27. K.D. Gardner Jr. and J. Bernstein (eds.): *The Cystic Kidney.* 1990
ISBN 0-7923-0392-X
28. M.E. de Broe and G.A. Verpooten (eds.): *Prevention in Nephrology.* 1991
ISBN 0-7923-0951-0
29. T.A. Depner (ed.): *Prescribing Hemodialysis.* A Guide to Urea Modeling. 1991
ISBN 0-7923-0833-6
30. V.E. Andreucci and A. Dal Canton (eds.): *New Therapeutic Strategies in Nephrology.*
Proceedings of the 3rd International Meeting on Current Therapy in Nephropology
(Sorrento, Italy, 1990). 1991
ISBN 0-7923-1199-X
31. A. Amerio, P. Coratelli and S.G. Massry (eds.): *Turbulo-Interstitial Nephropathies.*
Proceedings of the 4th Bari Seminar in Nephrology (April 1990). 1991
ISBN 0-7923-1200-7
32. M.G. McGeown (ed.): *Clinical Management of Renal Transplantation.* 1992
ISBN 0-7923-1604-5
33. C.M. Kjellstrand and J.B. Dossetor (eds.): *Ethical Problems in Dialysis and Transplan-
tation.* 1992
ISBN 0-7923-1625-8
34. D.G. Oreopoulos, M.F. Michelis and S. Herschorn (eds.): *Nephrology and Urology in
the Aged Patient.* 1993
ISBN 0-7923-2019-0
35. E.A. Friedman (ed.): *Death on Hemodialysis: Preventable or Inevitable?* 1994
ISBN 0-7923-2652-0
36. L.W. Henderson and R.S. Thuma (eds.): *Quality Assurance in Dialysis.* 1994
ISBN 0-7923-2723-3
37. J.G. Abuelo (ed.): *Renal Failure: Diagnosis and Treatment.* 1995
ISBN 0-7923-3438-8

Kluwer Academic Publishers – Dordrecht / Boston / London